Insane Society: A Sociology of Mental Health

T0076672

This book critiques the connection between Western society and madness, scrutinizing if and how societal insanity affects the cause, construction, and consequence of madness.

Looking beyond the affected individual to their social, political, economic, ecological, and cultural context, this book examines whether society itself, and its institutions, divisions, practices, and values, is mad. That society's insanity is relevant to the sanity and insanity of its citizens has been argued by Fromm in *The Sane Society*, but also by a host of sociologists, social thinkers, epidemiologists and biologists. This book builds on classic texts such as Foucault's *History of Madness*, Scull's Marxist-oriented works and more recent publications which have arisen from a range of socio-political and patient-orientated movements. Chapters in this book draw on biology, psychology, sociological and anthropological thinking that argues that where madness is concerned, *society* matters.

Providing an extended case study of how the sociological imagination should operate in a contemporary setting, this book draws on genetics, neuroscience, cognitive science, radical psychology, and evolutionary psychology/ psychiatry. It is an important read for students and scholars of sociology, anthropology, social policy, criminology, health, and mental health.

Peter Morrall has an academic background in medical/health sociology. He is currently Visiting Associate Professor in Health Sociology, University of Leeds, and Tutor at the Centre for Lifelong Learning, University of York, UK. Morrall has been steeped in the field of 'madness' for decades. He has worked in large mental hospitals and small psychiatric units, and has taught, researched, and written about madness (including 'madness and murder', 'the trouble with psychotherapy', and the insanity of society). Morrall's other interests beyond madness are music and motorcycling.

Routledge Studies in the Sociology of Health and Illness

For more information about this series, please visit: https://www.routledge.com/
Routledge-Studies-in-the-Sociology-of-Health-and-Illness/book-series/RSSHI

Insane Society: A Sociology of Mental Health

Peter Morrall

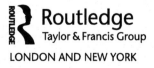

Routledge
Taylor & Francis Group

LONDON AND NEW YORK

First published 2020
by Routledge
4 Park Square, Milton Park, Abingdon, Oxon OX14 4RN
605 Third Avenue, New York, NY 10017

First issued in paperback 2023

Routledge is an imprint of the Taylor & Francis Group, an informa business

© 2020 Peter Morrall

British Library Cataloguing-in-Publication Data
A catalogue record for this book is available from the British Library

Library of Congress Cataloging-in-Publication Data
A catalog record has been requested for this book

ISBN: 978-1-03-257015-0 (pbk)
ISBN: 978-1-138-57607-0 (hbk)
ISBN: 978-1-351-27116-5 (ebk)

DOI: 10.4324/9781351271165

Typeset in Times New Roman
by Taylor & Francis Books

Contents

Introduction
Imagine

Imagine you (the reader) have an appointment with your medical practitioner concerning a difficulty you are having breathing, and a tendency to fall asleep particularly after meals. The medical practitioner notes that you drink far more units of alcohol than the recommended limit, take exercise only when it's unavoidable, have a very sweet tooth and eat mainly 'convenience' foods, and you are overweight. When questioned about these lifestyle habits of yours you explain that you are also 'stressed' and frequently feel 'down'. Moreover, when particularly frazzled and sad you feel that your family, friends, and work colleagues not only don't appreciate how you are feeling but you suspect many of them are also 'out to get you'. Alcohol, cigarettes, laziness, sweets, cake, and highly processed food are attempts, you claim, to 'de-stress'.

Following a few simple physical tests, your medical practitioner diagnoses early-onset asthma and type 2 diabetes, and prescribes anti-inflammatory and hypoglycaemic drugs as well as offering advice about a healthier diet, exercise, and alcohol consumption. Following a few simple psychological tests, she also diagnoses 'anxiety' and 'depression' whilst reserving a diagnosis of psychosis. The good doctor, and for sure she is well-qualified and is trying her best to help you, prescribes anti-anxiety and anti-depression drugs as well as recommending a course in cognitive therapy, basic relaxation techniques, and joining a gym. These standard medical interventions seem to be well researched and effective. Asthma and diabetes can be stabilised, misery managed, apprehension assuaged, and (if it should be necessary in your case) paranoia quelled. More sophisticated testing which examines in minute detail the genetic, biochemical, and anatomical make-up of every bit of your body may soon become *de rigour* in medical practice. This may involve identifying the molecular substance of every cell of every organ, including the brain and its associated somatic systems. What could then be offered as medical interventions are genetically-specific pharmaceuticals, precise gene-editing procedures, nanochip insertions, robotic attachments, and neurologically-founded psychotherapy. Within the next hundred years such developments, according to historian Yuval Harari (2017), offer the possibility of homo-sapiens overcoming morbidity and mortality, thereby transforming into 'homo-Deus'. That is, evolving from the animalistic to the godly.

What is not offered in medical practice, and there is no indication that it will ever be offered, is the testing and treatment of social disorder. Neither your physical nor your psychological condition is assessed for the effects of society. There may be an acknowledgement, particularly if you are referred to a specialist, of connections between your lifestyle habits, sorrow, unease and suspiciousness, and localised situation. But, medical tools equivalent to those which assess heart rate, blood pressure, extent of sweating, hormone and endocrine levels, and genomic makeup, are not employed. Medical scrutiny is already narrow and, aided by truly incredible technological visualisation and biological excavation, will become more and more focused on the infinitesimal. The star aspiration of natural science is to unify the miniscule with the massive, the subatomic with the cosmos. Medicine is not staring at the stars.

This medical appointment of yours has taken only 15 minutes from review to remedy. Society has not been reviewed and therefore not remedied. Should society also have been at the appointment then it would have needed to last more than 15 minutes.

Sociology

Society, however, is not just relevant to your (imaginary) medical scenario. No personal problem – I repeat *no* personal problem – is only personal. All personal problems, whether about money, relationships, holidays, gender and sexual orientation, intelligence, morality, food, alcohol, exercise, asthma, diabetes, body mass, anxiety, depression, or delusions, are both personal and social.

Every issue concerning an individual and every issue about which an individual is concerned is connectable to a social context. So far, the imaginary story described above has been primarily if not solely about you. The dialogue with the medical practitioner has covered your health deficits, your daily routines, your diagnosis, and treatments for you. What is missing is the realisation and reification of the persistent, potent, and possibly pestilential influences on you originating not in your biological or psychological dispositions but in the social (as well physical) environment. These influences external to you have, are, and will continue to contour your lifestyle, physical and psychological states, and interactions with medical practice. The conduct of the food, alcohol, and advertising and media industries, the norms and values of your kinfolk and peers, your level of education, income, gender, and age, the history, creeds, goals, status, and competency of the profession of medicine and allied occupations, and the financial interests of the drug companies, are just some of the social factors shaping your situation. What effects the situation of these factors is society's principles and provisions.

This is not to suggest that either you or the medical practitioner are unaware of at least some of the social factors affecting your situation. One does not need a PhD in sociology to spot that, for example, networks of family, friends and colleagues, the circumstances of home, neighbourhood, work, and leisure, influence both physical and mental well-being. The difference is understanding the scale, density, and altitude of that complexity. This is where both your imagination and the medical imagination require the supplement of the sociological imagination.

The sociological imagination, applied to madness, furnishes the thesis of this book. The thesis has three parts:

1   madness and society are interconnected;
2   'insane' aspects of society are linkable to psychological distress in individuals;
3   society itself may be insane.

This book revitalises and augments a perspective about madness which has been downgraded dramatically due to an intensifying emphasis on biological conceptualisations with those emanating from psychology increasingly biologically orientated. Such rampant biological reductionism has led to a near total fixation on biological treatments alongside biologically orientated psychological therapies.

Whilst biological disposition is undoubtedly bound-up with states of insanity and sanity, society impacts powerfully the minds and brains of individuals and therefore needs to be incorporated into the discourses of psychiatry and allied professions as well as public perspectives. Intellectual gazing at madness needs to be drawn back to a position whereby wider influences are incorporated or in some instances supersede the understanding of madness.

However, I argue that understanding, no matter how well infused with the imagination of sociology, is not enough. Remedial endeavours are required.

Terms

So far in this introduction, the term 'insanity' has been used when referring to certain societal conditions or the condition of society, and the term 'madness' used when referring to certain conditions of the mind.[1] Yet the title refers to 'mental health' (and by implication the terms 'mental illness' or 'mental disorder' are available for use). These expressions need to be clarified especially as they are both contentious and partisan. Indeed, the language concerning 'psychological ease' and 'psychological unease' (or equivalent euphemistic idioms) has become a minefield of contentiousness and partisanship. What is acceptable and unacceptable to the public, professionals, and patients ('patient' being yet another divisive appellation) is muddled, mutable, and narrow-minded.

First, there is not an agreed term for what I am referring to here as 'insanity' and 'madness' or any one definition that is agreed across academic and clinical disciplines, in the media, historically and trans-culturally, in formal and social media, and in everyday talk. There may never be agreement and maybe there never should.

'Insanity', from ancient Latin, is a combination of '*in*' meaning 'not' and '*sanus*' meaning general healthiness with the specific targeting of the mind occurring in the middle-ages (Onions, 1966). It was used as a legal term in Greco-Roman societies (Simon and Ahn-Redding, 2008). It is still used, mainly as a defence, in a wide range of countries including India, most states in the USA, Australia, and England (Math et al., 2015; Robinson and Williams, 2017; Loughnan, 2015; National Archives, 2018). Andrew Scull is a sociologist who specialises in the history of madness. He accepts that the term 'madness' is regarded today by many as politically incorrect (Scull, 2015). However, as with 'insanity' (and other now out-of-favour terms such as 'lunacy') it was the accepted descriptor until relatively recently for what has become described medically as mental disorder/illness. For Scull it remains a common-sense designation and one which is decoupled from medicalisation. The decoupling from medicalisation is important as the medical approach (mostly through its psychiatric subsidiary), although foremost in the field of madness, is only one of a plethora of available ideas (Morrall, 2017).

Attempts to register and temper psychiatric dominance as well generalised and persistent prejudice, have been made by other clinicians, academics, and activists, by promoting forms of de-medicalised and de-stigmatised language (Diana Rose[2] et al. 2007; Levine, 2016; Bupa/Mental Health First Aid, 2018; Time to Change, 2018). The suggested acceptable language includes the conflicting phrase 'mental health problem' (why have 'health' in that phrase at all?) and the substitution of 'patient' for the misleading descriptor 'service user' or worse still 'mental health consumer' (the implicit notion of empowerment in both descriptions is despoiled by the possibility of legally enforceable incarceration and treatment).

It is debatable if merely making linguistic readjustments will recalibrate the professional hierarchy or eradicate prejudice (Ruscio, 2004; Morrall, 2017). For that reason, but primarily to avoid implied acceptance of either medical or vogue jargon, for the most part 'madness' is employed in this book when referring to a state of mind and 'insanity' when referring to the state of society. 'Mental disorder' (or 'mental illness') and 'mental health' will be utilised in the main only when referring to medicalised notions. Moreover, references to 'mental disorder', especially where 'epidemics' are the topic, will be couched cautiously in phraseology such as 'a diagnosis of mental disorder' so as not to infer unqualified acceptance of medical accuracy or legitimacy.

'Madness', therefore, is my descriptor for a pre-medicalisation or non-medicalised signing of irregular and undesirable elements of human performance. 'Human performance' refers to all the behaviours, thoughts, and feelings which constitute an individual's, to borrow a phrase coined by the sociologist Erving Goffman (1959), 'presentation of self in everyday life'. There is no consistency in the medical or social science literature over what states of human performance 'madness' embraces (Morrall, 2017). At times the medicalised states of schizophrenia and manic-depression are recurrently considered 'real' madness, but at other times it the term is used arbitrarily. Apart from the obvious alliterative value of 'insane' coinciding with 'society' in the title of this book, the expression 'insane society' is an express connection I am making with Erich Fromm's book *The Sane Society* (see below).

There is an obvious inconsistency in having 'mental health' in the title instead of 'madness'. However, if the latter had been used it may have led to confusion over the substance of the book. That is, 'Insane Society: A Sociology of Madness' could suggest that the content was (only) about society rather than about people and their social settings.

Ideas[3]

Terminology is only one muddled matter concerning madness. Another, as has been alluded to above, is that of 'ideas'. There is no one position which is uncontroversial and irrefutable. Every idea about madness is contestable and thereby the divisions between madness, badness, and normality, cannot be established firmly.

Understanding the scale, density, and altitude of madness is certainly complex. Who is trying to understand, to which 'tribe' does he/she belong, why is an understanding being sought, needs to be understood first. This is because there is no agreed definition, let alone approach, across or even within academic and clinical disciplines, or one putative idea amongst the public (Morrall, 2017).

As already mentioned, there is a dominant idea emanating from contemporary 'scientific' psychiatry which for the most part psychiatry fixes its gaze on the brain and related somatic systems to find the cause of mental disorder, and in so doing asserts its status as a legitimate (scientific) branch of medicine. These biological factors include the neuro-genetic, neuro-chemical, and neuro-anatomic make-up of an individual. The corollary of this focus on physical causation is a preoccupation on physical remedies for the individual. There is also an acceptance, but to a much lesser extent, of psychological therapies especially if biological impairment is implicated and both cause and remedy can be endorsed scientifically. The core curricula of contemporary clinical psychology centres on categories of 'disorder' which have been conceived by either a medical-orientated early psychology or borrowed directly from psychiatry.[4] These include mood, eating, developmental, and sexual disorders. Whilst psychologists are manifestly interested in the thoughts, behaviours, and emotions of *individuals*, these features have biological connotations which are incorporated into psychological discernments and procedures (especially its cognitive and evolutionary divisions).

Ideas from sociology, anthropology, social history, 'anti' and critical psychiatry, some quarters of social psychology and radical psychology, however, contest the justification for biology's epistemological ascent and propose ideas of their own. Those ideas propose that madness is only understandable (and thus ameliorated credibly), when underlying social processes and configurations are accommodated. These processes and configurations include:

- *societal* variations in cultural and historical norms, values, beliefs, and physical environments;
- the distribution in *society* of power, wealth, resources, and prejudice.

Understanding madness necessitates fathoming which biological, psychological, and social factors are more involved than others, which ones are not involved, how each interrelates with each other one or interrelate with a collection of other factors, and how much research, the quality and status of that research, and the degree and effectiveness of its dissemination. Moreover, there will be factors not yet identified and even if identified they may not be accepted as relevant for social reasons.

One such reason is the continued commitment of professionals, corporations, and politicians to presiding knowledge. That commitment (for example, to biological causation) mitigates a move to a new way of thinking about and handling madness (for example, towards societal explanations). There are formidable economic, philosophical, occupational forces promoting and protecting 'biologism' (Stier et al., 2014; Goldacre, 2012; 2014). The profits of the entire pharmaceutical industry and careers of countless academics rely on biological reductionism in the construction, cause, and treatment of ill-health.

A consequence of formidable biologism increasingly adopted to support the science of psychiatry and associated occupations is not only the displacement of alternative ideas but the abandonment of the 'mind'. Harari (2015) observes that there has been a steady and forceful move by geneticists and neuroscientists to have the mind subsumed by the brain to the point that an individual's thoughts, feelings, and behaviours, along with all elements of consciousness, self-identity, personality, and 'soul', are nothing more than synaptic and neuro-chemical interactions. Molecular biologist and co-discoverer of the structure of DNA Francis Crick's comment that everything human is consignable to 'neurons' sums-up the ultimate position of biologism (Crick, 1995).

The upshot of biological reductionism, therefore, is at the downgrading or complete dumping of both society and what humans regard as inherent to their 'self', that is their mind. However, sociology, as well as social-psychology, philosophy, and anthropology, has a tradition of acknowledging integral and inevitable connections between society and the self.[5] The imagination of sociology is – or should be – unbounded. Therefore, a sociological account of madness whilst combating reductionism of any hue must engage with and where it is justifiable entertain other forms of knowledge.

Positivity

The original entertainment of this book originates from engaging with the imaginative thinking of sociologist C Wright Mills, medical practitioner and anthropologists Cecil Helman, and especially Erich Fromm. What had entertained Fromm's imagination was engagement with social psychology, psychoanalysis, philosophy, humanism, and sociology.

Mills (1959) points to the connection between 'private troubles' and 'public issues'. He proposes that no matter how we perform as individuals (what we feel, how we act, and what we think), our social experiences shape that performance. Seemingly exclusive personal states such as happiness, self-identity, volition, desire, empowerment, miserableness, and apprehensiveness, are linked inexorably to social factors. This linkage, however, is not unidirectional. For Fromm there is a reflexive interrelationship between the 'self' and society and between personal and social normalities and pathologies. Individuals are 'free' to operate how they wish but this apparent freedom is conditional on how society operates. How society operates is conditional on how individuals, either separately or grouped, think, feel, and act. Thus, individual volition and societal pressure are in a push-and-pull myriad of processes.

Sociologist Nikolas Rose and science historian Joelle Abi-Rached (2013) point out that individuals are also involved in a similarly intricate interplay with their biology. Their neuro-genes, brain anatomy, and neuro-chemistry cavort with their psychological dispositions and societal experiences. Neuroplasticity along with the interplay between the psyche and society furnish the notion of the mutable bio-psycho-social being affected by both nature and nurture.

Untangling the multifarious bio-psycho-social entanglements is problematic if not inviable in most instances although this hasn't prevented the regular proclamation, notably from those investigating biological causation, of this having been accomplished or at least close to accomplishment. For example:

Strongest single gene conclusively implicated in schizophrenia: Single-letter changes to the DNA code of one gene have been shown to have a substantial effect on the risk of schizophrenia.

(Sanger Media Team, 2016)

A Novel Rare Variant R292H in RTN4R Affects Growth Cone Formations and Possibly Contributes to Schizophrenia Susceptibility.

(Kimura et al., 2017)

Any proclamation of having unravelled the entanglements, and thus indicating a solution to private madness or public insanity, should be considered very cautiously.

For Helman 'culture' is entangled in the roots and display of all aspects of health and illness, and therefore should be considered in all aspects of health promotion and illness demotion. In his seminal text *Culture, Health and Illness* he promotes the insertion of culture into medical practice, and he inserted. Helman describes the combination of medical and anthropological knowledge and practices thus:

[Medical anthropology] is about how people in different cultures and social groups explain the causes of ill health, the types of treatment they believe in, and to whom they turn if they do get ill … [and] how these beliefs and practices relate to biological, psychological and social changes in the human organism.

(Helman, 2007, p. 2)

Acknowledging the relevance of culture identifies a fundamental knot concerning the conception and fixing of private madness and public insanity, that of cultural relativity. These two questions summarise the problem: a) can madness be categorised as universal or only related to a specific culture? b) are particular cultures insane or is the insanity globalised? The dominant idea (scientific-psychiatry) gives weight to universalism regarding mental disorder.

Whilst Mills and Helman helped seed this book's thesis, its main theoretical thrust (that is, society matters where madness is concerned) springs from the work of Fromm. His 1955 book titled *The Sane Society* is a springboard for understanding the social context of madness today. Fromm's perspective is not taken wholly in what appears in this book. Indeed, Fromm's analysis of humanity and social systems, and what should be done about both, cannot easily be considered as a synthesised whole. This is not just because there are inconsistencies, but his work contains unresolved dilemmas about the nature of society, and sanity and insanity. Nevertheless, the conceptualisation of some societal systems as essentially insane and provision of specific exemplars which perhaps have more resonance today than they did when he was writing in the mid-twentieth century, is both innovative and suitable as an intellectual instrument. This instrument, despite its imprecision, is used to initiate the process of excavating the underpinnings of substantive societal insanities and provide a base for consequential social reform, and thereby understand better the root causes and cures of some forms of personal madness. A more detailed examination of Fromm appears in Chapter 2.

What Fromm also contributes to my way of thinking is to think 'positively'. Such a way of thinking does not equate to the 'positive psychology' meaning of pursuing happiness rather than dwelling on calamities (Seligman, 2003). What I mean by thinking positively is enacting scepticism rather than cynicism. Cynicism is a frequent criticism of sociology and one I have made (Inglis, 2015; Morrall, 2009). My intention is to be both deconstructive and constructive. Therefore, the book contains specific suggestions for seeking a saner society.

Furthermore, I am not disregarding the progress made already by humanity. The psychologist Stephen Pinker (2018) posits that humans now have lives that are longer, healthier, safer and more peaceful, more prosperous, more stimulating, and more satisfying, than at any previous point in their history. That is, he admits, they have never had it so good except for inequality, the threats from nuclear weapons, climate change, and artificial Intelligence, and an undermining of Enlightenment ideals such as reason, science, and humanism. These exceptions alone qualify for regarding society as still less than *compos mentis*. There are many other extant and impending destructive and deadly societal insanities that Pinker does not concede. Dozens of severe unresolved global issues are listed by the United Nations (2018), most if not all are major obstacles to an individual's and society's well-being. Moreover, if we have never had it some good why, if measured medically, is mental disorder mounting.

There is, however, an overriding constructive proposal: practitioners and academics have a social responsibility to act as part of their professional role. Practitioners – as well as sociologists – and their institutions have an ethical onus to engage in the discourse(s) and implementation of improvements in society at clinical and collective levels.

Society

But what is meant by 'society'. Is there a 'global society'? Is there a society at all?

For sociologist Émile Durkheim (2013) there are two species of society: 'mechanical' and 'organic'. Mechanical society is largely based on a rudimentary agrarian economy. There is homogeneity amongst individuals in agrarian economic systems regarding work. Gender roles, however, are distinct with women working less on the land and more in the home than men. Kinship and local community ties are strong, and knowledge of and travel in the wider world limited. According to Durkheim, the development of organic society was kindled by industrialisation. Industrialisation required a high degree of specialisation and sophisticated interconnectedness in the division of labour, and this produced along weaker but more varied social ties within and external to the family. Inherent to notions of 'post-industrial', 'post-modern', 'digital', and 'data' society, is further specialisation and interconnectedness with relatively superficial but multi-faceted human identities and relationships globally (Kumar, 2004; Isin and Ruppert, 2015; Harari, 2017).

Harari (2015) argues that although human cultures (which he is equating for the most part with societies) are always in a state of flux they do have a common direction. That direction is a coalescence from simpler to more complex social systems. These complex systems may then turn into mega-cultures. For Hariri 'mega-culture' equates to an 'empire' social system. Examples include Akkadian, Han, Mogul, Inca, Roman, and British empires. These mega-cultures eventually disintegrate. In the main these complex systems are held together through the inculcation of the rulers' norms and values into the conquered population's culture with some degree of modifying effect on the formers by the latter. Harari (2017) argues that today's mega-culture is globalised capitalism, and all humans now belong to what he refers to as a 'global village'. Globalised capitalism is largely based on financial institutional and interpersonal relationships with such concomitant norms and values as democracy and human rights.

The notion of a globalised society has legitimacy therefore because the economic base of most countries is either already well on the way to be capitalistic (Bieler and Morton, 2018). Novelist and essayist Rana Dasgupta (2018) argues that notwithstanding resurgent nationalistic, consumer, and protest movements, the globalisation of capitalism, and its communicative and cultural concomitants, is indeed in command as the consolidating economic force of contemporary society. Furthermore, for Dasgupta, the core components of globalisation are furnishing conformity. Transnational inter-connectivity through digital systems of trade and transmission of related values is a constricting not a liberating force (Harari, 2017).

Notwithstanding its contradictions, crises, and divergencies, at present there is no other system of economic arrangements challenging capitalism's supre-macy. Economically-driven cultural homogeneity is not fully universal and there are counter-vailing pressures (Dunne and Reus-Smit, 2017). But many of the fundamental norms, values, and mores associated with capitalism have become internalised internationally and the political campaigner George Monbiot (2017) argues there are few 'countervailing voices'.

The internationalisation of capitalism has been instigated by a process associated with the operations of large corporations globally which sociologist George Ritzer (2018) describes as 'McDonaldization'. McDonaldization is characterised by mundane, and dehumanising 'rationalised' routines across all social institutions but markedly so in the work-place and in schools and universities. Moreover, human progress is 'rationally' measured by 'growth domestic product'. Pointedly, Ritzer claims that the McDonaldization of society is irrational because of this qualitative evaluation of social develop-ment rather than quantitively assessing human happiness.

One irrationally threatens the very sustainability of humanity (examined in Chapter 8), is that of global warming (Houghton, 2015; Intergovernmental Panel on Climate Change, 2018). Environmental and human rights activist Rebecca Solnit (2016) refers to the tremendous ecological destruction, and personal suffering because of climate change. Global society is in danger of disintegration because of unprecedented flooding and tsunamis, food and water shortages because of rises in temperatures and droughts, the increase of disease and the occurrence of old and new diseases in places previously unaffected. Solnit blames this destruction on the global application of 'neo-liberal' economic policy. She defines neoliberalism thus:

> [T]he cult of unfettered international capitalism and privatization of goods and services behind what gets called globalization – and might more accurately be called corporate globalization and the commodifica-tion of absolutely everything.
>
> (Solnit, 2016, pp. 10–11)

Put plainly, today's globalised economic system has an inherent and intensely insane contradiction. Put metaphorically, to sustain itself, neoliberal capital-ism isn't just biting the hand that feeds it but swallowing itself in an auto-cannibalistic feast.

But it's not only at the level of the 'system' that such inherent and intensely insane contradictions are to be found. For example, whilst intending to combat disease, health care professionals and patrons continue to contravene counselling about the inappropriate use of antibiotics. This has resulted in the growth of uncontainable pathogens which is argued to be a greater threat to the survival of the world's financial apparatuses supporting neoliberal capitalism than was the 2007–2008 economic crisis, and more worryingly, the survival of the earth's life forms than is climate change. Moreover, climate change and the increase in drug-resistant germs are interrelated, as may be the spread of novel diseases (World Health Organisation, 2019; Department of Health and Social Care [UK], 2019; Benton, 2020). One such novel disease is COVID-19. In the early months of 2020 this virus was undermining the health of the world's population and global economic and social systems (Gurria, 2020). 'Thanatos' from Greek mythology is the daemonic representation of death (Christou and Ramenah, 2019). In psychoanalytical terms, humans have a deep-rooted 'death wish' which is in a paradoxical position to their deep-rooted pursuance of pleasure (Ikonen and Rechardt, 1978). Applying Thanatos to the non-mythical superbug situation, humanity could be regarded as engaging in a struggle between survival and self-annihilation concerning the use and abuse of antibiotics and constructing societal conditions which concede the easy transmission of lethal viruses globally.

But might globalisation be reversing? Brexit and the election of Donald Trump as President of the USA, the trade feuds between China and the USA, the rise of political popularism in Europe, past and potential world-wide financial crises, and commerce refocusing on the local rather than international, may indicate that the spread of unfettered (neoliberal) capitalism as an economic system along with its cultural accoutrements of individualism, materialism, commodification, and consumerism is floundering, fragmenting, or fading (Foroohar, 2018; Hammes, 2019). Rather than globalisation enduring or expiring, there may be a moulding of the two processes into an economic form yet unknowable (Talani and Roccu, 2019). What is also unknowable is how sane or insane might be that system.

Content

Physician and former Director-General of the World Health Organisation (WHO) Margaret Chan stated bluntly that our irrationalities have led to a mess of global proportions:

> The world is in a mess, and much of this mess is of our own making…. We have made this mess, and mistakes today are highly contagious.
>
> (Chan, 2009)

A selection of 'irrationalities' which are part of this societal mess are covered in this book. They are selected because linkage can be made with the madness of people. The first two chapters, however, examine ideas which underpin the 'faulty individual' (Chapter 1) and 'faulty society' (Chapter 2). Ideas for these two chapters are extracted from psychiatry, biology, psychology, anthropology, users of mental disorder services, and sociology. The sociological side of Fromm is posited in Chapter 2 as the most appropriate idea(s) for identifying the connection between society and the individual where madness is concerned. Five societal insanities are covered in Chapters 3–7. Each chapter deals with one topic, but each chapter has many cross-over points with the other chapters. In combination they point to the insanity of our present society and to the pointlessness of any change other than that which is formidable if it is ever to become sane. The action can be individual, but the change must be societal. In every chapter the thoughts of Fromm make an appearance.

The five insanities are: violence; inequality; selfishness; insecurity; and stupidity.

In the book's conclusion there is a *précis* of this sociological critique of personal madness and societal insanity. There is re-emphasis of the need for dramatic transformations in society to minimise the occurrences of personal madness and for humanity is to survive sanely. There is also a warning of the ultimate insanity, the madness of humanity allowing the cataclysmic collapse of its habitation and hence society.

Summary

To summarise the thesis of the book: personal madness and society are inseparable and to ignore their inseparability is intellectually and ethically irresponsible. What is offered in this book is a sociological critique of that inseparability and a plea for 'moral action' to rectify madness and make society saner.

This book exhibits and debates the bonds madness has with society by gazing beyond the individual at the wider picture (social, political, economic, ecological, and cultural contexts) as a corrective to the current torrent of reductionist ideas emanating from, for example, genetics, neuroscience, and cognitive and evolutionary psychology. The focus of the analysis will be on questioning whether it is society (its institutions, divisions, practices, and values) which is 'mad' not, or as well as, its citizens.

Let us return to your imagined medical scenario described at the beginning of this Introduction. The factors not accommodated by the medical practitioner in your imaginary case is that you live close to a chemical plant and a main road, convenience foods are just that because your busy family and work life means you do not have the time or the energy to shop for healthier options or take regular exercise, all your income is taken-up paying for a mortgage, pensions, household amenities, food, and travelling, for you and your family. Your partner is unemployed, and the relationship is strained. At work your performance has deteriorated because you are distracted by these difficulties at home, and this deterioration has been noticed by your colleagues.

Some aspects of your messy life may have been noted during your medical assessment but, no matter that they are relevant and may be the root of your physical and psychological troubles, almost certainly they will not be treated. It is the only the symptoms of these societal disorders which are addressed, and *ipso facto* for many individuals and in epidemiological terms, routine medical practice is palliative not curative, tokenistic not corrective.

There is more to madness than the personal (biological/psychological) constituents of any individual. There is society to consider; that is, society matters in the making and mending of madness. The more sane society is, the less the psyche suffers.

Notes

1 The question of whether there is such an entity as the 'mind' is addressed later.
2 There are many 'Roses' referred to in this book (social scientist Diana Rose, neuro-biologist Steven Rose, feminist sociologist Hilary Rose, and sociologist Nikolas Rose). To avoid confusion, the first name will be included whenever one is mentioned.
3 The empirical data presented in the book to support the ideas at times is inconsistent. This is because different sources have been used and these sources have compiled their data in different ways.
4 See, for example: Jones T (2014) *Psychology Express – Abnormal and Clinical Psychology*, Cambridge, UK: Pearson; Davey G (2014) (second edition) *Psychopathology – Research, Assessment and Treatment in Clinical Psychology*, Chichester, UK: Wiley; Skuse D, Bruce H and Dowdney L (2017) (editors) *Child Psychology and Psychiatry: Frameworks for Clinical Training and Practice*, Chichester, UK: Wiley; Shephard S (2017) (editor) *The Wiley Handbook of Evolutionary Neuroscience*, Chichester, UK: Wiley; Weyandt L (2018) (second edition) *Clinical Neuroscience: Foundations of Psychological and Neurodegenerative Disorders*, New York, USA: Routledge.
5 See, for example: Mead, 1934; Hirst and Woolley, 1982; McGuire et al., 1986; Giddens, 1991; Rynkiewich, 2012; May, 2013.

References

Alzheimer's Society (2019) Social care training. www.alzheimers.org.uk/dementia-professionals/training-consultancy/training-organisations/social-care-training [accessed 7 January, 2020].
Baudrillard J (2013) *The Intelligence of Evil*. London: Bloomsbury.
Beck U (1992) *Risk Society*. London: Sage.
Bieler A and Morton A (2018) *Global Capitalism, Global War, Global Crisis*. Cambridge: Cambridge University Press.
Boseley S, Collyns D, Lamb K and Dhillon A (2018) How children around the world are exposed to cigarette advertising. *The Guardian*, 9 March.
Benton T (2020) *Coronavirus: Why Are We Catching More Diseases From Animals*. BBC News, 31 January [accessed 9 February, 2020]
Bull H and Watson A (eds) (1985) *The Expansion of International Society*. Oxford: Oxford University Press.
Bupa/Mental Health First Aid (2018) *Mind Your Language: Mental Health Terminology Being Misused Despite Growing Awareness*. www.bupa.co.uk/newsroom/ourviews/language-of-mental-health [accessed 23 April, 2018].

Burstow B (2015) *Psychiatry and the Business of Madness. An Ethical and Epistemological Accounting.* London: Palgrave.

Campaign for Tobacco-Free Kids (2019) Tobacco and kids: Marketing. www.tobacco freekids.org/fact-sheets/tobaccos-toll-health-harms-and-cost/tobacco-and-kids-marketing [accessed 7 January, 2020]

Chan M (2009) The impact of global crises on health. Address at the 23rd Forum on Global Issues. www.who.int/dg/speeches/2009/financial_crisis_20090318/en/ [accessed 28 May, 2018].

Christou M and Ramenah D (2019) *Greek Mythology Explained: A Deeper Look at Classical Greek Lore and Myth.* Miami, FL: Mango.

Cohen B (2016) *Psychiatric Hegemony: Marxism and Mental Health.* London: Palgrave.

Cohen B (2018) (editor) *Routledge International Handbook of Critical Mental Health.* London: Routledge.

Crick F (1995) *The Astonishing Hypothesis: The Scientific Search for the Soul.* London: Simon & Schuster.

Dasgupta R (2018) *The Demise of the Nation State. The Guardian,* 5 April.

Department of Health and Social Care [UK] (2019) Antimicrobial resistance: UK launches 5-year action plan and 20-year vision. www.gov.uk/government/news/a ntimicrobial-resistance-uk-launches-5-year-action-plan-and-20-year-vision [accessed 26th January, 2019].

Dunne T and Reus-Smit C (eds) (2017) *The Globalization of International Society.* Oxford: Oxford University Press.

Durkheim E (2013) *Durkheim: The Division of Labour in Society.* London: Palgrave. Original 1893: *De la Division Du Travail Social.* Paris: Presses Universitaires de France.

Foroohar R (2018) Corporate elites are overlooking deglobalisation. *Financial Times,* 14 October. www.ft.com/content/df3ded82-ce32-11e8-b276-b9069bde0956 [accessed 24 February, 2019].

Foucault M (1961) *Folie et Déraison: Histoire de la folie à l'âge classique* [Madness and Civilization]. Paris: Librarie Plon.

Foucault M (2006) *Psychiatric Power: Lectures at the Collège de France.* Basingstoke: Palgrave MacMillan.

Fromm F (1955) *The Sane Society.* New York: Rinehart.

Giddens A (1991) *Modernity and Self-identity: Self and Society in the Late Modern Age.* Cambridge: Polity Press.

Goffman E (1959) *The Presentation of Self in Everyday Life.* New York: Anchor.

Goldacre B (2012) *Bad Pharma: How Drug Companies Mislead Doctors and Harm Patients.* London: Fourth Estate.

Goldacre B (2014) *I Think You'll Find It's a bit More Complicated Than That.* London: Fourth Estate.

Gurría A (2020) COVID-19: Joint Actions to Win the War. The Organisation for Economic Co-operation and Development. http://www.oecd.org/coronavirus/ [accessed 23 March, 2020].

Hammes T X (2019) *Deglobalization: The Fragmenting World Economy and the Impact on International Security.* Annapolis, MA: Naval Institute Press.

Harari Y (2015) *Sapiens: A Brief History of Humankind.* London: Vintage.

Harari Y (2017) *Homo Deus: A brief History of Tomorrow.* London: Vintage.

Helman C (2006) *Suburban Shaman: Tales from Medicine's Front Line.* London: Hammersmith Press.

Helman C (2007) *Culture, Health and Illness,* 5th edn. London: Hodder Arnold.

Hirst P and Woolley P (1982) *Social Relations and Human Attributes.* London: Tavistock.

Houghton J (2015) *Global Warming: The Complete Briefing.* Cambridge: Cambridge University Press.

Hutton W (2016) Only fundamental social change can defeat the anxiety epidemic. *The Observer*, 8 May.

Ikonen P and Rechardt E (1978) The vicissitudes of thanatos: On the place of aggression and destructiveness in psychoanalytic interpretation. *Scandinavian Psychoanalytic Review*, 1(1), pp. 79–114.

Inglis D (2015) Cynical sociology? No, kynical sociology! *Australian Sociological association*, 15 April. https://tasa.org.au/blog/2015/04/15/cynical-sociology-no-kynical-sociology/ [accessed 11 May 2018].

Intergovernmental Panel on Climate Change (IPCC) (2018) Global Warming of 1.5c. Geneva: World Meteorological Organization/United Nations.

Isin I and Ruppert E (2015). *Being Digital Citizens.* London: Rowman & Littlefield.

Kimura H, Fujita Y, Kawabata T, Ishizuka K, Wang C, Iwayama Y, Okahisa Y, Kushima I, Morikawa M, Uno Y, Okada T, Ikeda M, Inada T, Branko A, Mori D, Yoshikawa T, Iwata N, Nakamura H, Yamashita T and Ozaki N (2017). A novel rare variant R292H in RTN4R affects growth cone formations and possibly contributes to schizophrenia susceptibility. *Translational Psychiatry*, 7, p.e1214. www.nature.com/articles/tp2017170 [accessed 24 May, 2018].

Kumar K (2004) *From Post-Industrial to Post-Modern Society: New Theories of the Contemporary World*, 2nd edn. Chichester: Wiley-Blackwell.

Levine S (2016) Insulting words with a psychiatric twist. *Psychology Today*, 9 June. www.psychologytoday.com/us/blog/our-emotional-footprint/201606/insulting-words-psychiatric-twist [accessed 23 April, 2018].

Liddle R (2014) *Selfish Whining Monkeys: How We Ended Up Greedy, Narcissistic and Unhappy.* London: Fourth Estate.

Loughnan A (2015) How the insanity defence against a murder charge works. *The Conversation*. 6 November. http://theconversation.com/how-the-insanity-defence-against-a-murder-charge-works-50188 [accessed 26 April, 2018].

Math S, Kumar C and Moirangthem S (2015) Insanity defense: Past, present, and future. *Indian Journal of Psychological Medicine*, 37(4), pp. 381–387.

May V (2013) *Connecting Self to Society: Belonging in a Changing World.* London: Palgrave.

McGuire W J, McGuire C V and Cheever J. (1986) The self in society: Effects of social contexts on the sense of self. *British Journal of Social Psychology*, 25(3), pp. 259–270.

Mead, G H (1934). *Mind, Self, and Society: From the Standpoint of a Social Behaviorist.* Chicago: University of Chicago Press.

Mental Health Foundation (2015) *Dementia, Rights, and the Social Model of Disability: A New Direction for Policy and Practice?* London: Mental Health Foundation.

Mills C W (1959) *The Sociological Imagination.* New York: Oxford University Press.

Monbiot G (2017) *How Did We Get into This Mess?: Politics, Equality, Nature.* London: Verso.

Morrall P (2009) *Sociology and Health: An Introduction*, 2nd edn. London: Routledge.

Morrall P (2017) *Madness: Ideas about Insanity.* Abingdon-on-Thames: Routledge.

National Archives [British] (2018) *Criminal Procedure (Insanity and Unfitness to Plead) Act 1991.* www.legislation.gov.uk/ukpga/1991/25/section/1

Onions C (1966) *Oxford Dictionary of English Etymology.* Oxford: Oxford University Press.

Pink Floyd (1973) *Dark Side of the Moon* (track 3 'Time'). London: Harvest Records/EMI.

Pinker S (2018) *Enlightenment Now: The Case for Reason, Science, Humanism, and Progress.* London: Allen Lane.

Ritzer G (2018) *The McDonaldization of Society: Into the Digital Age*, 9th edn. London: Sage.

Robinson P and Williams T (2017) Insanity defense. In *Mapping American Criminal Law: Variations Across the 50 States.* University of Pennsylvania Law School Scholarship Repository 1718. http://scholarship.law.upenn.edu/faculty_scholarship/1718 [accessed 24 April, 2018]

Rose D, Thornicroft G, Pinfold V and Kassam A (2007) 250 labels used to stigmatise people with mental illness. *BMC Health Services Research*, 7(97). www.ncbi.nlm.nih.gov/pmc/articles/PMC1925070/ [accessed 23rd April, 2018].

Rose N and Abi-Rached J (2013) *Neuro: The New Brain Sciences and the Management of the Mind.* Princeton, NJ: Princeton University Press.

Rogers A and Pilgrim D A (2014) *Sociology of Mental Health and Illness*, 5th edn. Chichester: McGraw-Hill.

Ruscio J (2004) Diagnoses and the behaviors they denote: A critical evaluation of the labeling theory of mental illness. *The Scientific Review of Mental Health Practice*, 3 (1). www.srmhp.org/0301/labels.html [accessed 5th August, 2015].

Rynkiewich M (2012) *Soul, Self, and Society: A Postmodern Anthropology for Mission in a Postcolonial World.* Eugene, OR: Wipf and Stock.

Sanger Media Team (2016) Strongest single gene conclusively implicated in schizophrenia: Single-letter changes to the DNA code of one gene have been shown to have a substantial effect on the risk of schizophrenia. Welcome Sanger Institute, 14 March. www.sanger.ac.uk/news/view/strongest-single-gene-conclusively-implicated-schizophrenia [accessed 24 May, 2018].

Scull A (1977) *Decarceration: Community Treatment and the Deviant – A Radical View.* Upper Saddle River, NJ: Prentice Hall.

Scull A (2015) *Madness in Civilization: A Cultural History of Insanity.* London: Thames & Hudson.

Seligman M (2003) *Authentic Happiness: Using the New Positive Psychology to Realise your Potential for Lasting Fulfilment.* Boston, MA: Nicholas Brealey.

Simon J and Ahn-Redding H (2008) *The Insanity Defense the World Over.* Lanham, MA: Lexington.

Solnit R (2016) *Hope in the Dark: Untold Histories and Wild Possibilities.* Edinburgh: Canongate.

Stier S, Schoene-Seifert B, Rüther R and Muders S (2014) The philosophy of psychiatry and biologism. *Frontiers in Psychology*, 25(5), p. 1032. www.ncbi.nlm.nih.gov/pmc/articles/PMC4166893/ [accessed 24 February, 2019].

Talani L and Roccu R (2019) (eds) *The Dark Side of Globalisation.* Basel, Switzerland: Springer

Time to Change (2018) Mind your language!www.time-to-change.org.uk/media-centre/responsible-reporting/mind-your-language [accessed 23rd April, 2018].

United Nations (2018) www.un.org/en/sections/issues-depth/global-issues-overview/index.html [accessed 16th April, 2018].

Wilkinson R and Pickett K (2010) *The Spirit Level: Why Equality is Better for Everyone.* London: Penguin.

World Health Organisation (2019) *A Global Health Guardian: Climate Change, Air Pollution, and Antimicrobial Resistance.* Geneva: World Health Organisation. www.who.int/publications/10-year-review/health-guardian/en/index3.html [accessed 26 January, 2019].

1 Faulty individual

To remind the reader, the idea of this book is that society matters to madness,[1] in terms of how it is considered and how it should be resolved (or even respected), and ideas from sociology and accordant disciplines are crucial in understanding society's connection to personal madness. Moreover, that society matters to madness should not be an addendum to or adornment of biological ideas. Society should be at the forefront of understanding insanity.

Medical considerations about madness have dominated the understanding and management of madness for centuries. Notwithstanding many challenges and challengers, this dominance is in the ascendant and not in retreat. There is a refurbishment of psychiatry's scientific credentials based largely on biological propositions and related remedies (both physical and psychological). There is an alternative to gazing into the brains and at implicated genes and neurological processes. Rather than focusing on faults in the individual, the alternative gaze is to look outwards at the faults in society (Chapter 2). The focus then shifts to social processes, structures, and institutions. Furthermore, just as the biological gaze has intensified, the societal gaze increasingly must extend beyond the local towards the global.

Paralleling today's invigorated biologism is the proclaiming of mental disorder 'epidemics' amongst adults and children globally, notably anxiety and depression ((Plant and Stephenson, 2009; WHO, 2017; American Psychiatric Association, 2018). But are these diagnoses justified or the consequence of commercial and professional interests which seeks to medicalise normality and personal problems (Whitaker, 2011; Allen, 2014; Pies, 2016)? Conventional psychiatrists, most psychologists and psychotherapists, and 'structuralist' sociologists, accept that psychological distress really does exist (although not all accept this should be medicalised as 'mental disorder'), and that some aspects of this distress have reached plague proportions. However, there is a fundamental conundrum for those with fundamentalist conviction about biological causation. If any epidemic of any mental disorder has occurred over a somewhat short period of time (a matter of decades), how can this be attributed to biological faults let alone evolutionary maladaptation? Biology does not change that fast. But society can change that fast. Moreover, society can and does change biology (Nikolas Rose, 2018).

It is also important to point out that alternative modes of thinking and practicing are not wholly excluded by the supremacy of the biological paradigm. For sociologist Nikolas Rose (2018) There is no one 'psychiatry'. Psychiatry, whilst dominated by biology, is heterogeneous in the sense that non-biological 'talking treatments' are prescribed (for example, cognitive behaviour therapy and mindfulness), and social factors in causation and recovery are not proscribed. Neuroscience has a social offshoot. 'Social neuroscience' acknowledges that humans are social species (Cacioppo and Decety, 2011). However, the goal of social neuroscience is to investigate the biological mechanisms which buttress the framework of society rather that how social structures, processes, and institutions might buttress biology. Western psychiatry, as with all medical specialities, legitimises its practices more-and-more on 'scientifically valid and reliable evidence, frequently at the insistence of governments attempting to reign-in expenditure on health care (Cairney and Oliver, 2017; Parkhurst, 2017). Today most of the evidence being sought by psychiatry is biological not social.

'Social prescribing' refers to the formal recommendation by medical practitioners for their patients to engage in volunteering, art, sports, dancing, singing, gardening, cooking, eating healthy food, talking to friends and making fresh friends, walking and cycling. Environmental psychologists (Hunter et al., 2019) have monitored a reduction in stress hormones such as cortisol after at least 20mins a day walking in a park or garden. Their research underscores social prescribing in form of 'nature pills' to improve mental well-being. The prescribing of activities is intended to replace or supplement surgical interventions and drug treatments (Department of Health, 2006; King's Fund, 2019). The UK government, therefore, is supporting social prescribing on the basis that it can reduce the occurrence of hypertension, diabetes, depression, and 'complex social needs' such as loneliness. There is also an economic saving compared with surgery and drugs (National Health Service England, 2019). Social prescribing is promoted as a 'holistic' approach to dealing with or preventing disease. It is also promoted as a variant of 'personalised' medicine with an emphasis on the patient taking control of her/his own health and ill-health. There is criticism of social prescribing for being more 'rhetorical' than justifiable based on empirical evidence (Bickerdike et al., 2017). Public health researcher Glen Stewart (2019), writing in the British Medical Journal, notes that social prescribing may distract attention from the 'wider determinants' of ill-health. Chapter 2 notes some of these wider social determinants.

This chapter is compiled of a series of biological and concomitant ideas (for example, from evolutionary psychology). These ideas arise in the main from empirical evidence (the notable exception is evolutionary psychology). Where it is obvious so to do, a critique of the idea in question is offered within this chapter. However, more attention is paid to critiquing the faulty individual approach in Chapter 2. Apart from that critique, Chapter 2 presents ideas resulting from gazing at the faults in society. These ideas arise from both empirical evidence and theoretical reasoning. As mentioned in the Introduction to the book, it is Fromm's 'insane society' idea which forms much of the theoretical backdrop to the proposition of this book. It is his sociologically informed stance on psychological states and the state of society which informs this sociological examination of madness. Hence, Chapter 2 highlights Fromm as the principal counterpoint to gazing at faults in the individual.

Neuro everything

Sociologist Hilary Rose and neuroscientist Steven Rose comment on the infiltration of neurological notions in scientific endeavour generally:

> Neuro occupies more and more space within mainstream science.
> (Hilary Rose and Steven Rose, 2016, p. 1)

'Neuro' has assuredly infiltrated contemporary scientific discourse focused on the making and mending of madness. Neuroscientists, neurogeneticists, neuroendocrinologists, neuroimmunologists, neuropsychiatrists, psychoneuroimmunologists, neuropsychologists, cognitive neuropsychiatrists, and cognitive neuropsychologists, along with evolutionary psychologists, are offering abundant claims of actual or potential cause and thereby assuagement for many forms of madness.

Focusing on biological faults in the individual to fathom and mitigate madness has a long history and powerful presence presently in psychiatry (Jasanoff, 2018). For example, a founder of psychiatry as a medical speciality in nineteenth-century France Jean-Etienne Esquirol and his German equivalent Wilhelm Griesinger, were both convinced that the brain was the locus for much of madness (Morrall, 2017).

Early in the twenty-first century psychiatrist and geneticist Peter McGuffin was to argue that a 'revitalised' and more scientific psychiatry infused with and enthused by the empirical outpourings of neurotechnology, and neuroscientific and genetic research could secure the future of psychiatry (Rose and McGuffin, 2005; McGuffin and Murray, 2014). The number of diagnostic technologies is expanding and their scrutiny intensifying. Examples are computerised axial tomography, magnetic resonance imaging, functional magnetic resonance imaging, positron emission tomography, and gene mapping. There is now a disparate array of old, refurbished, novel, and prospective physical methods of treatment such as: anti-psychotic, antidepressant, mood stabilising, anxiolytic, and hypnotic drugs; electroconvulsive therapy; repetitive transcranial magnetic stimulation; deep brain stimulation; and gene editing (Gargiulo and Mesones-Arroyo, 2018; Higgins, 2018; Doudna and Sternberg, 2017; Kozubek, 2018). Psychiatry, psychotherapy, and clinical psychology are justifying some psychotherapies as neurologically remedial (Grawe, 2005; Cozolino, 2010).

The promise of technology, genomics, and neuroscience is that in-depth imaging can show neurological 'functional' changes rather than just physical pathology when the subject is experiencing hallucinations or delusions, and physical treatments can reverse some these brain aberrations. Sets of genes implicated in the cause of schizophrenia and manic-depression have been identified, and a further promise is that responsible mix of faulty genes for many other disorders will eventually be found and fixed. Neuropathological sites, it is prophesied could be normalised by inserting freshly brain material or chemicals, stimulating undamaged neurons to form new pathways, or reassembling damaged neurological matrixes (Heinrich et al. 2014; Greenfield, 2016; Amen, 2020).

The Maudsley Biological Research Centre (2018) is partner to the Institute of Psychiatry, Psychology & Neuroscience at King's College London. This centre is a prime example of this shift in psychiatric theory and practice, and the expansion of psychiatry's 'neuro' domain. Its research endeavours cover: depression; manic-depression: anxiety disorders: schizophrenia, and 'other psychotic disorders and neurological diseases of the brain'; dementia and 'related disorders'; child and neurodevelopmental disorders including autism, attention deficit hyperactivity disorder, and 'other mental disorders which occur in children' such as anxiety, depression, and conduct disorder; use and abuse of tobacco, alcohol and 'illegal substances'; obesity; pain associated with mental disorder. There are displays of scanned brains and neurological structures in the link webpages to some research themes designed presumably purporting tangible or conceivable sites of neurologically-based mental malfunction.

What is also portended, mainly from researching rats, is that all aspects of the mind and madness can be pinned to brain activity. For example, neuroscientist Susan Greenfield (2016) proposes that the link between objective experience and subjective experience is the formation in the brain of neuronal 'assemblies' of varying sizes. Similarly, the proposition of neuropsychologists Peter Halligan and David Oakley (2018) is that both subjective experience of consciousness (personal awareness) and associated psychological processes (thoughts, beliefs, ideas, intentions and more) are products of non-conscious processes as are core biological processes (such as respiration and digestion). Human performance relies on 'unconscious authoring'. Complex and intelligent design in living come from naturally selected adaptations. Consciousness (and free-will) is contained (only) in neurological activity, and certain assemblies of such activity can be correlated with certain types of madness.

The inference is that the mind and madness are only a matter of matter, and hence humans are afflicted with what sociologist Hilary Rose and neuroscientist Steven Rose describe as a 'user illusion':

> For the neuroscientists of the twenty-first century, mental activity can be reduced to brain processes.... [I]n doing so, to make the mind, and the person it inhabits, merely 'a user illusion', fooling people into thinking that they are making decisions whereas it is really the brain that is doing it.
>
> (Hilary Rose and Steven Rose, 2016, p. 19)

Similarly, behavioural psychologist Nick Chater's (2018) proposition is that 'the mind is flat'. That is, the mind has no inner life, there is no unconscious or even subconscious, no 'personality', human perceptions of the external world are a mere mélange of guesses and insubstantial and disputable formulations, memory is mutable not meticulous, and emotions are merely reactions to external environmental stimuli and internal somatic movement. Again, 'the self' in the sense of a distinct, persistent, dispositional, knowable, determining human quality, is a hoax played on our 'selves'. From this perception, there is nothing sound in conceptions of sanity or insanity. Nor can there be in Charter's presumed perceptiveness.

For psychiatrist Barbara Schildkrout (2017) understanding of the brain is fundamental knowledge for all psychiatrists, claiming that the brain is the organ of psychiatry. What Schildkrout also makes the case for is recognising that understandings of the brain depend on what technological devices are used. Advances in technology have made it possible to investigate brain function in a living human and to study neurological links between genes, molecules, and the circuits, and human performance. However, Schildkrout points out that the underlying organisation of the brain is not clear. Different approaches are used to define and differentiate areas of the brain and their function. These include focusing on anatomical pathology of the cortex, pathological processes in cells, and on how various structures in the brain interrelate. Comprehending the brain, let alone connecting its activities to either normal or abnormal thoughts, emotions, and behaviours, is hampered severely, realises Schildkrout, by incomprehension between approaches. Moreover, even within one approach what is seen, and therefore what may become understood, will depend on the level of magnification. Cells, circuits, chemicals, or connecting configurations, will furnish diverse impressions depending on the parameters of the gaze which will also depend on which device is operated. Added to these factors framing what can be understood about the brain identified by Schildkrout, is the problem of partisanship. That is, what is looked for, what is perceived, and what then is made of that perception, depend on what professional discourse has been embraced, and what resources and requirements there are for research.

Psychiatric revolutions

Apart from the re-engineering of genes, the psychiatric revolution based on biology has been promised by advances in synthetic and systems biology (Tretter and Albus, 2008), robotic nanoscience/nanotechnology (Fond et al., 2013), humanised robots and artificial intelligence (Luxton, 2015). Moreover, apart from the long-term omnipresence of psycho-pharmaceuticals, another enduring physical method of treatment has been retained. Electroconvulsive therapy is as, if not more, controversial as the use of drugs in psychiatry, but it still has its ardent supporters such as the psychiatrist George Kirov (2017).

Other committed biologists join McGuffin in his prediction and celebration of neuroscience in psychiatry. Thomas Insel is presently (2018) head of a healthcare company and past director of the research organisation Verily (formerly Google Life Sciences) and previously head of the American [USA] National Institute of Mental Health. In the latter post he argued that advances in biological research had allowed psychiatry to be reinvented:

> A REVOLUTION is under way in psychiatry.... We are starting to build it on genomics and neuroscience, thanks to advances in DNA sequencing and functional imaging.
>
> (upper-case in the original, Insel, 2015)

He claims that the ideological and practical armaments for the impending transformation of psychiatry are the diagnostic and curative bullets being generated by genomics and neuroscience to combat, he cites, depression and schizophrenia. Insel is in no doubt that mental disorder is disorder of the brain and a consequence of 'connectopathies', that is problems in neurological circuits. The limited success so far in finding biological markers and related cures is merely a 'teething problem'.

A host of neuroscientists authoring a publication in the internationally renowned scientific journal 'Science' are enthusiastic about the promise of genetic analysis and investigative machinery in the search for biological causation:

> We're on the threshold to using genomics and molecular technology to look at [mental illness] in a way we've never been able to do before. Psychiatric disorders have no obvious pathology in the brain, but now we have the genomic tools to ask what actually goes awry in these brains.
>
> (Gandal et al., 2018)

These 74 researchers compare this research with genetic breakthroughs occurring in cancer studies.

Breakthroughs in psychiatry have happened, two of which are most apparent: the discovery in the 1880s of the responsible bacterium for general paralysis of the insane and the invention of curative antibiotic medication in 1940s; the production of a multitude of anti-psychotic, anti-anxiety, and anti-depression drugs for the mid-twentieth to the late-twentieth century (Shorter, 1997; Lieberman, 2015). Genetic and neuroscientific breakthroughs which are influencing psychiatry arrived during this latter period and have continued. The mapping of the human genome at the beginning of the twenty-first century was predicted at that point to be the most dramatic of revolutions for psychiatry (Insel and Collins, 2003). Psychologist and geneticist Robert Plomin (2018) claims that the evidence implicating 'nature' in determining the facets of an individual's mind, including his her/his susceptibility to mental disorder, is persuasive. For Plomin it is nature which regulates intelligence, levels of empathy and sociability. Societal and material circumstances do have an effect, but their potency is mediated markedly by genes. Moreover, Plomin further claims that the many major mental disorders cannot be categorised as unitary entities, but that genes are responsible for mental disorder 'spectrums'. These include 'depression spectrum' and 'schizophrenia spectrum'. Plomin's claims about the dominance of nature over human performance, however, are regarded as 'outlandish' and 'only half the story' by fellow psychologist and geneticist Kathryn Harden (2018).

Taking advantage of genomic scientific advances, the Psychiatric Genomics Consortium (2018) was set up in 2007. The Psychiatric Genomics Consortium comprises hundreds of researchers from around the world who by ten years later had collected samples of genes from nearly one billion people. Subdivided into 'work groups', it is investigating the causal biomarkers of a wide range of diagnostic categories. These include: schizophrenia, depression, manic-depression (bi-polar disorder), anxiety, Alzheimer's disease, post-traumatic-stress disorder, substance use, obsessional-compulsive disorder, attention-deficit disorder, autism spectrum, and eating disorders. It is also attempting to establish genetic influences which transcend diagnostic boundaries. Funders of the Psychiatric Genomics Consortium include national and international agencies and business organisations.

There is parallel research in genomics attending to physical disorder. For example, in 2018 'Genomics England', an agency of the British Government, announced the successful sequencing of 100,000 genomes of patients with rare diseases and cancer and aims increase this number to millions in the coming years. Geneticists working on the project accept that, except for a few, most diseases are the caused by a complexity of genes (and the DNA between genes), and complexity of environmental factors. The aim of the agency is to improve diagnosis, prevention, and treatment by targeting the complex mix of genes associated with these diseases. There is not an equivalent targeting of the environmental complexity.

The Schizophrenia Working Group of the Psychiatric Genomics Consortium (2014) has declared success in establishing inherited 'polygenetic risk' for schizophrenia. Over one hundred-and-forty variants of DNA are claimed to be responsible. A possible link between the immune system and schizophrenia was also given support. The Major Depressive Disorders Workgroup of the Psychiatric Genomics Consortium (2018) has identified forty-four 'independent and significant loci' associated with increased risk of major depressive disorder.

Psychiatric and genetic researchers Thomas Schulze and Kristina Adorjan (2018) describe developments in genomics as revolutionary since the mapping of the human genome which have direct relevance to mental disorder as 'amazing'. They refer to the century-long accumulation of evidence from twin and adoption studies indicating the familial and hereditary basis of some mental disorders. But, they argue, a 'paradigm shift' is occurring now that hundreds of genetic loci are connectable with the cause of schizophrenia and scores with depression and bipolar disorder, through the work, for example, of the Psychiatric Genomics Consortium. Despite revolutions, paradigm shifts, and being amazed, Schulze and Adorjan present a cautionary missive:

> One has to admit that these approaches are still in their infancy, we have not yet delivered clues that can allow for a rapid translation into the clinical world.
>
> (Schulze and Adorjan, 2018)

Aspirant transformations in psychiatric knowledge and practice continue to appear in the academic and professional journals and in the media.

A second case in point is the reporting of a Swedish study by the BBC in which there is there is the suggestion of the 'enormous potential' of treating of 'severe mental disorders' such as schizophrenia and manic-depression with cheap and already widely available medications (Gallagher, 2019). The drugs in question are those used for diabetes, hypertension, and high cholesterol. Significant reductions in hospital admissions and in self-harming. The report of the study in the journal concludes:

> If substantiated, this study has *considerable implications for clinical practice* and drug development.... Understanding their [the drugs] mode of action on the central nervous system may facilitate better understanding of the pathophysiology of SMI [sever mental illness] and offer opportunities for *innovative pharmacotherapy* development. [emphases added]
>
> (Hayes, et al., 2019)

Further on in the BBC article psychiatrist James MacCabe is quoted: 'These findings are very compelling' (Gallagher, 2019). The researchers in the BBC article and their formal report, and in the BBC article an expert in cardio-metabolic medicine, Naveed Sattar, advise caution about their results, and both want further and more robust clinical trials to be conducted.

Although there are non-chemical alternative treatments for depression (for example, cognitive-behavioural therapy), pharmaceuticals remain the most common medical intervention. Antidepressants, of which there are about 40 from which to choose, are amongst the most commonly prescribed group of drugs in developed countries (Wilson, 2018). More than 70 million antidepressant prescriptions were dispensed in England by the National Health Service during the year 2018, double the number since 2008. The cost for 2018 antidepressant prescriptions was nearly £9 billion. Private prescriptions and those dispensed in hospitals are not included in these figures. (NHS Digital, 2019). Despite this high usage, the efficacy of anti-depressants is disputed.

In 2018 the results of a meta-analysis of extant research into the effectiveness of prescribed anti-depressant drugs was published in the medical journal *The Lancet* (Cipriani et al., 2018). The authors claimed that the antidepressants covered in study were more efficacious than placebos for moderate to severe depression and that the results should be to guide 'evidence-based' medical practice and health policy. The study was quoted widely in the media under headlines and subsequent explanatory text such as this one from the British newspaper *The Guardian*:

> The drugs do work: antidepressants are effective, study shows. Doctors hope study will put to rest doubts about the medicine, and help to address global under-treatment of depression. It's official: antidepressants are not snake oil or a conspiracy.

> (Boseley, 2018)

Biological psychiatrist Carmine Pariante, is quoted as saying that the study 'finally puts to bed the controversy on anti-depressants', and his opinion is accredited to the Royal College of Psychiatrists (Therrien, 2018).

Medical journalist Clare Wilson (2018) commented that almost every headline published about the study was wrong. The study was not original research but a meta-analysis of extant studies. Many of the included studies, the authors accept, could have been biased for example by financial association with pharmaceutical companies, and some relevant research has not published and therefore was not included in their meta-analysis. They did, they argue, attempt to control for these weaknesses in their research.

But these weaknesses may not have been controlled fully, and other weaknesses were left uncontrolled (McCormack and Korownyk, 2018). The study did not focus on mild depression, which is by far the most common type whereby anti-depressant medication is prescribed. Only an eight-week use of anti-depressants was examined. It did not highlight the dangers of anti-depressant usage which can increase the likelihood of suicide and homicide. There is no accounting for the 'epidemic' of diagnosis relating to depression. Nor is there exploration of the societal causation. These weaknesses led to the Council for Evidence-based Psychiatry (2018) to exclaim that not only does the study prove anything new, but the above statement attributed to the Royal College of Psychiatrists is 'irresponsible and unsubstantiated'. Danish physician and leader of the Nordic Cochrane Center Copenhagen Peter Gøtzsche (2018) declared that the results of the study 'should not be trusted'.

Inflamed brain

Caution about other aspects of psychiatric success is also expressed by neuropsychiatrist Edward Bullmore (2018a). Commenting on detection of genes for depression, affirms the heritability of such mental disorders Bullmore suggests that the case for genetic causation remains incomplete. Bullmore observes that 44 'independent and significant loci' (out of the twenty-thousand genes which comprise the human genome) carry only a small amount of the genetic risk let alone the risk carried from other influences. It is the cumulative impact from a complexity of factors which makes depression more likely not a few dozen genes. Bullmore maintains that the mix of 'genes for depression' has not yet been found despite inflammatory pronouncements by international researchers.

> There a hundreds of thousands of biomarkers, and they are rapidly growing in number sophistication, in all areas of medicine … except psychiatry, which doesn't currently have a single blood test or biomarker to in name.
>
> (Bullmore, 2018b, p. 107)

It is inflammation that Bullmore pronounces as a the major 'other influence' in the complex mix which causes depression.

For Bullmore, an inflamed brain is directly related to depressive episodes and genes do play a part in the triggering of inflammatory responses by the immune system. There are, he argues, also more obvious somatic, psychological, and social 'stress' triggers. Infection anywhere in the body, surgery to any part of the body, and any of countless major and minor personal and social problems (from bereavement, abuse, and assault, to public speaking and dental surgery) may lead to mental disorder, notably depression but possible schizophrenia and dementia. What these any or all these triggers do is incite inflammation by provoking the immunological system. When the brain is not the immediate target of inflammation, it inevitably becomes a secondary one due to the interlinking of somatic systems.

Bullmore's acceptance that vulnerability to a detrimental inflammatory response to stress must be looked for in nature and nurture does not detract from his desire to trigger a revolution in psychiatry. The focus of the revolution must be on inflammation and one which targets not just depression but other major mental disorders such as schizophrenia, dementia, and obsessive-compulsive disorder, and *Gilles de la Tourette's* syndrome (Bullmore, 2018a; 2018b). In terms of future treatments, Bullmore proposes that his inflammatory revolution should aim to break what he describes as the 'vicious cycle' in which 'stress' leads to inflammation which then leads to depression, and then back to 'stress'.

Despite Bullmore's recognition of 'nurture' in the causation of mental disorder, and the possible need for interventions which modify the mind or the environmental, his emphasis is on biological intervention. New drugs are needed to break the 'vicious cycle'. Alongside academic positions, Bullmore works for the pharmaceutical company GlaxoSmithKline assisting in the search for anti-inflammatory pharmaceutical interventions for depression.

That the brain and mind of an individual can be undermined through the 'autoimmunological' dispersal of inflammation is certainly gaining in popularity both in neuroscience and psychiatry. Psychiatrist Belinda Lennox and her colleagues suggest that some patients diagnosed with schizophrenia or bipolar disorder may have an immune disorder (Lennox et al., 2017). They recommend that anyone with a first episode of psychosis should be screened for potentially pathogenic antibodies. Neurologist Souhel Najjar and his colleagues claims that there is evidence linking psychosis and autoimmune pathological reaction particularly misplaced or excessive inflammation (Najjar et al., 2018) They claim, for example, that antibodies released by the immune system can harm synaptic and neuronal cell membrane proteins, and this can lead to subtype of psychosis which they describe as 'autoimmune psychosis'. Najjar states his belief in the possibilities that neurology[2] can offer to understand psychosis:

> If an autoimmune disease can create symptoms that look exactly like schizophrenia, that raises the question, what is schizophrenia? And are there forms of schizophrenia that are caused by other types of auto-immune disease? Or other [physical] diseases that we haven't discovered yet? *It's all neurological.* [emphasis added]
>
> (Najjar quoted in Cadwalladr, 2013)

Other apparent psychiatric-neuroscientific discoveries orientated to inflammation include the benefits of nutrition. A healthy 'anti-inflammatory' diet, especially one based on traditional Mediterranean ingredients, may offer confer protection against depression (Lassale et al., 2018). Microbe perturbances in the gut may have a role in inflaming the brain. If the trillions of microbes in the gut become out of balance, or if the gut is invaded by pathogens, then because of the immunologically connected 'gut-brain-axis' and the spreading of inflammation, depression, anxiety, autism, and neurodegenerative, may be the result (Clapp, et al., 2017; Rieder et al., 2017; Liu and Zhu, 2018).

It is worth remembering, however, that inflammation because of immunological reactions is in the main not malevolent but beneficial in the fight against disease. Inflammation is a vital element of the body's immunological processes and the latter is vital to survival. Moreover, the beneficence of the immune system can be augmented through medical manipulation Immunologists James Allison and Tasuku Honjo were awarded a Nobel Prize in 2018 for establishing a new approach to containing and possibly curing cancer. They had demonstrated how stimulating the immune system in specific ways destroyed tumour cells (Nobel Assembly at Karolinska Institute, 2018).

Brain anatomical pathology is also implicated in the causation of the diagnosis of a series of mental disorders according to a series of neuroscientists, psychiatrists, and psychologists. The amygdala is a bilateral cluster of neurons found deep in the temporal lobe of the brain which is probably part of the limbic system and is associated particularly with regulating emotions, the management of memory, and decisions-making. Dysfunction of the amygdala is associated with, for example, anxiety and phobias, depression, schizophrenia, autism, schizophrenia, manic-depression, post-traumatic stress disorder, and psychopathy (Fudge et al., 1998; Schumann et al., 2011; Marsh, 2017; Ewbank et al., 2018).

Psychology evolution

Evolution has also been impugned with selecting certain features of human performance which may become diagnosed as mental disorder. Evolutionary psychologists and their epistemological twins in psychiatry have attempted to align the past biological evolution of humans with present emotional states, patterns of thinking, and modes of behaviour.

The origins of evolutionary psychology and evolutionary psychiatry arise from the 'sociobiology' of biologist Edward Osborne Wilson (1975). Wilson formed his ideas about humans from studying non-humans (he had a special interest in ants), and contended that nature (that is, genes) was the foundation for human performance not nurture. For all forms of life, including humans, psychological and psychiatric evolutionists accept that the drive for genetic survival and reproduction is primary (Andrews and Thompson, 2009; Buss, 2017; Stevens and Price, 2000; Abed and St John-Smith, 2016). Sociobiology was rebranded as evolutionary psychology in the 1990s, and evolutionary psychiatry was to follow although it remains a fringe medical sub-discipline (Hilary Rose and Steven Rose, 2016; Abed and St John-Smith, 2016; Brune, 2008).

But for genetic survival and reproduction, are those elements of human performance which are susceptible to a mental disorder diagnosis maladaptive and adaptive? For example, is human existence endangered or ameliorated by exaggerated angst, elevated excitement, severe sadness, bogus beliefs, specious sensations, and excessive egocentrism? Some supposed symptoms of mental disorder, propose the neo-evolutionists, may be either or both dysfunctional or functional for the individual and/or society. They may either be an inherited process which may lead to an individual experiencing emotional turmoil and physical harm or prove a challenge to the normalcy and efficiency of society. However, they may also warn of danger, the need to rest, to enable artistic, musical, and comedic creativity, academic ingenuity, commercial success and corporate growth, and political contrivance and endurance (Stevens and Price, 1996; Brune, 2008; Andrews and Thomson, 2009).

For both evolutionary biologists and evolutionary psychologists/psychiatrists of either the soft or hard deterministic kind there is a major theoretical and empirical glitch in their respective propositions. For the hard determinist biology directs all or most of human performance without the assistance of society and psychological factors such conscious free-will. For the soft determinist biology directs all or most of human performance with the assistance of society and psychological factors such a conscious free-will. How then are the accoutrements of culture and personal disposition transmitted and transmuted so swiftly from generation to generation, within a generation, or individual? How is it that some cultural constitutions and personal performances are so patently and dramatically different when compared to those in the immediate past of a society and to proximate progenitors? The protracted pace of natural selection, as it is customarily compiled, cannot account for the relatively recent global spread of neoliberal capitalism and a culture of narcissism, the shift in the homicide rate of

New York over a few years, the burgeoning of women's rights during the early parts of the twenty-first century, the election as President of the United States of Donald Trump, personal and societal shifts in tastes regarding music, and latter-day epidemics in anxiety and depression? How might a future society imbued with artificial intelligence and future robotically readapted be explained by evolutionary adaptation, or the self and societal insanity that might lead to ecocide and anthropocide?

Another glitch in the submissions of evolutionary psychology/psychiatry appertains to the function of social institutions. A mixture of biological and psychological evolutionism can be applied to how human performance (especially cognitive capacities and partialities) helps to develop and modify social intuitions (Lewis and Steinmo, 2012; Boyer and Peterson, 2012). But is the social institution of psychiatry, given it has varied societal formations (but which are increasingly galvanising globally into biologism) adaptive or maladaptive? Madness has become medicalised and thereby the mad are de facto framed as maladapted by psychiatry. However, if, as is argued by some evolutionary psychologists/psychiatrists, madness may be adaptive then is psychiatry itself not an adaptive social institution but societally maladaptive? That is, if psychiatry (except for its few 'evolutionary' practitioners) is not recognising the personal and cultural purposefulness of what it brands as depression, anxiety, schizophrenia, and psychopathy, then rather than helping individuals and being socially useful is it not hindering genetic and societal evolution?

Notwithstanding these glitches (more compelling condemnation appears in Chapter 2), sociobiology still has adherents. For example, behavioural ecologist John Alcock (2003) uses case-studies which purport to provide 'triumphant' sociobiological answers to human mating conduct such as sexual jealousy, underhand copulation, and rape.

Violence, murder, and war all have evolutionary psychological perspectives (Shackelford and Weekes-Shackelford, 2012). Psychologist Glenn Geher's enthusiasm for the evolutionary branch of his discipline is unmistakable:

> Evolutionary psychology is a powerful approach to understanding human behavior and mental processes – leading to advancements in such important domains as education … physical health … and mental health.
>
> (Geher, 2015)

Biological evolutionary theory is hailed as a unifying foundation to support the future of psychology. It should be taught not just to psychologists but to those studying all social sciences (Buss et al., 2009). Presumably, the intention behind that suggestion is to 'Darwinise' the ideas of, for example, sociologists and anthropologists, thereby refocusing their gaze from the outward to the inward. Understandings of 'social' conditions such as socio-economic position, gender performance, norms, and mores, would then be sought primarily in genes, biochemistry, and brains, and only secondarily (if at all) in social structures, institutions, and processes.

Psychology has not evolved only into a variant of evolutionary biology. Research into 'conduct disorder led by psychologists with neuro-biological rather than evolutionary biological proclivities indicates that those with this diagnosis have faults in the 'structural wiring' of their brains (Rogers, et al., 2019; Birmingham University, 2019). This claim is striking because, as these researchers point out, one in twenty children teenagers are diagnosed in the UK and other European countries with 'conduct disorder'. Furthermore, they highlight that conduct disorder covers severe anti-social behaviours ranging from violence and vandalism, and a diagnosis of attention-deficit/hyperactivity disorder (ADHD), anxiety, and depression. The research also indicated, that those with conduct disorder are more have reduced empathy. However, the legitimacy of conduct disorder as a psychiatric category is questioned. It is argued that this diagnosis along with a host of others including depression, anxiety and ADHD, is part of the 'mental illness industry' medicalising normality (Appignanesi, 2011).

Psychology without the imposition of evolutionary or biological variants still steers its gaze towards the inner functions and failings of the mind for an explanation of such relevant questions as asked by 'spiritual' psychologist Steve Taylor:

> Why do we find it impossible to live in harmony with each other, with the natural world, or even with our own selves? Why is human history an endless, depressing saga of warfare, conflict, oppression? Why are do we seem impelled to destroy our environment and hence ourselves as a species?
>
> (Taylor, 2012, p. xi)

Taylor determines that the insanity of society is rooted in a basic psychological disorder form which all humans suffer. Madness is intrinsic to the psychological makeup of humans for Taylor because the ego is faulty or rather 'over-developed' through historical happenchance. His solution to what he fortuitously accedes is societally produced pervasive personal madness is swimming, contemplation, singing and dancing, and generally 'going inside yourself' and to reach 'inner harmony'. It would seem the resolution to poverty, prejudice, and persecution, is to admire but also adjust one's 'self'. This, as Taylor identifies, is also the premise of the popular contemporary cognitive-behavioural psychotherapies.

Anthropology evolution

As already indicated, social science subjects other than sociology contribute ideas about the influence of society on human performance, the most pertinent of which in relation to perceptions and productions of madness is anthropology. Anthropologists acclaim the influence of society on human performance (and vice versa), but spotlight the 'cultural' aspects of society.

The contention of anthropology is that culture (the beliefs, norms, mores, and value-laden artefacts of human social groupings) affect the chances of being classified as mad, and influences how madness is regarded and regulated. Culture shapes societal attitudes towards what may be construed as madness, such as hearing voices or believing in spirits and monsters, and the meaning of these experiences to those affected. Everyday environmental experiences mould what is considered normal or abnormal human performance (Helman, 2007; Jones and Luhrmann, 2016; Luhrmann; and Marrow, 2016). However, powerful social institutions can mould cultural attributions above and beyond local experiences. In a globalised society in which the culture originating from one location (Western neoliberalism) has become dominant, concomitant conceptualisation from the powerful institution of psychiatry have permeated cultures which previously had their own categories of madness (Kleiman, 1988). For example, hearing voices or believing in spirit possession in sole cultures is not unusual but may be in Western terms viewed as signs of severe mental disorder if not severe disturbance of the brain.

Anthropology, however, has also undergone an epistemological turn whereby biology and culture are viewed as interconnected. That is, anthropological firm adherence to the notion that culture is predominant in the shaping of human performance has become less firm with the advent of 'evolutionary anthropology' (Jolly, 2016; Gibson and Lawson, 2015). This approach accepts that the evolution of human biology and human cultural evolution cannot be disconnected.

As with evolutionary psychology and psychiatry, neuroscience, and parts of sociology, there are disagreements amongst evolutionary anthropologists about which drives the other more (Richerson and Boyd 2005). That is, do genes shape culture, does culture shapes genes, is it a bit of both, and if it is a bit of both can this be measured or is the interplay between genetics and culture again too complex to be disentangled?

Anthropological thinking about evolution contains the same glitches found in the thoughts of evolutionary psychologists. It also leads straight back to the nature-nurture debate, and to where in that debate can an understanding of madness be disentangled.

Memetics and epigenetics

A study by international examining continued human susceptibility to the pressures of natural selection concluded that specific traits such as body mass, in humans are being passed from one generation to the next, but these are 'quite weak'. That is, these traits are affected strongly by changes in society and medical interventions (Sanjak et al., 2018). In another study a team of geneticists attempting to identity genetic mutations which threaten survival admit:

> while there is overwhelming evidence for human evolution and unequi-
> vocal footprints of adaptation in the genome, rarely have scientists been

able to directly observe natural selection operating in people. As a result, biologists still understand very little about the workings of natural selection in humans.

(Mostafavi et al., 2017)

Notwithstanding the apparent faintness of natural selection on contemporary humans the evolutionary biologists Richard Dawkins (1976; 2018) has offered the concept of the 'meme' to explain how elements of culture and human performance such as specific rules and ideas about morality might be passed from one generation to another. The meme is meant not to be just a metaphor but have an existence like that of a virus (Brodie, 2009). Psychologist Susan Blackmore (2000) attempts to constitute memetics as a science. For Blackmore memes are replicate cultural and personal facets independently from selfish genetic programming of natural selection. Such independence leads to deviation from pure survival and reproduction

Blackmore's hope is that memetics will explain the aspects of culture and personal disposition left unexplained by genomics. A core part of memetics is this issue of consciousness (and free-will). Similarly to Greenfield (op. cit.), philosopher and cognitive scientist Daniel Dennett (2017) thinks that our mental capabilities are nothing more than a by-product of the brain's physical processes. We simply evolved the how and why of human consciousness, which gave rise to thinking and the ability to think about thinking and memes assisted this process. Blackmore (2017) proposes that consciousness is a memetically transmuted delusion.

However, the idea of a biologically-driven conduit as instigated by Dawkins (his idea of 'memes') for personal and cultural attributes, is highly controversial (Nikolas Rose, 1998; Dupre, 2014). Theologian and essayist David Hart (2017) and philosopher Mary Midgely (2011) attack the teleological and illogical thinking at the heart of the idea that humans do not think for themselves. He asks how could humans develop thinking without first having the ability, or at least proto-thinking abilities, to think? For Hart and Midgely, the notion of consciousness as an illusion is an illusion and the notion of memes is illusory. That is, existence of either proposition is unsubstantiated by the very type of (empirical) evidence that those who have invented or are promoting them usually demand before the status of 'scientific' can be attributed.

The second offering purporting to be connected to personal and societal transmutations and transmissions which do not seem to accord easily with sheer natural selection or any crude distinction between nature and nurture is 'epigenetics'. Epigenetics is the study of the ways in which the 'phenotype' aspects of genetic material are altered in individuals and passed on from one generation to the next without discernible changes occurring in the 'genotypes'. The genotype is the observable presentation of genetic influences and the 'genotype' is the actual gene material within which the phenotypical presentations such as behaviour are stored (Carey, 2012). Epigeneticists argue that phenotypical change which does not correspond to genotypical change happens regularly because of conditions in the social and physical environment which furnish 'stress' (from, for example, childhood trauma, famine, armed conflict, and pollution), as well as personal disposition, habits, and disease, such as aggressiveness, smoking, and diabetes, all of which are also swayed by society (Francis, 2012; Palumbo et al., 2018). Darwinian evolutionary mechanisms associated with natural selection, argue epigeneticists, are therefore not the only means of biological adaptation (and maladaptation) taking place in humans. Moreover, rather than changes taking perhaps thousands of generations to take effect epigenetic mechanisms within the lifetime of the affected person and subsequently her/his offspring. There is the suggestion by epigeneticists that mental disorders such as schizophrenia and depression are connectable to environmental stress and sway (Akbarian, 2014; Dalton et al., 2014).

However, both the idea of epigenetics and the notion that any one gene or mix of genes decide the whole destiny of all humanity or of any one human is rejected by most mainstream geneticists. Medical practitioner and educator John Launer (2016) notes that the epigenetics has inherited a high level of hype. Historian of biology Nathaniel Comfort (2018) notes that simplistic reasoning determines the idea that nature is indomitable.

Neurology and psychiatry

Ironically, the proposition that many mental disorders are caused by neurological disturbances, immunologically inflammatory or not, seems to underscore the argument of renegade psychiatrist Thomas Szasz's (1970; 2010) idea that if there is no neurological pathology present then mental disorder is a myth. If there is a neurological pathology, then it is not mental disorder but neurological disorder.

Szasz's idea that madness is metaphorical not medical had an exclusionary clause (1961; 1994): Some forms of madness are medical not mythical. These were those with identifiable biological (genetic, neuroanatomical, neurochemical) faults affecting the brain. But these, to date, remain few and far between. Crucially for consistency in this contention of Szasz, is that if biological fault is proven, this does not mean schizophrenia and manic-depression will thereby become authentic mental disorders. He reasons that if there is a recognisable organic malfunction in the brain, then it is to the neurologists that the patient should be referred.

Neurological disorders should, continues Szasz, be dealt with by neurologists not psychiatrists.

Psychiatrist Mike Fitzgerald (2015) maintains advances in neuroscience in recent years have blurred the boundaries between psychiatry and neurology. For Fitzgerald psychiatrists should return home to neurology and medicine and leave non-medical interventions to non-medical practitioners, for example in relation to specialist or long-term psychotherapy. Neurologists and psychiatrists need to merge into neuropsychiatry or some acceptable title.

Szasz (2009) argues that the merger of psychiatry with neurology has a decisive deficiency and implies that he is therefore against the merger of neurology with psychiatry as opposed to the complete dissolution of the latter as a medical speciality along with its legal powers. It will not, he suggests, eliminate stigma. Paradoxically, it may increase stigma. That is, stigmatisation may be amplified not abridged if a patient's brain, DNA, or biochemistry, is identified authoritatively as faulty.

What also could ensue is a return to 'listening' for symptoms rather than 'hearing' the meaning given by the individual to the meaning of her/his narrative. The forging medical managing of madness into purely neurological disorder once again creates a clear gulf between expert knowledge and the expressed experience of the patient. The power imbalance in the patient-clinician relationship would also return to one of professional dominance and patient disempowerment. Furthermore, the proposal of medical anthropologist Cecil Helman (2007) is that medical practice is both a science and an art. The key to effective treatment is the scientific monitoring of the workings of the patient's body together attending to the workings of her/his mind. But, for Helman both must be situated in the patient's culture. Hence mind-body duality is medically inappropriate, as the separation of the individual from societal beliefs, norms, and mores, and value-laden artefacts.

The Royal Australian and New Zealand College of Psychiatrists (2019) describes the focus of neuropsychiatry as the interrelation of psychiatric disorders and neurology'. The (British) Royal College of Psychiatrists does have a faculty of neuropsychiatry which does not mention specifically the amalgamation of neurology with psychiatry. It does set out its aim as improving understandings of brain disorders by promoting the integration of psychiatry with neuroscience. Its Chair is Eileen Joyce is described as a neuropsychiatrist on the website of her place of work, which is the National Hospital for Neurology and Neurosurgery in London (University College London Hospitals, 2019).

Psychiatry's re-established predilection for biological vindication is stumbling over the seemingly smatter of its brand name, but also representation. There are competitors for 'neuropsychiatry'. One is the World Federation of Societies of Biological Psychiatry (2019). Founded in 1974, it claims to be composed of 63 psychiatric organisations from over seventy countries, and to have key opinion-leaders in the practice of biological psychiatry. The American Neuropsychiatric Association (2016), claims 500 members from around the world. Founded in 1988, it contends to be the 'premier' 'unique', 'diverse', and vibrant' international organisation' of clinicians and researchers for neurology and neuropsychiatry. There is also the 'International Neuropsychiatric Association' with claimed commitment from organisations across the Americas, Europe, Asia, and Oceania, and psychiatrists, neurologists, neurosurgeons, neuroscientists, nurses, and social workers, as members. It was formed in 1996, with the more modest aim of sharing a 'unique perspective' on what it deems to be a 'burgeoning discipline'.

So is it neuropsychiatry, 'biological psychiatry', or perhaps 'biopsychiatry, or possibly 'psychobiology'? Can one organisation assert to be 'unique', another to be fomenting a viewpoint which 'unique', and yet another to be key in leading opinion? Confusion over a name and disputation over representation are not inconsequential. They imply either epistemological immaturity or an epistemological cul-de-sac, the chance to burgeon or to fade. Moreover, the intellectual and empirical fodder for neuropsychiatry (or whatever) has its own administrative muddles with which to contend. Neuroscience is not a united discipline. There are intellectual and institutional rivalries between the various subdivisions of neuroscience with no common language (Hilary Rose and Steven Rose, 2016). Of course, neuropsychiatry and neuroscience are the only disunited disciplines in the field of madness. Psychotherapy suffers from similar divisions regarding its knowledge, practices, and accomplishments (Morrall, 2008).

Schildkrout (2017) advocates a form of neuropsychiatry which embraces environmental and interpersonal influences on the brain and vice versa (Schildkrout and Frankel, 2016). Integrating these multilayer factors whilst maintaining the brain as the organ of psychiatry is a prospect yet to be promised. Psychiatry is not dissolving into neurology but is refurbished by neuroscience and revitalising itself as a speciality and either advertently or inadvertently merging with neurology (Arzy and Danziger, 2014; Schildkrout and Frankel, 2016; Arciniegas et al., 2018). The 'faulty individual' gaze is neither dimming nor visualising wider sightings but becoming more myopic.

Summary

This chapter has provided coverage of a selection of biological and allied psychological justifications for an approach to comprehending madness which attends to faults in the individual. For the most psychiatry, psychology, and psychotherapy only look for faults in the individual. Her/his close social groupings are given an occasion glance in clinical practice, and in the academic and professional literature 'society' is mentioned but intermittently and without epistemological gravitas or practical uptake. The plethora of pharmaceuticals and psychotherapies, and prospective catalogue of neuro-genetic manipulations, are intended to abate, correct, or prevent these faults in the individual not those of society.

The focus on the faulty individual through the narrowest of epistemological lenses relies heavily on empirical evidence, which then steers clinical practice if not for the psychiatry of today, then that of tomorrow, and accentuates its scientific status (Morrall, 2017). However, scepticism has long surrounded empiricism and scientism, with claims of epistemological over-reach, dogmatisms, and tyranny (Quine, 1951; Feyerabend, 1970; 2011; Williams and Robinson (2014); de Ridder et al., 2018). Chapter 2 sets out to temper these excesses.

Except where censure is too manifest and pronounced to be avoided, the presentational tone of this chapter is intended to be as neutral as is likely in a book which from the outset declares its intention to be a corrective to the overwhelming sway of the biological paradigm for madness. That changes in Chapter 2 where the critique of finding faults only in the individual and looking only at genes, brains, and biochemicals to explain madness is itself considered a sort of insanity. Chapter 2 also makes mention of the equally unreasoned configuring of madness as contrived wholly by society. That society matters in the making and mending of madness, does not mean forgetting that there may be faults in the individual.

Notes

1 As mentioned in the Introduction, I am usually using the idiom 'madness' to refer to personal psychological states and 'insanity' to refer to the state of society. The term 'psychological distress' is adopted on occasion as an alternative phrase to madness. 'Mental disorder' (or 'mental illness') is utilised when madness is configured medically.
2 The distinction between neurology and neuroscience is habitually blurred in the clinical literature. However, the tendency is to consider the former as a medical speciality which is supported by the concepts and data arising from the latter. Moreover, neuroscience embraces many practices and practitioners other than those with a background or interest in neurology (Martin, 2002).

References

Abed R and St John-Smith P (2016) Evolutionary psychiatry: A new college special interest group. *British Journal of Psychiatry Bulletin*, 40(5), pp. 233–236.
Akbarian S (2014) Epigenetic mechanisms in schizophrenia. *Dialogues in Clinical Neuroscience*, 16(3), pp. 405–417.
Alcock J (2003) *The Triumph of Sociobiology*, 2nd edn. New York: Oxford University Press.
Allen F (2014) *Saving Normal: An Insider's Revolt against Out-of-Control Psychiatric Diagnosis, DSM-5, Big Pharma, and the Medicalization of Ordinary Life*. New York: William Morrow.
American Neuropsychiatric Association (2016) About American Neuropsychiatric Association. www.anpaonline.org/About-Us [accessed 30 January, 2019].
Amen D (2020) *The End of Mental Illness*. Carol Stream, Illinois, USA: Tyndale Momentum.
American Psychiatric Association (2013) *Diagnostic and Statistical Manual of Mental Disorders, Fifth Edition (DSM-5)*. Arlington, VA: American Psychiatric Association.
American Psychiatric Association (2018) Americans say they are more anxious than a year ago: Baby boomers report greatest increase in anxiety. American Psychiatric Association. www.psychiatry.org/newsroom/news-releases/americans-say-they-are-more-anxious-than-a-year-ago-baby-boomers-report-greatest-increase-in-anxiety.
Andrews P and Thomson A (2009) The bright side of being blue: Depression as an adaptation for analyzing complex problems. *Psychological Review*, 116(3), pp. 620–654.

Appignanesi L (2011) The mental illness industry is medicalising normality. *The Guardian*, 6 September.

Arciniegas D, Yudofsky S and Hales R (2018) *Textbook of Neuropsychiatry and Clinical Neurosciences*, 6th edn. Washington, DC: American Psychiatric Association.

Arscott J (2018) Eight ways you can help women's rights. *The Conversation*, 6 March http://theconversation.com/eight-ways-you-can-help-womens-rights-88113 [accessed 4 February, 2019].

Arzy S and Danziger S (2014) The science of neuropsychiatry: Past, present, and future shahar. *Journal of Neuropsychiatry and Clinical Neurosciences*, 26(4), pp. 392–395.

Baggini J (2017) *A Short History of Truth: Consolations for a Post-Truth World*. London: Quercus.

Barrett L (2017) *How Emotions are Made: The Secret Life of the Brain*. London: Macmillan

BBC News (2018) Prime Minister appoints minister for suicide prevention. 10 October. www.bbc.co.uk/news/health-45804225 [accessed 10 October, 2018].

Bateson G, Jackson D, Haley J and Weakland J (1956) Toward a theory of schizophrenia. *Behavioral Science*, 1(4), 251–264.

Bentall R (2003) *Madness Explained: Psychosis and Human Nature*. London: Allen Lane.

Bentall R (2009a) *Doctoring the Mind: Why Psychiatric Treatments Fail*. London: Penguin.

Bentall R (2009b) Formulating Zeppi. In Sturmey P (ed.) *Clinical Case Formulation: Varieties of Approaches*. Chichester: Wiley, pp. 119–131.

Bentall R (2016) Mental illness is a result of misery, yet still we stigmatise it. *The Guardian*, 26 February.

Bentall R and Pilgrim D (2016) There are no 'schizophrenia genes': Here's why. *The Conversation*, 8 April. https://theconversation.com/there-are-no-schizophrenia-genes-heres-why-57294 [accessed 24 May 2018].

Best B, Bonefeld W and O'Kane C (eds) (2018) *The Sage Handbook of Frankfurt School Critical Theory*. London: Sage.

Bhugra D et al. [40 co-authors]. (2017) The World Psychiatric Association-Lancet Psychiatry Commission on the future of psychiatry. *The Lancet*, 4(10), pp. 775–818.

Bickerdike L, Booth A, Wilson P, Farley K and Wright K (2017) Social prescribing: Less rhetoric and more reality. A systematic review of the evidence. *British Medical Journal*, 7(4). https://bmjopen.bmj.com/content/7/4/e013384 [accessed 19 May, 2019].

Birmingham University (2019) Brain wiring differences identified in children with conduct disorder. www.birmingham.ac.uk/news/latest/2019/04/brain-wiring-differences-in-children-with-conduct-disorder.aspx [accessed 20 May, 2019].

Blackmore S (2000) *The Meme Machine*. Oxford: Oxford University Press.

Blackmore S (2017) *Consciousness: A Very Short Introduction*. Oxford: Oxford University Press.

Bocock R, 1978, *Freud and Modern Society: The Making of Sociology*, Nelson.

Boseley S (2018) The drugs do work: Antidepressants are effective, study shows. *The Guardian*, 21 February.

Boyer P and Peterson M (2012) The naturalness of (many) social institutions: Evolved cognition as their foundation. *Journal of Institutional Economic*, 8(1), pp. 1–25.

Brodie R (2009) *Virus of the Mind: The Revolutionary New Science of the Meme and How it Can Help You*. London: Hay House.

Brown G W (1959) Experiences of discharged chronic schizophrenic patients in various types of living group. *Milbank Memorial Fund Quarterly*, 37(2), pp. 105–131.

Brune M (2008) *Textbook of Evolutionary Psychiatry*. Oxford: Oxford University Press.

Buller D (2012) Four fallacies of pop evolutionary psychology. *Scientific American, Special Editions*, 22(1s), pp. 44–51.

Bullmore E (2018a) This revolution in our understanding of depression will be life-transforming. *The Observer*, 29 April.

Bullmore E (2018b) *The Inflamed Mind: A Radical New Approach to Depression*. London: Short Books.

Buss D (2017) *Evolutionary Psychology: The New Science of the Mind*, 5th edn. Abingdon: Routledge.

Buss D, Kruger D and Kurzban R (2009) Evolutionary theory and psychology. Psychological science agenda [Science Briefs]. *American Psychological Association*. www.apa.org/science/about/psa/2009/05/scibrief.aspx#Povinelli,%20Penn,%20and%20Holyoak [accessed 22 January, 2019].

Cacioppo J and Berntson G (1992) Social psychological contributions to the decade of the brain: Doctrine of multilevel analysis. *American Psychologist*, 47(8), pp. 1019–1028.

Cacioppo J and Decety J (2011) Challenges and opportunities in social neuroscience. *Ann N Y Acad Sci*, 1224(1), pp. 162–173.

Cacioppo J and Patrick W (2009) *Loneliness: Human Nature and the Need for Social Connection*. London: W W Norton & Company.

Cadwalladr S (2013) Susannah Cahalan: 'What I remember most vividly are the fear and anger'. *The Guardian*, 13 January.

Cahalan S (2012) *Brain on Fire: My Month of Madness*. London: Penguin.

Cairney P and Oliver K (2017) Evidence-based policymaking is not like evidence-based medicine, so how far should you go to bridge the divide between evidence and policy? *Health Research Policy and Systems*, 15(35). https://health-policy-systems.biomedcentral.com/articles/10.1186/s12961-017-0192-x [accessed 21 January, 2019].

Carey N (2012) *The Epigenetics Revolution: How Modern Biology is Rewriting our Understanding of Genetics, Disease and Inheritance*. London: Icon.

Chater N (2018) *The Mind Is Flat*. London: Allen Lane.

Chomsky N (2007) *Failed States: The Abuse of Power and the Assault on Democracy*. London: Penguin.

Cipriani A, Furukawa, T, Salanti G, Chaimani A, Atkinson L, Ogawa Y, Leucht L, Ruhe H, Turner E, Higgins J, Egger M, Takeshima N, Hayasaka Y, Imai H, Shinohara K, Tajika A, Ioannidis J, Geddes J (2018) Comparative efficacy and acceptability of 21 antidepressant drugs for the acute treatment of adults with major depressive disorder: a systematic review and network meta-analysis. *The Lancet*, 391(10128), pp. 1357–1366.

Clapp M, Aurora N, Herrera L, Bhatia M, Wilen E and Sarah Wakefield (2017) Gut microbiota's effect on mental health: The gut-brain axis. *Clinical Practice*, 7(4), p. 987. www.ncbi.nlm.nih.gov/pmc/articles/PMC5641835/ [accessed 29 November, 2018].

Cohen B (2016) *Psychiatric Hegemony: A Marxist Theory of Mental Illness*. London: Palgrave McMillan.

Comfort N (2018) Genetic determinism rides again: Nathaniel Comfort questions a psychologist's troubling claims about genes and behaviour. *Nature*, 561, pp. 461–463.

Connor S (2015) Many people have genes missing but are still fit and healthy. *The Guardian*, 1 October.

Council for Evidence-based Psychiatry (2018) Do antidepressants work? The new research proves nothing new. http://cepuk.org/2018/02/22/antidepressants-work-ne w-research-proves-nothing-new/ [accessed 24 February, 2018].

Cozolino L (2010) *The Neuroscience of Psychotherapy: Healing the Social Brain*, 2nd edn. London: W W Norton & Company.

Dalton V, Kolshush E and McLoughlin D (2014) Review: Epigenetics and depression: return of the repressed. *Journal of Affective Disorders*, 155(1), pp. 1–12.

Davis E (2017) *Post-Truth: Why We Have Reached Peak Bullshit and What We Can Do About It*. London: Little Brown.

Dawkins R (1976) *The Selfish Gene*. Oxford: Oxford University Press.

Dawkins R (2018) *Science in the Soul: Selected Writings of a Passionate Rationalist*. London: Black Swan.

Dempsey-Jones H (2018) Neuroscientists put the dubious theory of 'phrenology' through rigorous testing for the first time. *The Conversation*, 22 January.

Dennett D (2017) *From Bacteria to Bach and Back: The Evolution of Minds*. London: W W Norton & Company.

Department of Health [UK]. (2006) *Our Health, Our Care, Our Say: A New Direction for Community Services*. London: Department of Health [UK].

de Ridder J, Peels R and van Woudenberg R (eds) (2018) *Scientism: Prospects and Problems*. Oxford: Oxford University Press.

Dorling D (2015) *Inequality and the 1%*. London: Verso.

Doudna J and Charpentier E (2014) The new frontier of genome engineering with CRISPR-Cas9. *Science*, 346(6213), 28 November. http://science.sciencemag.org/ content/346/6213/1258096 [accessed 29 June 2018].

Doudna J and Sternberg S (2017) *A Crack in Creation: The New Power to Control Evolution*. London: Bodley Head.

Dunt I (2016) *Brexit: What the Hell Happens Now?* Tonbridge: Canbury.

Dupre J (2014) *Processes of Life: Essays in the Philosophy of Biology*. New York: Oxford University Press.

Eagleman D (2015) *The Brain: The Story of You*. Edinburgh: Canongate.

Edgerton R (1992) *Sick Societies: Challenging the Myth of Primitive Harmony*. New York: Free Press.

Eisenberg L and Kleinman A (eds) (1980) *The Relevance of Social Science for Medicine*. New York: Springer.

Ewbank M, Passamonti L, Hagan C, Goodyer I, Calder A and Fairchild G (2018) Psychopathic traits influence amygdala–anterior cingulate cortex connectivity during facial emotion processing. *Social Cognitive and Affective Neuroscience*, 13(5), pp. 525–534.

Fallon J (2014) *The Psychopath Inside: A Neuroscientist's Personal Journey into the Dark Side of the Brain*. London: Current.

Feyerabend P (1970) Against method: Outline of an anarchistic theory of knowledge. Minnesota Center for Philosophy of Science (University of Minnesota). http://mcps. umn.edu/assets/pdf/4.2.1_Feyerabend.pdf [accessed 15 January, 2019].

Feyerabend P (2011) *The Tyranny of Science*. Cambridge University Press: Polity

Fitz N (2015) Economic inequality: It's far worse than you think. *Scientific American*, 31 March. www.scientificamerican.com/article/economic-inequality-it-s-far-worse-tha n-you-think/ [accessed 27 September, 2018].

Fitzgerald M (2015) Do psychiatry and neurology need a close partnership or a merger? *British Journal of Psychiatry*, 39(3), pp. 105–107.

Fond G, Macgregor A and Miot S (2013) Nanopsychiatry, the potential role of nanotechnologies in the future of psychiatry: A systematic review. *European Neuropsychopharmacology*, 23(9), pp. 1067–1071.

Foucault M (1961) *Folie et Déraison: Histoire de la folie à l'âge classique* [Madness and Civilization]. Paris: Librarie Plon.

Foucault M (1963) *Naissance de la Clinique* [Birth of the Clinic]. Paris: Universitaires de France.

Foucault M (1966) *Les mots et les choses: Une archéologie des science* [The Order of Things: An Archaeology of the Human Sciences]. Paris: Gillimard.

Foucault M (2006) *Psychiatric Power: Lectures at the Collège de France.* Basingstoke: Palgrave MacMillan.

Francis C (2012) *Epigenetics: How Environment Shapes Our Genes.* London: W W Norton & Company.

Fudge J, Powers J, Haber S, and Caine E (1998) Considering the role of the amygdala in psychotic illness: A clinicopathological correlation. *Journal of Neuropsychiatry Clinical Neuroscience*, 10(4), pp. 383–394.

Fund for Peace (2018) *Fragile States Index 2018 – Annual Report.* Fund for Peace. http://fundforpeace.org/fsi/2018/04/24/fragile-states-index-2018-annual-report/ [accessed 4 February, 2019].

Gallagher J (2019) Cheap common drugs may help mental illness. *BBC.* www.bbc.co.uk/news/health-46809517 [accessed 9 January, 2019].

Gallop (2019) *Gallup 2019 Global Emotions Report.* www.gallup.com/analytics/248906/gallup-global-emotions-report-2019.aspx [accessed 21 May, 2019].

Gandal M, Haney J, Parikshak N, Leppa V, Ramaswami G, Hartl C, Schork AJ, Appadurai V, Buil A, Werge T, Liu C, White K, Horvath S and Geschwind D, CommonMind Consortium, PsychENCODE Consortium, iPSYCH-BROAD Working Group (2018), Shared Molecular Neuropathology Across Major Psychiatric Disorders Parallels Polygenic Overlap. *Science*, 359(6376), pp. 693–697.

Gargiulo P and Mesones-Arroyo H (eds) (2018) *Psychiatry and Neuroscience Update –Vol. II: A Translational Approach.* New York: Springer.

Gates B (2017) Bill Gates's 7 predictions for our future. World Economic Forum, 8 May. www.weforum.org/agenda/2017/05/bill-gates-is-pretty-good-at-predicting-the-future-this-is-what-he-thinks-will-happen-next1 [accessed 9 July, 2018].

Gates S, Nygård H, Strand H and Urdal H (2014) *Trends in Armed Conflict, 1946–2014.* Peace Research Institute Oslo. www.prio.org/utility/DownloadFile.ashx?id=8&type=publicationfile [accessed 4 February, 2019].

Geher G (2015) What is evolutionary psychology? 5 foundational concepts for understanding evolutionary psychology. *Psychology Today*, 18 August. www.psychologytoday.com/us/blog/darwins-subterranean-world/201508/what-is-evolutionary-psychology [accessed 22 January, 2019].

Genomics England (2018) The UK has sequenced 100,000 whole genomes in the NHS. www.genomicsengland.co.uk/the-uk-has-sequenced-100000-whole-genomes-in-the-nhs/ [accessed 8 December, 2018].

Gibson M and Lawson D (2015) Applying evol anthropol. *Evolutionary Anthropology*, 24(1), pp. 3–14.

Goffman E (1961) *Asylums: Essays on the Social Situation of Mental Patients and Other Inmates.* New York: Anchor.

Goldacre B (2009) *Bad Science.* London: Harper Perennial.

Goldacre B (2012) *Bad Pharma: How Drug Companies Mislead Doctors and Harm Patients.* London: Fourth Estate.

Goldacre B (2015) *I Think You'll Find It's a Bit More Complicated Than That.* London: Allen Lane.

Gøtzsche P (2015) *Deadly Psychiatry and Organised Denial.* Copenhagen, Denmark: People's Press.

Gøtzsche P (2018) Cipriani review does not add anything. Council for Evidence-based Psychiatry. http://cepuk.org/2018/02/22/peter-gotzsche-cipriani-review-not-add-anything/. [accessed 24 February, 2018].

Gould S J (1997) Darwinian fundamentalism. *New York Review of Books*, 12 June. www.nybooks.com/articles/archives/1997/jun/12/darwinian-fundamentalism/?page=1. [accessed 12 December, 2018].

Grawe K (2005) *Neuropsychotherapy: How the Neurosciences Inform Effective Psychotherapy.* Abingdon: Routledge.

Greenfield S (2016) *Day in the Life of the Brain: The Neuroscience of Consciousness from Dawn Till Dusk*: London: Allen Lane.

Greenhill K (2011) *Weapons of Mass Migration: Forced Displacement, Coercion, and Foreign Policy.* New York: Cornell University Press.

Haas B and Reuters (2017) China's Shanghai sets population at 25 million to avoid 'big city disease'. *The Guardian*, 26 December.

Hacker P (2015) Philosophy and scientism: What cognitive neuroscience can and cannot explain. In Robinson D and Williams R (eds) *Scientism: The New Orthodoxy.* London: Bloomsbury, pp. 97–116.

Hallowell E (2018) *Because I Come from A Crazy Family: The Making of a Psychiatrist.* London: Bloomsbury.

Harari Y (2015) *Sapiens.* London: Vintage.

Harari Y (2017) *Homo Deus: A Brief History of Tomorrow.* London: Vintage.

Hart D (2017) 'The Illusionist'. *The New Atlantis*, 53, pp. 109–121. www.thenewatlantis.com/publications/the-illusionist [accessed 1 November, 2018].

Harden K (2018) Heredity is only half the story. www.spectator.co.uk/2018/10/heredity-is-only-half-the-story/ [accessed 10 December, 2018].

Hayes J, Lundin A, Wick S, Lewis G, Wong I, Osborn D and Dalman C (2019) Association of hydroxylmethyl glutaryl coenzyme a reductase inhibitors, l-type calcium channel antagonists, and biguanides with rates of psychiatric hospitalization and self-harm in individuals with serious mental illness. *JAMA Psychiatry*, 9 January. https://jamanetwork.com/journals/jamapsychiatry/fullarticle/2719703. [accessed 10 January, 2019].

Heinrich C, Bergami M, Gascón S, Lepier A, Viganò F, Dimou L, Sutor B, Berninger B and Götz M (2014) Sox2-mediated conversion of ng2 glia into induced neurons in the injured adult cerebral cortex. *Stem Cell Reports*, 3(6), pp. 1000–1014.

Helliwell J, Layard R and Sachs J (eds) (2019) *World Happiness Report (2019).* New York: Sustainable Development Solutions Network.

Helman C (2007) *Culture, Health and Illness*, 5th edn. London: Hodder Arnold.

Herriot P (2008) *Religious Fundamentalism: Global, Local and Personal.* Abingdon: Routledge.

Higgins E (2018) *The Neuroscience of Clinical Psychiatry*, 3rd edn. Philadelphia, PA: Lippincott Williams and Wilkins.

Hossain N, Byrne B, Campbell A, Harrison E, McKinley B and Shah P (2011) *The Impact of The Global Economic Downturn on Communities and Poverty in the UK.* York: Joseph Rowntree Trust.

Hunter M, Gillespie B and Yu-Pu Chen S (2019) Urban nature experiences reduce stress in the context of daily life based on salivary biomarkers. *Frontiers Psychology*, 4 April. www.frontiersin.org/articles/10.3389/fpsyg.2019.00722/full [accessed 11 April, 2019].

Insel T (2015) Psychiatry is reinventing itself thanks to advances in biology. *New Sci*, 3035, 19 August. www.newscientist.com/article/mg22730353-000-psychiatry-is-reinventing-itself-thanks-to-advances-in-biology/ [accessed 13 November 2015].

Insel T and Collins F (2003) Psychiatry in the genomics era. *Am J Psychiatry*, 160(4), pp. 616–620.

Institute for Economics and Peace (2017) *Global Terrorism Index 2017*. Sydney, Australia: Institute for Economics and Peace.

Institute for Policy Studies (2018) Inequality and health. https://inequality.org/facts/inequality-and-health/ [accessed 27 September, 2018].

International Neuropsychiatric Association. About the International Neuropsychiatric Association. www.inawebsite.org/about-ina [accessed 30 January, 2019].

James O (2016) *Not in Your Genes: The Real Reasons Children are Like Their Parents*. London: Vermillion.

Jasanoff A (2018) *The Biological Mind: How Brain, Body, and Environment Collaborate to Make Us Who We Are*. New York: Basic Books.

Jenkins P (2018) *Minding Our Future*. London: Universities UK Task Group on Student Mental Health Services, Universities UK.

Johnstone L (2014) *A Straight Talking Introduction to Psychiatric Diagnosis*. Ross-on-Wye: PCCS.

Johnstone L and Boyle M (2018) The power threat meaning framework: an alternative nondiagnostic conceptual system. *Humanistic Psychology*, 5 August. http://journals.sagepub.com/doi/abs/10.1177/0022167818793289?journalCode=jhpa [accessed 30 October, 2018].

Johnstone L and Dallos R (eds) (2013) *Formulation in Psychology and Psychotherapy*, 2nd edn. Abingdon: Routledge

Jolly C (2016) A life in evol anthropol. *Annual Review of Anthropology*, 45, pp. 1–15. www.annualreviews.org/doi/10.1146/annurev-anthro-102215-095835 [accessed 16 January, 2019].

Jones J (1993) *Bad Blood: Tuskegee Syphilis Experiment*. New York: Free Press.

Jones N and Luhrmann T (2016) Providing Culturally Competent Care: Understanding the Context of Psychosis. *Psychiatric Times*, 33(10), 31 October. www.psychiatrictimes.com/special-reports/providing-culturally-competent-care-understanding-context-psychosis [accessed 28 June 2018].

Kallert T, Mezzich J and Monahan J (eds) (2011) *Coercive Treatment in Psychiatry: Clinical, Legal and Ethical Aspects*. Chichester: Wiley-Blackwell.

Kaltwasser C, Taggart P, Espejo P and Ostiguy P (eds) (2017) *The Oxford Handbook of Populism*. Oxford: Oxford University.

Keane J (2018) Post-truth politics and why the antidote isn't simply 'fact-checking' and truth. *The Conversation*, 23 March. http://theconversation.com/post-truth-politics-and-why-the-antidote-isnt-simply-fact-checking-and-truth-87364 [accessed 27 September, 2018].

King's Fund (2019) What is social prescribing?www.kingsfund.org.uk/publications/social-prescribing [accessed January 28, 2019].

Kirov G (2017) Electroconvulsive therapy does work – and it can be miraculous. *The Conversation*, 20 April. https://theconversation.com/electroconvulsive-therapy-does-work-and-it-can-be-miraculous-76381.

Kleiman A (1988) *Rethinking Psychiatry: From Cultural Category to Personal Experience.* New York: Free Press.

Kozubek J (2018) *Modern Prometheus: Editing the Human Genome with Crispr-Cas9.* Cambridge: Cambridge University Press.

Krishnamurti J (2017) *Krishnamurti: The Essential Collection. Common Ground:* Champaign, IL: University of Illinois Research Park.

Kuma K (2004) *From Post-Industrial to Post-Modern Society: New Theories of the Contemporary.* Chichester: Wiley-Blackwell.

Kynge J and Jonathan Wheatley (2015) Emerging markets: Redrawing the world map. *Financial Times,* 3 August.

Laing R D (1960) *The Divided Self: An Existential Study in Sanity and Madness.* London: Tavistock.

Lassale C, Batty G, Baghdadli B, Jacka F, Sánchez-Villegas A, Kivimäki M and Akbaraly T (2018) Healthy dietary indices and risk of depressive outcomes: A systematic review and meta-analysis of observational studies. *Nature, Molecular Psychiatry,* 26 September, pp. 1–22. www.nature.com/articles/s41380-018-0237-8 [accessed 26 September, 2018].

Launer J (2016) Epigenetics for Dummies. *Postgraduate Medical Journal (British Medical Journal),* 92(1085), 183–184.

Lennox B, Palmer-Cooper E, Pollak T, Hainsworth J, Marks J, Jacobson L, Lang B, Fox H, Ferry B, Scoriels L, Crowley H, Jones P, Harrison P and Vincent A (2017). Prevalence and clinical characteristics of serum neuronal cell surface antibodies in first-episode psychosis: A case-control study. *The Lancet (Psychiatry),* 4(1), pp. 42–48.

Lessenich S, Dörre K and Rosa R (2015) *Sociology, Capitalism, Critique.* London: Verso.

Lewis O and Steinmo S (2012) How institutions evolve: Evolutionary theory and institutional change. *Polity,* 44(3), pp 314–339.

Lewontin R (2001) *It Ain't Necessarily So: The Dream of the Human Genome and Other Illusions.* New York: New York Review of Books.

Lewontin R, Rose S and Kamin L (1984) *Not in Our Genes: Biology, Ideology, and Human Nature.* New York: Pantheon.

Lieberman J (2015) *Shrinks: The Untold Story of Psychiatry.* Weidenfeld & Nicolson.

Liu L and Zhu G (2018) Gut–brain axis and mood disorder. *Frontiers in Psychiatry,* 9, p. 223. www.frontiersin.org/articles/10.3389/fpsyt.2018.00223/full. [accessed 29th November, 2018].

Luhrmann T and Marrow J (2016) *Our Most Troubling Madness: Case Studies in Schizophrenia across Cultures* (Ethnographic Studies in Subjectivity). Oakland, CA: University of California.

Luxton D (ed.) (2015) *Artificial Intelligence in Behavioral and Mental Health.* Cambridge, Massachusetts: Elsevier Academic.

Lyons S (2018) Wall Street at 30: Is greed still good? *The Conversation,* 8 December. http://theconversation.com/wall-street-at-30-is-greed-still-good-87612 [accessed 4 February, 2019].

Major Depressive Disorder Working Group of the Psychiatric Genomics Consortium (2018) Genome-wide association analyses identify 44 risk variants and refine the genetic architecture of major depression. *Nature Genetics,* 50(5), pp. 668–681.

Marmot M (2016) *The Health Gap: The Challenge of an Unequal World.* London: Bloomsbury.

Marsh A (2017) *Good for Nothing: From Altruists to Psychopaths and Everyone in Between*. London: Robinson.

Martin J (2002) The integration of neurology, psychiatry, and neuroscience in the 21st century. *American Journal of Psychiatry*, 159(5), pp. 695–704.

Maudsley Biol Res Centre (2018) Clinical disorders and health behaviours cluster. www.maudsleybrc.nihr.ac.uk/research/clinical-disorders-and-health-behaviours/ [accessed 31 January, 2019].

Mazower M (2018) Fascism revisited? A warning about the rise of populism. *Financial Times*, 11 April. www.ft.com/content/6d57a338-3be9-11e8-bcc8-cebcb81f1f90 [accessed 4 February, 2019].

McCarthy-Jones S (2017) The concept of schizophrenia is coming to an end – here's why. *The Conversation*, 24 August. https://theconversation.com/the-concept-of-schizophrenia-is-coming-to-an-end-heres-why-82775 [accessed 25 September, 2018].

McCormack J and Korownyk C (2018) Effectiveness of antidepressants. Lots of useful data but many important questions remain. *British Medical Journal*, 9 March. www.bmj.com/content/360/bmj.k1073 [accessed 13 January, 2019].

McGuffin P and Murray R (eds) (2014) *The New Genetics of Mental Illness*. Oxford: Butterworth-Heinemann

McIntyre L (2018) *Post-Truth*. Cambridge, MA: MIT.

Megget K (2016) Crispr goes commercial. Royal Society of Chemistry. www.chemistryworld.com/news/crispr-goes-commercial/9359.article [accessed 20 August, 2018].

Midgely M (2011) *The Myths We Live By*. Abingdon: Routledge.

Midgely M (2014) *Are You an Illusion?* Abingdon: Routledge.

Mill J S (1869) *The Subjugation of Women*. London: Longmans, Green, Reader, and Dyer.

Mills C (2014) *Decolonizing Global Mental Health: The Psychiatrization of the Majority World*. Abingdon: Routledge.

Monbiot G (2016) Neoliberalism is creating loneliness. That's what's wrenching society apart. *The Guardian*, 12 October.

Moncrieff J (2013) *The Bitterest Pills: The Troubling Story of Antipsychotic Drugs*. London: Palgrave Macmillan.

Moncrieff J (2014) A Critique of genetic research on schizophrenia – expensive castles in the air. *Critical Psychiatry, Mad in America: Science, Psychiatry and Social Justice*, 1 September. www.madinamerica.com/2014/09/critique-genetic-research-schizophrenia-expensive-castles-air/ [accessed 11 July, 2018].

Moncrieff J and Middleton H (2015) Schizophrenia: A critical psychiatry perspective. *Current Opinion Psychiatry*, 28(3), pp. 264–268.

Morrall P (2008) *The Trouble with Therapy: Sociology and Psychotherapy*. Chichester: Open University Press/McGraw-Hill.

Morrall P (2017) *Madness: Ideas about Insanity*. Abingdon-on-Thames: Routledge.

Morrall P, Worton K and Antony D (2018) Why is murder fascinating and why does it matter to mental health professionals? *Mental Health Practice*, 23 April. https://journals.rcni.com/mental-health-practice/evidence-and-practice/why-is-murder-fascinating-and-why-does-it-matter-to-mental-health-professionals-mhp.2018.e1249/abs [accessed 4 February, 2019].

Morrison A, Renton J, Dunn J, Williams S and Bentall R (2003) *Cognitive Therapy for Psychosis: A Formulation-Based Approach*. Abingdon: Routledge.

Mosley I (ed.) (2000) *Dumbing Down: Culture, Politics and the Mass Media*. Exeter: Imprint Academic.

Mostafavi, H, Pickrell J and Przeworski M (2017) Evolutionary geneticists spot natural selection happening now in people. *The Conversation*, 12 September. http://theconversa tion.com/evolutionary-geneticists-spot-natural-selection-happening-now-in-people-836 21 [accessed 5 December, 2018].

Mukherjee S (2017) *The Gene: An Intimate History*. London: Vintage.

Müller J (2017) *What is Populism?* London: Penguin.

Najjar S, Steiner J, Najjar A and Bechter K (2018) A clinical approach to new-onset psychosis associated with immune dysregulation: The concept of autoimmune psychosis. *Journal of Neuroinflammation*, 15(50). www.ncbi.nlm.nih.gov/pmc/articles/ PMC5809809/ [accessed 26 July, 2018].

National Aeronautics and Space Administration [NASA]. (2018) Long-term warming trend continued in 2017. NASA and Goddard Institute for Space Studies. www.giss. nasa.gov/research/news/20180118/ [accessed 27 September, 2018].

National Health Service England (2019) Social prescribing. www.england.nhs.uk/p ersonalisedcare/social-prescribing/ [accessed 28 January, 2019].

NHS Digital (2019) The Prescription Cost Analysis, England 2018. Leeds: NHS Digital.

Nobel Assembly at Karolinska Institute (2018) 2018 Nobel Prize in Physiology or Medicine – Press Release. www.nobelprize.org/uploads/2018/10/press-medicine2018. pdf [accessed 1 October, 2018].

O'Connor C and Weatherall J (2018) *The Misinformation Age: How False Beliefs Spread*. New Haven, CT: Yale University Press.

Office of National Statistics (UK) Suicides in the UK: 2017 Registrations. www.ons. gov.uk/peoplepopulationandcommunity/birthsdeathsandmarriages/deaths/bulletins/ suicidesintheunitedkingdom/2017registrations [accessed 10 October, 2018].

Palumbo P, Mariotti M, Iofrida C and Pellegrini S (2018) Genes and aggressive behavior: Epigenetic mechanisms underlying individual susceptibility to aversive environments. *Frontiers in Behav Neurosci*, 12, 117. www.ncbi.nlm.nih.gov/pmc/a rticles/PMC6008527/ [accessed 6 December, 2018].

Panksepp J and J B Panksepp (2000) The seven sins of evolutionary psychology. *Evolution and Cognition*, 6(2), pp. 108–131.

Parkhurst J (2017) *The Politics of Evidence*. Abingdon: Routledge.

Pies R (2016) The astonishing non-epidemic of mental illness. *Psychiatric Times*, 1 November. www.psychiatrictimes.com/blogs/astonishing-non-epidemic-mental-illness.

Pinker S (2018) *Enlightenment Now: The Case for Science, Reason, Humanism and Progress*. London: Allen Lane.

Plant J and Stephenson J (2009) *Beating Stress, Anxiety and Depression: Groundbreaking Ways to Help You Feel Better*. London: Little, Brown.

Plomin R (2018) *Blueprint: How DNA Makes Us Who We Are*. London: Allen Lane.

Psychiatric Genomics Consortium (2018) What is the PGC?www.med.unc.edu/pgc. [accessed 10 July, 2018].

Quine W (1951) Two dogmas of empiricism. *Philosophical Review*, 60(1), pp. 20–43.

Richerson P and Boyd R (2005) *Not by Genes Alone: How Culture Transformed Human Evolution*. Chicago, IL: University of Chicago Press.

Rieder R, Wisniewski P, Alderman B and Campbell S (2017) Microbes and mental health: A review. *Brain Behavior and Immunity*, 66, pp. 9–17.

Rogers J, Gonzalez-Madruga K, Kohls G, Baker R, Clanton R, Pauli R, Birch P, Chowdhury A, Kirchner M, Andersson J, Smaragdi A, Puzzo I, Baumann S, Raschle N, Fehlbaum L, Menks W, Steppan M, Stadler C, Konrad K, Freitag C, Fairchild G and De Brito S (2019) White matter microstructure in youths with conduct disorder: Effects of sex and variation in callous traits. *J Am Acad Child Adolesc Psychiatry*, S0890–8567(19), pp. 30251–30255.

Rose H and Rose S (2014) *Genes, Cells and Brains: The Promethean Promises of the New Biology.* London: Verso.

Rose H and Rose S (2016) *Can Neuroscience Change Our Minds?* Cambridge: Polity.

Rose N (1998) Controversies in meme theory. *Journal of Memetics. Evolutionary Models of Information Transmission*, 2. http://cfpm.org/jom-emit/1998/vol2/rose_n.html [accessed 21 April, 2015].

Rose N (2018) *Our Psychiatric Future: The Politics of Mental Health.* Cambridge: Polity.

Rose N and Abi-Rached J (2013) *Neuro: The New Brain Sciences and the Management of the Mind.* Princeton, NJ: Princeton University Press.

Rose N and McGuffin P (2005) Will science explain mental illness? *Prospect Magazine*, October, pp. 28–32.

Rosenhan, D L (1973) On being sane in insane places. *Science*, 179, pp. 250–258.

Royal Australian and New Zealand College of Psychiatrists (2019) Section of Neuropsychiatry. www.ranzcp.org/membership/faculties-sections/neuropsychiatry [accessed 14 January, 2019].

Royal College of Psychiatrists (2019) Faculty of Neuropsychiatry. www.rcpsych.ac.uk/members/your-faculties/neuropsychiatry. [accessed 14 January, 2019].

Russo J and Sweeney A (eds) (2016) *Searching for a Rose Garden: Challenging Psychiatry, Fostering Mad Studies.* Ross-on-Wye: PCCS.

Sanjak J, Sidorenko J, Robinson M, Thornton K and Visscher P (2018) Evidence of directional and stabilizing selection in contemporary humans. *Proceedings of the National Academy of Sciences*, 115(1), pp. 151–156.

Scheff T (1966) *Being Mentally Ill: A Sociological Theory.* Chicago: Aldine.

Schildkrout B (2016) How to move beyond the diagnostic and statistical manual of mental disorders/international classification of diseases. *Journal of Nervous and Mental Disease*, 204(10), pp. 723–727.

Schildkrout B (2017) Neuroanatomy and the 21st century psychiatrist. *Psychiatric Times*, 34(3), 21 March. www.psychiatrictimes.com/neuropsychiatry/neuroanatomy-and-21st-century-psychiatrist/page/0/1?GUID=EBC79EE0-EC28-48F7-A99F%2029CB7FE8DC6E&rememberme=1&ts=11042017 [accessed 28 June, 2018].

Schildkrout B and Frankel M (2016) Neuropsychiatry: Toward solving the mysteries that animate psychiatry. *Psychiatric Times*, 33(12), 15 December. www.psychiatrictimes.com/neuropsychiatry/neuropsychiatry-toward-solving-mysteries-animate-psychiatry?GUID=EBC79EE0-EC28-48F7-A99F-29CB7FE8DC6E&rememberme=1&ts=29122016 [accessed 5 July, 2018].

Schizophrenia Working Group of the Psychiatric Genomics Consortium (2014) Biological insights from 108 schizophrenia-associated genetic loci. *Nature*, 511(7510), pp. 421–427.

Schizophrenia Working Group of the Psychiatric Genomics Consortium (2016) Schizophrenia risk from complex variation of complement component 4, *Nature*, 530 (7589), pp. 177–183.

Schulze T and Adorjan K (2018) From the genomic revolution to friendly data sharing and global partnerships. *Psychiatric Times*, 35(8), pp. 1–4. www.psychiatrictimes.com/genetic-disorders/psychiatric-genetics-2018-genomic-revolution-friendly-data-sharing-and-global-partnerships [accessed 13 December, 2018].

Schumann C, Bauman M and Amaral D (2011) Abnormal structure or function of the amygdala is a common component of neurodevelopmental disorders. *Neuropsychologia*, 49(4), pp. 745–759.

Scull A (2007a) Scholarship of fools. The frail foundations of Foucault's monument. *The Time Literary Supplement*, March 23 pp. 3–4.

Scull A (2007b) Mind, brain, law and culture – Book reviews by Andrew Scull. *Brain*, 130, pp. 585–591.

Scull A (2011) *Madness: A Very Short Introduction*. Oxford: Oxford University Press.

Shackelford T and Weekes-Shackelford V (eds) (2012) *The Oxford Handbook of Evolutionary Perspectives on Violence, Homicide, and War*. New York: Oxford University Press.

Shorter E (1997) *A History of Psychiatry: From the Era of the Asylum to the Age of Prozac. A History of Psychiatry*. New York: Wiley.

Stier, M, Schoene-Seifert B, Rüther M and Muders S (2014) The philosophy of psychiatry and biologism. *Frontiers in Psychology*, 5(1032). www.ncbi.nlm.nih.gov/pmc/articles/PMC4166893/ [accessed 12 December, 2018].

Stevens A and Price J (2000) *Evolutionary Psychiatry: A New Beginning*, 2nd edn. London: Routledge.

Stewart G (2019) Social prescribing. *British Medical Journal*, 28 March, 364(1285). www.bmj.com/content/364/bmj.l1285/rr [accessed May 19, 2019].

Strachey J (2001) *Complete Psychological Works of Sigmund Freud*. London: Vintage.

Sweeney E (2019) No-deal Brexit scenario would create serious traffic congestion and supply chain chaos. *The Conversation*, 8 January. https://theconversation.com/no-deal-brexit-scenario-would-create-serious-traffic-congestion-and-supply-chain-chaos-109480 [accessed 4 February, 2019].

Szasz T (1961) *The Myth of Mental Illness: Foundations of a Theory of Personal Conduct*. New York: Hoeber-Harper.

Szasz T (1970) *The Manufacture of Madness: A Comparative Study of the Inquisition and the Mental Health Movement*. New York: Harper and Row.

Szasz T (1977) *Psychiatric Slavery When Confinement and Coercion Masquerade as Cure*. New York: Free Press.

Szasz T (1994) Mental illness is still a myth. *Society*, 31(4), pp. 34–39.

Szasz T (2009) Merger of Psychiatry, Neurology [letter to the editor]. *Psychiatric News of the American Psychiatric Association*. https://psychnews.psychiatryonline.org/doi/10.1176/pn.44.5.0025 [accessed 31 October, 2018].

Szasz T (2010) The illegitimacy of the 'psychiatric bible'. *The Freeman*, 60, pp. 16–18.

Szasz T (2011) The myth of mental illness: 50 years later. *The Psychiatrist*, 35, pp. 179–182.

Szmolka I (ed.) (2017) *Political Change in the Middle East and North Africa: After the Arab Spring*. Edinburgh: Edinburgh University Press.

Tallis R (2004) *Why the Mind is Not a Computer: A Pocket Lexicon of Neuromythology*, 2nd edn. Exeter: Imprint Academic.

Tallis R (2016) *Aping Mankind*: Abingdon: Routledge.

Taylor S (2012) *Back to Sanity: Healing the Madness of Our Minds*. London: Hay House.

Therrien A (2018) Anti-depressants: Major study finds they work. *BBC*, 22 February. www.bbc.co.uk/news/health-43143889 [accessed 13 January, 2018].

Thorley C (2017) *Not By Degrees Improving Student Mental Health In The UK's Universities*. London: Institute for Public Policy Research.

Tretter F and, Albus M (2008) Pharmacopsychiatry. *Systems Biology and Psychiatry –Modeling Molecular and Cellular Networks of Mental Disorders*, 41(1), S2–S18. www.ncbi.nlm.nih.gov/pubmed/18756416 [accessed 2 November, 2018].

United Nations (2018) Global issues – Overview. www.un.org/en/sections/issues-depth/global-issues-overview/ [accessed 14 August, 2018].

University College London Hospitals (2019) Professor Eileen Joyce. www.uclh.nhs.uk/OurServices/Consultants/Pages/ProfEileenJoyce.aspx [accessed 14 January, 2019].

Verhaegue P (2014) *What About Me: The Struggle for Identity in a Market-based Society*. Melbourne, Australia: Scribe.

Wessely S (2016) A fuller picture of modern psychiatry. *The Guardian*, 26 February.

Wessely S and James O (2013) Do we need to change the way we are thinking about mental illness? *The Observer*, 12 May.

Whitaker R (2011) *Anatomy of an Epidemic: Magic Bullets, Psychiatric Drugs, and the Astonishing Rise of Mental Illness in America*. New York: Broadway.

Whitaker R and Cosgrave L (2015) *Psychiatry Under the Influence: Institutional Corruption, Social Injury, and Prescriptions for Reform*. London: Palgrave MacMillan.

Wiggershaus R (2010) *The Frankfurt School: Its History, Theory and Political Significance*. Cambridge: Polity.

Wilkinson R and Pickett K (2010) *The Sprit Level: Why More Equal Societies Almost Always Do Better*. London: Penguin.

Wilkinson R and Pickett K (2017) Inequality and mental illness. *The Lancet*, 4(7), 25 May, pp. 512–513.

Williams R and Robinson D (eds) (2014) *Scientism: The New Orthodoxy*. London: Bloomsbury.

Wilmott P and Young M (1957) *Family and Kinship in East London*. Harmondsworth: Penguin.

Wilson C (2018) Almost every antidepressant headline you'll read today is wrong. www.newscientist.com/article/2161911-almost-every-antidepressant-headline-youll-read-today-is-wrong/ [accessed 20 May, 2019].

Wilson E O (1975) *Sociobiology: The New Synthesis*. Cambridge, MA: Harvard University Press.

Wolff M (2018) Fire *and Fury: Inside the Trump White House*. London: Abacus.

Wolin R (2006) *The Frankfurt School Revisited*. Abingdon: Routledge.

Woolf S and Aron L (2013) *U.S. Health in International Perspective: Shorter Lives, Poorer Health*. Washington DC: National Academies of Science, Engineering, and Medicine.

Wootton D (2018) Comfort history. *The Times Literary Supplement*, 14 February. www.the-tls.co.uk/articles/public/comfort-history-enlightenment-now/ [accessed 9 July, 2018].

World Federation of Societies of Biological Psychiatry (2019) About the World Federation of Societies of Biological Psychiatry. www.wfsbp.org/about/ [accessed 30 January, 2019].

World Health Organisation (WHO) (2013) *Mental Health Action Plan 2013–2020*. Geneva: World Health Organisation.

World Health Organisation (WHO) (2017) *Depression and other Common Mental Disorders: Global Health Estimates.* Geneva: World Health Organisation.

World Health Organisation (WHO) (2014) *Social Determinants of Mental Health.* Geneva: World Health Organisation and the Calouste Gulbenkian Foundation.

World Health Organisation (WHO) (2017) *Depression and Other Common Mental Disorders: Global Health Estimates.* Geneva: World Health Organisation.

World Health Organisation (WHO) (2018a) *The International Statistical Classification of Diseases and Related Health Problems 11 Revision [ICD-11]. Mental, Behavioural or Neurodevelopmental Disorders.* Geneva: World Health Organisation.

World Health Organisation (WHO) (2018b) *Health Topics.* Geneva: World Health Organisation www.who.int/health-topics/ [accessed 14 August, 2018].

World Health Organisation (WHO) (2018c) *Schizophrenia: Key Facts [Causation].* Geneva: World Health Organisation. www.who.int/news-room/fact-sheets/detail/schizophrenia [accessed 28 September, 2018].

Žižek S (1989) *The Sublime Object of Ideology.* New York: Verso.

2 Faulty society

In Chapter 1 there is an account of a selection of ideas which are used to understand madness,[1] especially its cause(s), through gazing at what are construed as perceptible or potentially palpable personal impediments to normality. Whilst Chapter 1 contained several criticisms of these ideas, which largely flow from biology, this chapter covers core criticisms of the very nature of biological thinking concerning madness. What follows is coverage of selective sociological ideas about madness, culminating with Erich Fromm's proposition that the very sanity of society needs to be critiqued.

The fixation on the brain and all things neuroscientific fixates on finding faults in the individual to explain normality and madness, and by default or deliberately demotes much or for some all human performance to neurological processes including consciousness. Hilary Rose and Steven Rose (2016) comment that this fixation on finding faults in the individual (and on fixing him or her through physical methods of treatment), emphasised and legitimised through the' hype' surrounding 'big brain projects', relies on a 'crassly empiricist' epistemology. Observations of apparent material abnormalities in genes, biochemicals, and brain anatomy, are coupled with both cause and remedy of psychological distress. Neuroscience is, they argue, therefore rich with data but poor on theory. The absence of theory addressing the role of society is conspicuous.

Ideas which adhere to an outward gaze can be loosely corralled into two strands of critical thought. First, there is criticism of biological depictions and management of madness. Second, rather than focusing on the neuro-genetic, neuro-chemical, and neuro-physiological for answers to the riddles of madness, there is from many of these alternative standpoints the proposal that madness is only understandable and potentially ameliorated, when the configurations of society, rather than those associated with the brain, are accommodated. More credibly, a societal gaze rather than discounting the neurological should accommodate implication of pathology, in the main, as 'effects', but on occasion as a cause, of madness. Accommodation of the reverse is not forthcoming to any profound degree.

What is not claimed here is that society causes all forms of madness or is always the dominant causative feature of even when it is implicated. What is claimed here is that madness cannot be appreciated or alleviated by just auditing and editing neurogenetic, neuro-anatomical, and neuro-chemical events and entities. This is also so for ill-health which is regarded rightly as broadly biologically. For example, cancer and dementia have social connotations. Easy availability and inventive advertising of cigarettes heighten the uptake amongst certain social groups (notably young people) and thereby heightens the incidence of lung cancer (Boseley et al., 2018; Campaign for Tobacco-Free Kids, 2019). The family and the community of an individual suffering with Alzheimer's disease will be affected socially in the sense of the cost of providing care, and that care is likely to be based either tacitly or overtly on a 'social model' (Alzheimer's Society, 2019; Mental Health Foundation, 2015).

So, things are complicated. Fromm does not deliver a complete resolution to this complexity, but he does offer hope.

Flawed thinking

Psychiatry, by becoming more absorbed with the minutiae of the performance of the brain, is suffering from biologism. 'Biologism' refers to the unwarrantable reduction of most or all human emotions, behaviour, and thinking to biological processes (Steir et al., 2014; Tallis, 2016).

Sociologist Andrew Scull notes psychiatry's biological reductionists inclination:

> So far as psychiatry is concerned, we once again live in an era where simplistic and biologically reductionist accounts of mental disorder enjoy widespread currency. Patients and their families have learned to attribute their travails to biochemical abnormalities, to faulty neurotransmitters, and to genetic defects.
>
> (Scull, 2005)

But these claims are overblown, premature, or erroneous. Most of these claims do not incorporate adequate – if any – homage to the external impact of the social environment, including its physical aspects, on the internal mental workings of individuals. The environment impacts dramatically on physical and psychological health –shortcomings in society shorten lives (Woolf and Aron, 2013).

For Hilary Rose and Steven Rose (2016), this biological reductionist approach to understanding human mental faculties and failings is merely 'internal phrenology', that is the equivalent of 19th century scientifically suspect attempt to find personality signatures and signs of criminality and madness by the crudely empiricist tactile search for bumps and crevasses on the exterior of the skull. Replacing tactile testing with modern imaging devices has not afforded phenology scientific authenticity (Dempsey-Jones, 2018).

For sociologist Nikolas Rose along with Joelle Abi-Rached, an historian of science, a deepening of biological reductionism in psychiatry began in the 1960s. This new positioning in the study of human biology, which they term 'the neuromolecular gaze', is exceptionally reductionist because it moves scientific and psychiatric technology and thinking into looking at and conceptualising the most miniscule of workings in the body and especially the brain (Rose and Abi-Rached, 2013; Rose, 2018). Psychiatry's knowledge and practices have been re-positioned to be based on genetics and neuroscience. Genetic and neuroscience research attracts large-scale funding for, and gives scientific credibility to, psychiatry. Major psychiatric research institutions in many Western countries concentrate on this research, as do major commercial industries which intend benefiting from its outcomes.

Nikolas Rose and Abi-Rached (2013) explore the meaning of the neuro-molecular gaze for society and individuals, and ponder what exactly shapes human performance, whether that be classified as normal or abnormal. They reject the pretentious yet populist maxim espoused by purists of biological determinism that 'the mind is what brain does' (Nikolas Rose and Abi-Rached, 2013, p. 3). For them human performances such as falling in love, empathy, hostility, a fixation on material possessions, deviancy, and madness, cannot be summoned-up by mapping out and postulating on the intricacies of DNA, synapses, and compounds. In stark contrast to the claims of biological reductionists, Nikolas Rose and Abi-Rached, point out that notwithstanding all the funding and studies, and technologies associated with gazing deeper and deeper into the minutiae of the human gene and neurological processes, no specific biomarkers have been conclusively connected to specific disorders. Therefore, no specific treatments, beyond the palliative or placebic, have emerged:

> Despite the penetrating gaze of neuroscience … psychiatric classification remains superficial. This neuromolecular vision seems incapable of grounding the clinical work of psychiatry in a way that has become routine in other areas of medicine.
>
> (Rose and Abi-Rached, 2013, p. 138)

The DSM 5 (American Psychiatric Association, 2013) contains nearly 800 categories/sub-categories. There is also ICD-11 (World Health Organisation, 2018a). Transgender removed, 'Gaming Disorder' and 'Avoidant-Restrictive Food Intake Disorder' included in the DSM 5. There are no biomarkers to match against DSM diagnoses and very little if any success in the neuroscientific treatment of madness. There is no simple connection between neurons and madness and this includes much of dementia (Hilary Rose and Steven Rose, 2016).

Joanna Moncrieff (2014) is a 'critical psychiatrist'. That is, she is one in a network of psychiatrists who are critical of the reductionist approach in her profession. She also remarks on the discrepancy between, on the one hand, the vast amount of money spent on biological research, and the 'much trumpeted claims' and 'endless predictions' of her biologically-minded colleagues, and would-be commercial benefactors, and, on the other hand, a solution to such conditions as schizophrenia. Certain genes have been found to have 'weak associations' with schizophrenia. But, generalising to most let alone all of those diagnosed as schizophrenic has not and is extremely unlikely to happen. This is because the studies have not been repeatable, and the schizophrenia as a psychiatric category is unstable if not invalid.

Schizophrenia and depression have been heralded by biological determinists as mental disorders which are caused by faulty genes (see Chapter 1). Radical psychologist Richard Bentall along with clinical psychologist and medical sociologist David Pilgrim (2016) avow that there are no genes for schizophrenia. They trace theories of genetic to nineteenth century views about a host of physical and psychological aberrations. Madness, 'idiocy', epilepsy, alcoholism, prostitution, alcoholism, and criminality were all envisaged as manifestly biological. Equally manifestly, these personal faults needed to be controlled through eugenic policies such as social isolation and kerbing reproduction. In the twentieth century, genetics was taken to the extreme under the Nazis. During that century, although the explicit advocation of eugenics has not reoccurred, 'quantitative geneticists' studying of families, twins and adopted children, with their furthering of 'heritability' and 'polygenetic risk' concerning schizophrenia and depression, were inadvertently abetting eugenics or at least underscoring the notion that the individual has inbuilt imperfections which need perfecting. Bentall and Pilgrim are adamant that the geneticists' explanations and adjustments are not justified. For them there is scant evidence of genetic causation as there are no schizophrenic genes to be found.

Neurobiologist Steven Rose identifies defects in the thinking of biological reductionists. In his debate with neuroscientist Peter McGuffin (Steven Rose and McGuffin, 2005) he accedes that neurology and genetics may play a part in psychological distress. However, he argues it is wrong to ascribe biological states, whether or not pathological, to what technological devices appear to expose. It is, he points out, axiomatic that psychological states have corresponding brain states. An individual who is markedly anxious or hallucinating is likely to have different brain processes which are apparent in images of the brain when it is scanned compared with someone who is calm and not psychotic. An individual's thinking, emotions, or behaviour may alter after taking medication designed to interfere with neurochemistry.

But, argues Steven Rose, imaging and neurochemical alteration only provides evidence of association not proof of origin. Pictures of pathology and pharmaceutically-induced alterations to performance do not does not confirm that root of mental disorder is biological. Moreover, Stephen Rose attempts to measure scientifically what is not conceptually defined accurately, if it is definable at all, is at root illogical. Whilst there is ample precision in the technological tools used to study genetics and neurology, there is little precision in psychiatric categories. McGuffin, however, argues, that the science of psychiatry and the interconnectedness of technological tools and diagnostic categories needs to be advanced not abandoned (Stephen Rose and McGuffin, 2005). This is a fair defence of biologism, but fair rejoinders are to ask: how much longer will it take to find precise biological causation which then can lead to precise cures of any, some, most, or all of the hundreds of mental disorders in the psychiatric diagnostic lexicons'?; how much more research should be conducted and money spent on finding definitive biomarkers when none have been so far found after decades to searching?

Neuroscientist and philosopher Raymond Tallis (2004) reasons that what an individual interprets her/his sensory experiences, translates these into thoughts, emotions, and behaviours, and articulates these in highly unlikely to correspond to the conjectures of the evolutionary psychologist, the geneticist's DNA samples, or the neuroscientist's images. What is happening both within the 'self' of the individual, within the technologies and the gaze of the theorist and observer, are clashes and amasses of predisposed and generated realities. Put starkly, subjective experience and expression does not, indeed cannot, correspond with the avowed objective framing of geneticist and neuroscientist, or the perceptual paraphernalia of psychiatric practice (Morrall, 2017).

The imaging of the brain is never 'correct' as each type of scan and each new development in imaging reveals distinctive impressions (which then must be interpreted using other distinctive tools of analysis) relating to the functioning and framework of the brain's almost 'inconceivable complexity' (Hilary Rose and Steven Rose, 2016).

Furthermore, the assertion that neurological pathology and mental disorder are conjoint is a teleological proposition. That is, the description of genetic, brain, or immunological mishaps as the cause of one mental disorder does not actually explain that linkage. Philosopher Peter Hacker (Hacker 2015 in Robinson and Williams) focuses on yet another elementary lapse in logic when activities in the brain are not attributed to interactions with other biological systems and deportments of the mind or to the whole person. For Hacker the absence of accounting for interactions of society and the whole person, including his/her brain, is a further illogicality. Evolutionary biologist Richard Lewontin decries the 'biologizing' of the psyche and the social as 'simplistic scientism' and 'banal biologism'. The title of Lewontin's book in which the long history of biological ideological infiltration into would-be scientific thinking about the workings of the mind sums up his critical position:

'It Ain't Necessarily So'

(Lewontin, 2001)

Teleology is inherent to the (flawed) reasoning of evolutionary psychologists, denunciation of evolutionary psychology can be savage and emanate from a range of sources. These sources include sociology, neuroscience, and general medical practice (Panksepp and Panksepp, 2000; Hilary Rose and Steven

Rose, 2014; Tallis, 2016; Goldacre, 2015). There is, argue the critics little hard evidence to back psychology/psychiatry's adaptation of Darwinian biology. Nikolas Rose and Abi-Rached (2013) reject the 'simplifications' of socio-biology and evolutionary psychology as they do those of biological determinists. Palaeontologist Stephen Jay Gould (1997) describes evolutionary psychology (and by implication also evolutionary psychiatry) as a 'superficially attractive cult'. Lewontin argues that evolutionary psychologists and sociobiologists perpetuate the 'pervasive error' of completely conflating genetic forms of humans and other animals (from ants to primates), with human physical, psychological and social attributes (Lewontin et al., 1984).

Devotees of evolutionary psychology can produce, in the main, only post hoc theoretical suppositions evidence to support their claims. For Scull (2007b) human history is far too complex, and any evidence (for example, extracted from archaeological artefacts) far too flimsy, for anything other than conjecture. Claiming that the thoughts, behaviours, and feelings of contemporary humans can be traced though thousands if not millions of years is fascinating but fictitious. Moreover, evolutionary psychology has become popularised despite its fallacies. The claims of psychological evolutionists are perceived by the public as having legitimacy rather than being mere speculations (Hilary Rose and Steven Rose, 2016). The ideas of evolutionary psychologists are nothing more 'speculative'. 'deeply flawed' speculations (Buller, 2012).

Teleological rationalisation is at the heart of sociobiology and evolutionary psychology. There is a promiscuous obsessiveness to describe and thereby justify every element of human performance by an evolutionary 'function', and one's which may be ascribed to primates, no-matter that vital empirical evidence for such justification is absent, and no-matter that the underlying logic is circular. This is bad science and bad reasoning (Goldacre, 2009; 2015). To define intelligence, aggression, flirting, consciousness, or schizophrenia, by listing its characteristics, and to peer into the murkiness of human history through the disadvantage point of contemporary cultural lenses, or observe the demeanour and shenanigans of other species, and then claim to know about twenty-first century human thinking, emotions, and behaviours, is interesting but not ratifiable through reason or research (Lewontin, 2001).

When undertaking my bachelor's degree in sociology one of my lecturers (I can't remember whom) invented a phrase to summarise criticism of sociobiology. The following is my paraphrase of what for us sociology undergraduates become a popular line in intellectual hubris delivered whenever there was an opportunity to attempt to impress anyone unfortunate enough within earshot:

Biological ethological anthropomorphic teleological reductionism.

The phrase indicts sociobiology for making spurious claims about human performance from observing animal behaviour, and unevidenced claims over unidentifiable millennia which are assumed to give insight into the thoughts, feelings, and behaviours of contemporary humans. The latter is a criticism applicable to evolutionary psychology (and evolutionary psychiatry).

Flaky formulations

For Richard Bentall (2009a; 2016) rather using classifications such as 'schizophrenic' judgement about psychological distress should be led by listening to the patient's 'complaint'. Bentall and like-minded colleagues such as Johnstone campaign for alternative diagnostic systems to those used by psychiatry including 'Clinical Case Formulation' and 'Power Threat Meaning Framework' (Bentall, 2009b; Morrison et al., 2003; Johnstone and Dallos, 2013; Johnstone and Boyle, 2018). They argue that the DSM and ICD have two other major flaws besides the diagnostic flakiness of the psychiatric categories contained within them. The first of these added flaws is that they do not incorporate the specialness of the patient's story (that is, she/he is not properly 'heard').

Psychiatry has formulated hundreds of mental disorders (the sum of categories and subcategories in the DSM 5 is nearly 800 (American Psychiatric Association, 2013). Szasz (1970; 2010) takes the view that virtually all psychiatric classifications are not just flaky but false. For Szasz, diagnostic appellations are unduly and excessively attributed to aspects of human performance without corresponding linkage to tangible organic disease. Szasz suggests that psychiatry has contrived the whole paradigm of 'mental disorder', and supposed disorders such as depression, anxiety, depression, manic-depression, schizophrenia, and psychopathy, are manufactured medical 'metaphors' for madness. For sociologist Thomas Scheff (1966), madness fashioned as mental disorder is a metaphorical 'label' which is applied when all when all other categories of social deviance have been exhausted. For example, a criminal suspect brought before a court may have the label of 'psychopath' determined because the judiciary and jury cannot identify a motive or that the perpetrator committed the crime due to her/his inherent 'badness'. A further argument from Szasz is that the phrase 'mental illness' (or mental disorder) is oxymoronic. That is, the concepts of 'mental' and 'disorder' are mutually exclusive. 'Mental' denotes an abstract or unknowable state of mind whereas the term 'illness', as used in most areas of medical practice, implies a concrete and identifiable physical condition.

Madness, maintains Szasz, is merely a personal problem which may have significance for society, but which should not, unless there is known organic causation, involve the medical profession. Virtually all the vast array of mental disorders contained in the various editions of the two psychiatric lexicons (the DSM and ICD), therefore for Szasz, are categorisable as 'problems with living'. Szsaz is a radical libertarian. He promulgates freedom of choice for the individual and the minimum of State involvement in people's lives. Individuals, perhaps with the aid of their families, friends, colleagues, and communities, and possibly with the requested intervention of non-medical professionals or unrequested intervention of agents of the law, should take responsibility to sort out their problems with living.

Psychiatric categories are created by committees of the very professionals whose careers and status will benefit from their affirmation. There is also financial benefit from the affirmation of old and creation of new psychiatric categories for, for example, the technological and pharmaceutical companies which furnish the concomitant diagnostic equipment and chemical medications.

In the USA there is concomitance between biological research in psychiatry, some psychiatric professionals, and pharmaceutical companies. There is a host of opinion from various disciplines criticising this allegiance citing irregular scientific procedure and irrelevant diagnostic categorisation, financial and status profiteering, the generation of more harmful than beneficial effects, and for neglecting or minimising psychological and social factors. This host includes, journalist Robert Whitaker (2005; 2010), anthropologist and psychotherapist James Davis (2013), 'critical psychiatrist' Joanna Moncrief (Moncrieff, 2013; Moncrieff and Middleton, 2015), radical psychologist Lucy Johnstone (2000; 2014), medical practitioner and promoter of robust uncontaminated science Ben Goldacre (2009; 2012). A prominent and long-term critic of psychiatry for its biological and pharmaceutical linkage is another radical psychological Richard Bentall (2003; 2009a). Journalist Robert Whitaker and radical psychologist Lisa Cosgrove argue that the corrupting influence of the pharmaceutical industry and the bias and financial interests of the American Psychiatric Association, are paramount in what becomes accepted and acceptable knowledge by psychiatry especially in the USA. For them biological research is erroneously endorsed as providing solid support for intervening in the biology of the individual which may in the first place be erroneously diagnosed. Whilst most psychiatrists are well-meaning, the institution of psychiatry has failed on nearly all its undertakings regarding evidence and efficacy (Whitaker and Cosgrave, 2015).

> [T]he giants of the drug companies – Big Pharma – have been a potent source of funding for molecular neuroscience.
> (Hilary Rose and Steven Rose, 2016, p. 27)

Those arguing for an alternative system of classifying psychological distress which centres on hearing the patient's story rather than itemising 'symptoms' point to another flaw in psychiatric formulations. For them neither the DSM nor the ICD give proper weight to social contexts.

Bentall (2016) makes the point that large numbers of people manage to live productive lives despite experiencing symptoms of severe psychiatric disorders at some time or another, and without seeking help. Moreover, many of those with apparent biological defects show no signs of disorder. However, cognitive-behaviour-therapy is a form of treatment considered by several of the critics of biological thinking and formulations in psychiatry to be recommendable for those who are troubled psychologically (Bentall, 2009b; Johnstone, 2014; Johnstone and Dallos, 2013). Therefore, their 'hearing' may be faulty given their predispositions and their mindfulness of social causation flaky.

The very idea of truth and reality being truthful and real is challenged by philosopher Paul Michel Foucault. For Foucault (1966) reality and truth are sold as such by the powerful but countless other realities and truths are possible. Knowledge, therefore, is always contestable. Scientific and psychiatric 'facts' are always flaky because other 'facts' could be presented if alternative historical events had taken place. For example, the medical profession became powerful through occupational manoeuvrings over hundreds of years and has invented a way of viewing the human body, and health and disease which has become dominant. The 'mental' side of medical practice was able to flourish because of the opportunity afforded to the profession when in the nineteenth century it took over administering the asylums which were built on mass in North America, Europe, and in the colonies of countries such as Britain (Foucault, 1961; 2006)[2]. Moreover, the medicalising of madness, argues Szasz (1977) and Scull (1977; 1979) provides power for psychiatry and that power is legitimised by the State because psychiatrists enact the role of 'control agents' over social deviants – that is those designated mad.

Foucault is arguing that knowledge is 'made-up', and madness is manufactured. Science and psychiatry have also to be placed in time and space. They are social institutions staffed by social beings. What is also pertinent for how madness is manufactured for Foucault (1963) is the invention of the laboratory and 'birth of the clinic' and the tapering of the medical scrutiny. This tapering has moved from dissecting organs and tissues to gazing at neuromolecules.

Had the medical profession failed in its power-seeking endeavours, then other 'discourses' promulgated by other groups may have achieved dominance. To a limited degree medical dominance has diminished through increased authority of, for example, 'complementary therapies' and cynicism about experts which is a characteristic of what is claimed to be today's 'post-modern' society (Kuma, 2004). The dominance of psychiatry is disputed by, for example, the discourses of psychology psychotherapy, social work, and also 'survivors'.

There is a multitude of 'survivor' groups'[3] representing a section of patients who regard the power of psychiatry as abusive have sprung-up. Many of their aims chime with the positions of professional dissenters such as Laing and Szasz, and those associated with the 'Critical Psychiatry Network' (2018). The demands of survivor groups have been demanding is less or no coercion, greater diagnostic accuracy, and more effective, or at least less harmful, treatments. Nikolas Rose: The survivor movement has provided a challenge to psychiatric power.

> [F]undamental transformation in the power of psychiatry will not come about from the discovery of the genetic or neurobiological basis of mental illness, but because of the increasing recognition that the recipients of psychiatric ministrations ... are increasingly acquiring a voice, and some power, in the way they are treated.
>
> (Nikolas Rose, 2018, pp. ix-x)

Some survivor groups have argued for is a disengagement from, if not a dissolution of, the institution of psychiatry. Above all they are demanding to be 'heard' (Rissmiller and Rissmiller, 2006; Kallert et al., 2011; Russo and Sweeney, 2016).

Societal situations

Many of those mentioned above who criticise both biology and psychiatry for faulty thinking and faulty formulations accept that biology can play a part in making some people vulnerable to mental disorder. Bentall (2016), for example, accepts that faulty genes may lead to psychological distress, but possibly thousands of genes are involved, each conferring a tiny increase in risk. Biology acknowledges Stephen Rose (Steven Rose and McGuffin, 2005), is certainly involved in some conditions such as Alzheimer's Disorder.

However, much more potent in potentiating madness for the critics of biological-psychiatry are situations of society's making not that of biology. These include: abuse and neglect in childhood; cruelty, destitution; financial insecurity; the absence of, insecure, or degrading employment; living in slum housing, family discord; injustice, the celebration of egocentricity; marginalisation; discrimination; exposure to conflict and natural disasters; deficient nutrition; polluted or inadequate supply of water; low self-esteem because of distressing social circumstances such as those just mentioned (Moncrieff, 2014; Bentall and Pilgrim, 2016; Hilary Rose and Steven Rose, 2016; Nicklas Rose, 2018). These societal factors are associated a range of diagnosed mental disorders including depression, anxiety, panic and post-traumatic-stress, drug and alcohol dependency, and schizophrenia (World Health Organisation, 2014; Nikolas Rose, 2018).

A report on the happiness of 156 countries from 2005 to 2018 (Helliwell et al., 2019) consents that at a country level income growth correlates with an upsurge in self-reported happiness and economic slumps are associated with a rise in misery. But, the conclusions of the report are that long-term economic increases alone do not bring contentment, happiness world-wide is falling whilst worry, and sadness, anger in increasing, and certain other social factors mitigate happiness in countries in which income has risen over the long-term. In the USA a depletion in health within the overall population, a lowering of social trust (especially regarding politicians and political processes), and what the authors of the report describe as a 'mass addiction society', work against the positive effects on mood from increases in income. The addictions referred in the report arise from the use of opioids, the overuse of the internet (for example, social media and texting, and gaming), and the misuse of food. These addictions, which according to the authors of the report are presently 'epidemics', do more than temper happiness and foster misery but can trigger depression and suicide. The happiest country is Finland followed by Denmark, Norway, and Iceland, whilst the least happy are Yemen, Rwanda, Tanzania, Afghanistan, Central African Republic (3.083), and lastly South

Sudan. Despite being the richest country in the world, the USA is 19th in this report's ranking of happiness. Despite their growing economic prowess, China's happiness ranking is 93 and India 140.

Radical psychologist Oliver James (2016) puts the case against biologism succinctly when he discerns that genes do not explain why some people are rich and others are poor, genes do not explain social success, genes have not explained most of madness. For James, no genetic study so far has proven beyond reasoned doubt that any single gene or any combination of genes generate differences in intelligence, personality, or psychological sturdiness. He predicts that no unquestionable cause-and-effect relationship will ever be found for any of these aspects of human performance.

For Moncrieff (2014), there a glaring obvious corollary of finding only flimsy evidence for biological representation of madness, and one which is also the paramount denouement of this book: rather indulging in further and feasibly futile intellectual effort gazing at the no-doubt wondrous world of the neuromolecular, pouring more resources into the 'bottomless pit' of biological research, and pursing miracle antidotes to claimed somatic imperfections, instead fix the faults in society.

The recognition of societal linkage to psychological states isn't just the province of those directly critical of psychiatry's growing biological devotion. Epidemiologist Michael Marmot (2016) makes these linkages as does the World Health Organisation (2014). Medical Physician Margaret Chan is a former Director-General of the World Health Organisation. In her introduction to the WHO's (2013) long-term 'action plan' for mental health, she links the long-term 'macro-socioeconomic' effect on psychological stability of the 2007/8 global financial crisis. In the subsequent years rates of mental disorder diagnoses and suicide increased but funding for services offering support and preventative measures decreased. Moreover, Chan points out that people diagnosed with mental disorders such as depression and schizophrenia have between 40% and 60% of dying than the population average. This is a consequence of suicide or of contracting, for example, cancer, cardiovascular disease, diabetes and HIV infection, and then not either taking-up or having access to physical health services. WHO's objectives in the action plan refer to international efforts to strengthen leadership, governance, and research, and providing comprehensive, integrated and responsive services. What is does not recommend is serious solutions to the societal insanities it identifies as triggers for mental maladies.

Such plans as that of the WHO (2013) have a negative effect on global society according to radical psychologist China Mills (2014). The scaling-up of provision for those already diagnosed and those susceptible to a diagnosis of mental disorder is helping to 'psychiatrise' the world. For Mills this is the medical equivalent of military colonisation and isn't justified because the efficacy of psychiatric treatments is suspect whilst their side-effects are established. What psychiatry should be engaged with is remedying the social factors out of which psychological distress emerge not adding the subjugation of people already living in difficult circumstances. Psychiatry as an institution, and science as a conglomeration of specialties including a range of biological subjects, is also situated in certain social circumstances.

Psychiatry in society

Steven Rose along with feminist sociologist Hilary Rose (Hilary Rose and Stephen Rose, 2014) point out is that science itself has a social context. Politics, economics, interprofessional and interprofessional rivalry and hubris, amongst other social factors affect what is studied, what is published, what is considered important, and what is implemented. Regarding madness, there is no unqualified formulation of 'facts' whether this is relating to comprehension, causation, or cure. Neuroscience (including genetics relating to the brain) as with the brain is not an enterprise separate from society, and its promises are hyped hugely (Hilary Rose and Stephen Rose, 2016).

Preoccupation with all things neurological and biological reductionism in general, Hilary Rose and Steven Rose (2016) propose, is a consequence of social processes – specifically patriarchy, cultural imperialism, and neo-liberalism. Neither the science nor scientists can be separated from society.

Nikolas Rose and Abi-Rached (2013) specify the 'biopolitical' corollaries of focusing on biology to account for human performance. Issues of social power and individual freedom are affected by how much society, and behaviour, emotions, and feelings, and madness, are projected as being orchestrated by biology. For them madness is not a problem to be understood in the laboratory, but of the individual in his/her society's culture and history.

Neuroscientists have grasped that the brain is 'plastic', a reflexive organ. Nature and nurture interact and in doing so each can alter (Eagleman, 2015). However, Nikolas Rose and Abi-Rached (2013) point out that the biopolitical sequelae of accepting the occurrence of neuro-plasticity is an increase in the 'new-liberal' obligation for individuals to take more and more responsibility for their own self. If humans can modify their social as well as their physical environment and are not just irresolute brains, biochemistry, and sequences of DNA, then they can be blamed for their own deviancies including those concerning their psychological states and the State can opt out of its duties and put aside charges of incompetence or malevolence.

'Brain projects', observes Nikolas Rose (2018), are funded in Europe, North America, and Asia. Most psychological distress is handled by the affected person, their family, friends, or lay helpers. Psychiatry and its diagnostic classifications play a significant role in perceptions of madness and normality. This influence is growing globally.

However, Nikolas Rose (2018) questions whether there really is an epidemic (let alone an 'iceberg') of mental disorder or has 'psychiatrisation' of society increased substantially? More specifically, he is asking, has the medicalistion of madness reached global proportions whereby very high levels of mental disorder have already been diagnosed in many developed countries, but in developing countries[4] there is only an assumed diagnostic 'tip-of-the-iceberg' with most yet to be uncovered? He concludes that the numbers should be regarded cautiously.

What Nikolas Rose's questioning raises is the underlying issue of identifying causation. That is, if there is an epidemic can this be linked to a decline in the biological conditions of individuals or in the conditions of society? He asks, has neoliberal capitalism has created any of the epidemics in depression, anxiety, social phobia, eating disorders, loneliness, and self-harm. If living conditions are getting worse, then should certain aspects be tackled or the whole global system? Monbiot is in no doubt:

> What greater indictment of a [neoliberal] system could there be than an epidemic of mental illness? Yet plagues of anxiety, stress, depression, social phobia, eating disorders, self-harm and loneliness now strike people down all over the world.
>
> (Monbiot, 2016)

Rose concludes that it is more complicated than blaming neoliberalism. He points out that, loneliness, for example, has a longer history than neoliberalism. Also, for him the term neoliberalism is too vague and too extensive to be then attributed to the causes of psychological states such as anxiety and depression.

It's complicated

The title of a book written by medical practitioner and campaigner for scientific rigour Ben Goldacre (2015) is *I Think You'll Find It's a Bit More Complicated Than That*. This title applies to both biological and sociological thinking about madness.

To repeat, notwithstanding perpetual proclamations in academic journals and the media of important, innovative, and impending findings, biology has yet (at the time of writing – 2019) to provide evidence which incontrovertibly verifies single-gene or polygenic causation for most of mental disorder diagnosis (Verhaeghue, 2014; World Health Organisation, 2018a). To repeat, for finding the cause of most diagnoses of mental disorder most neuroscientists and geneticists accept that societal environmental factors must be taken into consideration (Rose and Abi-Rached, 2013; Gandal et al., 2018). As historian Yuval Harari notes:

> [M]ost biologists are not fanatics.
>
> (Harari, 2015, p. 434)

Alan Jasanoff (2018) is biological engineer who contends that the brain and the rest of the body along with the physical and social environment collaborate to make us who we are. Human experience of 'selfhood' doesn't just come from the brain, but also from the interactions of chemicals from our bodies and the environment. He argues that neuroscience has failed to make a real difference in anyone's life is because of its 'brain-centeredness'. That is, the neuroscientific gaze needs to be widened. Mental disorder is not only a consequence of genetics and brain structure but is affected by other parts of the body as well as society.

In contemporary scientific research the hunt for biological causation in the main concentrates on finding the bundle of genes, neurochemicals, and/or brain anatomical abnormalities which associable with a diagnosis of mental disorder. The hunt, however, is thwarted profoundly by the inherent complexity of such bundles, the complex intra and inter interconnections of human somatic and psychological systems, and the complex and perhaps incomparable philosophical, scientific, and technological, conceptualisations of the mind and body. Further thwarting is faced with the finding that some of those diagnosed with a mental disorder do not possess the supposed genetic/neurological fault, and those who are not so diagnosed who do (Connor, 2015). The latter includes neuroscientist, James Fallon (2014), whose expertise is the finding of biological causative factors in those classified in the USA criminal justice system as 'psychopathic serial killers' – factors he found he has.

The acceptance that the pursuit of causation regarding madness needs to accommodate both nature and nurture is thwarted by disproportionate consideration regarding research monies and media interest in favour of the former (Nikolas Rose, 2018). Accommodating both nature and nurture is also thwarted by those adhering to sociological reductionism. For example, James (2016) views such socialisation factors as, on the one hand, experiencing in childhood supportive and kindly parental input, and on the other, experiencing in childhood cruelty and neglect in child, transcend the effect of any positive or negative biological factor. Bruce Cohen (2016) provides a Marxist analysis with lays the blame for psychological distress, along with many other personal and societal ails, squarely on capitalism.

That madness is complicated is illustrated by neuropsychologist Simon McCarthy-Jones (2017) using the example of schizophrenia. McCarthy-Jones opines that despite the regular and vociferous of biological discoveries for scores of years the proportion of those people diagnosed with schizophrenia who 'recover' (never mind 'cured') has not changed. There are, acknowledges McCarthy-Jones, genetic and possibly inflammatory influences in the causation of schizophrenia, but these are minimal and must set alongside the hugely more potent effect of social factors such as abuse.

However, for McCarthy-Jones there is the confounding issue of schizophrenia as a concept. The category of schizophrenia, and other mental disorders such as manic-depression, is a spectrum of conditions, a spectrum of roots, and a spectrum of behavioural, emotional, and cognitive performances. That schizophrenia is not a single entity with a single cause means different treatments are required. Different people will display different symptoms the cause of which could be their dysfunctional biology or their dysfunctional social circumstances, or a combination of both. What comes to be diagnosed as schizophrenia may come from nature or nurture or the two may could be implicated, but whether one is responsible or there is collusion between the two, the route from defective DNA, biochemicals, or society, is certainly complex and maybe unfathomable.

Nikolas Rose, as stated above, accepts that both biological and social causative factors change the brain (Nikolas Rose, 2018). He provides the examples of schizophrenia and dementia, both of which he contends arise from 'complex interactions' between the individual's characteristics and the character of her/his societal circumstances. These interactions are fluid over a life-time (and arguably over the individual's ancestors' lifetimes). How these 'disorders' are characterised depends on the meanings a particular culture has at its disposal. Medical attributions of 'disorder' therefore are only of relevance if the cultural antecedents have relevance in the present.

A report by the World Psychiatric Association and the journal *The Lancet* on the future of psychiatry (Bhugra, 2017) does not expressly support combing the biological with the social (and psychological factors must not be forgotten) to form a 'holistic' synthesis. But it does recognise society in the perpetration and perpetration of mental disorder. The report pays homage to what it describes as 'technical advances' made in identifying biomarkers, which as previously mentioned is a contestable claim. However, the report also identifies the 'therapeutic alliance' between patient and practitioner as central to psychiatric practice, and the need be sensitive to her/his cultural identity. Furthermore, the report advocates the fostering of 'social interventions' and political involvement' for psychiatry. This report, concludes, necessitates the training of psychiatrists not just in biological sciences but those in the social sciences.

For Nikolas Rose (2018) the World Psychiatric Association-Lancet report into the future of psychiatry is at root recommending relatively superficial changes to the present condition of psychiatry. Rose is specifically advocating a much more fundamental coming together of social science and psychiatry than is, he claims, suggested in that report. There should be, he proposes, an epistemological and service delivery unification of biological (especially neurological) insights and practices with empirical and theoretical insights into societal influences on madness. But this unified approach must initiate its intellectual gaze not with the brain but the individual in her/his social milieu. Professionals, including psychiatrists, should be agents of social change. Psychiatry was and is powerfully political. Nikolas Rose (2018) wants psychiatry's political preference to be revamped radically. At present the mental health system does not tackle social problems, but he argues that psychiatry could lead the way to social change aimed at relieving social stress and psychological distress. This is where Fromm's idea is germane.

Finding Fromm

In terms of critiquing society, finding Fromm, for me, was revelatory, prescient, and productive. What Fromm offers in his commentary about the condition of individuals and society are ideas which arise from gazing inwards and outwards, and this provides a threefold contribution to sociological reasoning. First, Fromm examines human intra-action and interaction through a Freudian prism. Second, he looks beyond individuals to consider society overall. Third, he incorporates a scathing critique of how individuals are operating in certain societal set-ups with a constructive idea for a better world for humanity. There are faults in all three aspects of Fromm's reasoning, but that need not detract from the essence of what I argue is a remarkable, ethical, and utilitarian perspective and one that underpins this book.

Societal insanity in relation to personal madness has been observed in 'micro' social settings rather than the 'macro' social setting of the whole of society. These smaller situations, however, have connections are part of the culture and structure of society.

Sociologist Erving Goffman (1961) researched the culture of what he described as 'total institutions'. Whether this was a prison, nunnery, monastery, or asylum, all the needs of those living and working there were met. The asylum also had a contradictory component to its culture. Its residents, who may not have been mad or at least vividly abnormal on or following admission were obliged to become mad. Becoming mad was a prerequisite to being regarded by the staff as deserving the chance to normalised and hence warranting the opportunity for discharge arose. If there was resistance to this process, then the patient was considered deviant in the context of these implicit rules of the asylum.

Sociologist George Brown (1959) 'expressed emotion' in families was a predictor of relapse for those diagnosed with schizophrenia. If a patient's diagnosis of schizophrenia is considered in remission and is discharged from psychiatric care returns to a family in which there are open and voluble disputations, then the she/he is at risk of displaying the symptoms which had previously heralded psychiatric intervention. For biologist and anthropologist Gregory Bateson and his colleagues (Bateson et al., 1961) schizophrenia rather than caused by biology was a learned outcome of distorted interpersonal communications within families. Contrary verbal and non-verbal messages of, overt and veiled meanings such as love and hate, and respect and disdain, abounded in certain families. Noticeably, argued Bateson, these concerned mothers and sons. The mother' affection and disaffection with her son would put the latter in a 'double-bind', that is a state of emotional and cognitive confusion, not knowing which of the messages was meant and therefore not knowing how to react. The result could be a diagnosis of madness in the son. It was unorthodox psychiatrist Ronald David Laing who later borrowed Bateson's idea of 'double-bind' but proposed that it wasn't just certain families that furnished madness but the social institution of the modern nuclear family which was to blame. Laing expanded theorising on the effects of the double-bind, arguing that those who were diagnosed as mad were attempting to deal sanely with a mad situation. Listening to and hearing the patient's story is the corollary of the idea that she/he is in an untenable predicament. Listening and hearing is a diagnostic tool and the treatment of choice.

Steven Rose (Rose and McGuffin, 2005) is another advocate of listening to patients rather than allowing technology and physical methods to resolve the patient's psychological predicaments. The psychiatrist, and by implication any other clinician with a professional leaning towards neuroscience and genetics and their concomitant ingesting, implanting, and editing therapies, should be open to 'hear' the patient's story and allow that story to dictate the terms of assessment and remedy. However, there is a tendency in medical practice to listen for symptoms which match pre-set diagnostic categories, not to hear the idiosyncrasies embedded in each patient's story. Neuroscientific technology steers the diagnostician away from both listening and hearing the patient and towards only viewing the imagery of scans and microscopes.

Fromm extends the notion of attributing the cause of apparent madness to a fault in society (for example, the pathological connotations of contradictory messages in families) to the fault lying with the whole of society. Hs idea that virtually the entire population of certain societies is insane because those societies are insane. That is, there are not just aspects of society which cause madness, but society is completely mad, and this causes mass madness. Fromm, as sociologically informed psychoanalyst, is coupling psychological states with the state of society. What Fromm also does is offer a blueprint for a better society.

In Fromm's 1955 book titled *The Sane Society* he criticises the direction the Western world has taken. Accepting the Western world's insane values and means of achieving these values is, for Fromm, madness. The powerful in society foster this madness for their own ends and pacify the general population, helped by psychiatrists, by generating what he refers to as 'pathological conformity'. The non-powerful population of the West for Fromm have become automatons, submitting to, and mostly unaware of, the craziness of their way of life (except seemingly for Fromm). This way of life, argues from, is dehumanising. Humans in Western society have, for Fromm, become alienated from their authentic 'self'. It is postulates from the capitalist mode of economic production that have created a culture in which individuals have lost their humanness.

Fromm takes his notions of the psychology of normal and pathological human processes from Sigmund Freud, the founder of an innovative understanding of the workings of the mind. He takes his ideas about normal and pathological societal processes from Karl Marx, the founder of an innovative understanding of the workings of society. Marx's intellectual contribution to sociology is his perception of capitalism (and all previous economic systems) as having inherent contradictions. Alongside, the splitting of society into two opposing classes with marked differences in wealth and therefore power, the most pronounced feature of capitalism for Marx was its need to find more markets for which more goods had to be generated to keep the economics of the system working. The contradiction for Marx in this system was that no matter how sophisticated and opportunistic its propagators, eventually it would fail. Capitalism, in its endeavour to survive, has gone global, has become immersed in the infinitesimal, and extra-terrestrial. It has also, to assist its survival, spawned conflicts to protect markets, and intense individualism, egocentricity, and narcissism to spawn commodification and consumerism.

However, Fromm also took from one strand of Marxism the idea that other economic systems than capitalism can also produce social insanity. This other strand was the Frankfurt School of Critical Theory (Best et al., 2018). Critical theorists are vehement in their disapproval of capitalism, including its 'neoliberal' variant (Lessenich et al., 2015). But they likewise condemn the kind of socialist society which is dominated by the State or presided over by oligarchies or despots. All forms of fascism are condemned. What critical theorists are proposing is an economic system with political overseeing which is not totalitarian or libertarian, neither wholly by the cravings of the State or the individual.

Sociologist Bruce Cohen (2016) critique of psychiatry is informed by Marxism and its offshoot critical theory. He accuses psychiatry of 'victim blaming'. Psychiatry for Cohen supports capitalism by using what he claims to be pseudoscientific evidence to assist in legitimising madness based on personal defects rather than because of defectiveness in the disposition of society. In the process, Cohen suggests, real suffering, labelled erroneously as mental disorder, may well be increasing due to neoliberal excesses. Epidemics of mental disorder therefore are epidemics of a disordered society.

The suggestion that society is 'disordered' is paradoxical. The 'disorder' can be used in the strict meaning of that term to indicate the obvious societal, environmental, and interpersonal mess created by, for example, external and civil wars, proven political corruption, and climate change. 'Disorder' can be used in the sense implied by Fromm and Cohen, the debasement of humanity created by specific social systems such as capitalism and totalitarianism. But these systems are also 'ordered' in the sense that strict rules apply examples of which are the regulations of market economics and the regulating of the population by despotic regimes.

Fromm blames the cultural craziness of capitalism and totalitarian communism and fascism for much of the diagnoses of mental disorder. Fromm, however, accepts that mental disorder will be diagnosed in some people even if society becomes sane. The World Health Organisation (2017) claims one-in-four people will be diagnosed with a 'mental health problem' at some point in their lives. But this means that most people will not be diagnosed with such conditions no matter that globalisation has, using Fromm's approach, spread the 'insanity'.

Including and updating Fromm's examples of societal insanities are: a preponderance of banal and sadistic entertainment (Mosley, 2000: Morrall et al,. 2018); gratuitous avarice (Lyons, 2017); the rise of religious fundamentalism and intolerance (Herriot, 2008); the spread of political popularism and fascism (Kaltwasser, et al., 2017; Mazower, 2018); global financial crises, and economic and employment upturns and downturns (Hossain et al., 2011); the political upheavals in the middle-east and northern Africa (Szmolka, 2017); the fragmentation and failure of States (Chomsky, 2007; Fund For Peace, 2018); mass unmanaged migration into cities and across continents (Greenhill, 2011); fatalities and injuries from armed conflicts and terrorism (Gates, et al., 2014; Institute for Economics and Peace, 2017); the subjugation of women (Mill, 1869; Arscott, 2018; the political turmoil following the vote by the British in 2016 to leave the European Union (Dunt, 2016; Sweeney, 2019; the peculiarity of the eighteen-month long US Presidential race culminating in the election of billionaire and TV celebrity Donald J Trump and his subsequent time in office (Wolff, 2018); the intensified melting of Arctic/Antarctic ice-sheets associated with global warming caused by human activity (National Aeronautics and Space Administration, 2018); and the spread of what is or is construed as 'fake news', 'alternative facts', 'mis-speaking', and 'post-truth' (O'Connor and Weatherall, 2018; Davis, 2017; Baggini, 2017; McIntyre, 2018; Keane, 2018).

The United Nations (2018) and the World Health Organisation (2018b) collectively list hundreds of global problems. For example, approximately 830 women during pregnancy and childbirth die each day from preventable causes. Nearly half-a-million people die each year from Malaria. Global warming is the coming decades is predicted to cause 250,000 deaths from infectious diseases, malnutrition, and hyperthermia but disruption for disrupted food production and distribution and rising sea levels may lead to mobility and mortality catastrophe. Nearly 250 million children are affected by armed conflict many of whom experience separation from families. Annually approximately one billion children suffer from physical or sexual violence, and nearly 300 children die each day from violence. These significant and enduring societal dislocations and predicaments are occurring at the same time as there is a sizeable rise in the diagnosis of depression and anxiety as well as other serious mental illnesses/disorders.

According to a poll with a sample of populations from 140 countries conducted in 2018 by the global analytics and policy advice firm Gallop (2019), people there is increasing negativity around the world. The angriest populations were Armenians followed by Iraqis, Iranians, Palestinians and Moroccans, and the most anxious were Greeks. African countries had the highest levels of negative responses with Chad the worst followed by Niger, and Sierra Leone. The Gallop report links the negativity of Chadians to the exacerbation of violence and concomitant collapse of basic services in the country. The next most negative were Iraq, Iran, Benin, and Liberia. There is a general pattern globally, the report comments, of high levels of armed conflict concurring with negative emotions.

But, have all societies not been insane? Robert Edgerton in his book title Sick Societies contends that all societies are sick although some are sicker than others. Some of the sickest societies are not those with modern or even post-modern culture but pre-industrial and pre-colonial cultures. For Edgerton, in terms of violence, torture, human sacrifice, exploitation, witchcraft, greed, unstable mores, abusing and murdering children, misogyny, genital mutilation, physical ill-health, cannibalism, blood feuds, and unhappiness, the latter were more 'primitive' than the former.

Fromm in his thesis does not address a set of highly relevant questions. These are: in an insane society who is mad and who is normal? Is everybody in an insane society mad? Is everybody in an insane society 'normal' (except for a percentage who in any society are categorised as mad)? Does the insanity of society exacerbate considerably the diagnosis of mental disorder and the rest of the population escape the effects of the madness? How can biology be seated in the societal insanity thesis? Attempts will be made in this book to answer these questions.

Fromm therefore has his own faults. That admitted, his contribution to identifying insanities in today's (global), and his propositions for a saner society, have merit as highlighted in the ensuing chapters.

Summary

Biology is the present-day prescription permeating psychiatry for defining and dealing with madness. However, Stephen Rose (Steven Rose and McGuffin, 2005) to the conclusion that the answer to mental disorder may not lie with science, including that of biology. What Stephen Rose is intonating is that waiting for biological science to emancipate the mysteries of madness could be as fruitless as was for the two characters in Samuel Beckett's tragicomedy 'waiting for Godot'. The difference is that Beckett was a fictional allusion to the wretchedness of the human condition whereas madness, no matter how it is construed, is experienced by many as misery. The fabric of society needs to be studied not (just) the minutiae of the brain's workings. Structural reform of society is necessary not structural reform of the brain. (Hilary Rose and Steven Rose, 2016).

Specious societal situations are linkable to psychological distress. There is evidence of specific circumstances leading to a diagnosis of specific mental disorders such as anxiety and depression. In recognition of that evidence, in England medical practitioners and nurses along with hundreds of 'link workers' specially employed for the purpose, have been tasked by the government to prescribe non-biological 'social' treatments aimed at alleviating psychological distress (National Health Service England, 2019).

The next five chapters of this book, however, will assess the connection between personal madness and sizeable societal insanities. There is, however, need to be mindful that at least in part the huge rise in the diagnosis of mental disorders may indicate a huge rise in psycho-medicalisation and increased psychiatric imperialism rather than society being particularly insane. The first of the substantial insanities of society to be inspected for its union with personal madness is violence.

Notes

1 As discussed in the Introduction to the book, there is a lack of consistency in the literature and thinking about the meaning and appropriateness of the terms 'madness' and 'mental disorder'. That inconsistency occurs in this book but there is an

effort to apply the former term to denote social scientific and the latter term those of medical/psychiatric formulations.

2 Foucault wrongly identified the previous centuries as the era of mass incarceration of the mad (Scull, 2007; 2011).

3 For example: International Hearing Voices Network (2018) Intervoice and the Hearing Voices Movement www.intervoiceonline.org/about-intervoice [accessed 31 October, 2018]; Hearing Voices Network (2018) Hearing Voices Network: About Us www.hearing-voices.org/about-us/ [accessed 31 October, 2018]; Mindfreedom (2018) Mindfreedom: Who We Are. www.mindfreedom.org/who-we-are [accessed 31 October, 2018]; National [UK] Survivor User Network (2018) National [UK] Survivor User Network: History. www.nsun.org.uk/history [accessed 31 October 2018].

4 The notion of 'developing' and 'developed' (and 'non-developing' or 'undeveloped') refer to a country's trajectory towards or attainment of a high standard or productivity as measured by such economic factors as country's gross domestic product, and average income level. Also, what may be included are cultural properties such as the standard of health and education services. However, governments and international agencies do not provide a definitive designation for these terms, and there is confusion and conflation over these terms and alternative descriptions of economic positioning and cultural properties such as 'emerging' and 'emerged' (Kynge and Wheatley, 2015).

References

Abed R and St John-Smith P (2016) Evolutionary psychiatry: A new college special interest group. *British Journal of Psychiatry Bulletin*, 40(5), pp. 233–236.

Akbarian S (2014) Epigenetic mechanisms in schizophrenia. *Dialogues in Clinical Neuroscience*, 16(3), pp. 405–417.

Alcock J (2003) *The Triumph of Sociobiology*, 2nd edn. New York: Oxford University Press.

Allen F (2014) *Saving Normal: An Insider's Revolt against Out-of-Control Psychiatric Diagnosis, DSM-5, Big Pharma, and the Medicalization of Ordinary Life*. New York: William Morrow.

Alzheimer's Society (2019) Social care training. www.alzheimers.org.uk/dementia-professionals/training-consultancy/training-organisations/social-care-training [accessed 7 January, 2020].

American Neuropsychiatric Association (2016) About American Neuropsychiatric Association. www.anpaonline.org/About-Us [accessed 30 January, 2019].

American Psychiatric Association (2013) *Diagnostic and Statistical Manual of Mental Disorders, Fifth Edition (DSM-5)*. Arlington, VA: American Psychiatric Association.

American Psychiatric Association (2018) Americans say they are more anxious than a year ago; baby boomers report greatest increase in anxiety. American Psychiatric Association. www.psychiatry.org/newsroom/news-releases/americans-say-they-are-more-anxious-than-a-year-ago-baby-boomers-report-greatest-increase-in-anxiety.

Andrews P and Thomson A (2009) The bright side of being blue: Depression as an adaptation for analyzing complex problems. *Psychological Review*, 116(3), pp. 620–654.

Appignanesi L (2011) The mental illness industry is medicalising normality. *The Guardian*, 6 September.

Arciniegas D, Yudofsky S and Hales R (2018) *Textbook of Neuropsychiatry and Clinical Neurosciences*, 6th edn. Washington, DC: American Psychiatric Association.

Arscott J (2018) Eight ways you can help women's rights. *The Conversation*, 6 March http://theconversation.com/eight-ways-you-can-help-womens-rights-88113 [accessed 4 February, 2019].

Arzy S and Danziger S (2014) The science of neuropsychiatry: Past, present, and future shahar. *Journal of Neuropsychiatry and Clinical Neurosciences*, 26(4), pp. 392–395.

Baggini J (2017) *A Short History of Truth: Consolations for a Post-Truth World.* London: Quercus.

Barrett L (2017) *How Emotions are Made: The Secret Life of the Brain.* London: Macmillan.

BBC News (2018) Prime Minister appoints minister for suicide prevention. 10 October. www.bbc.co.uk/news/health-45804225 [accessed 10 October, 2018].

Bateson G, Jackson D, Haley J and Weakland J (1956) Toward a theory of schizophrenia. *Behavioral Science*, 1(4), 251–264.

Bentall R (2003) *Madness Explained: Psychosis and Human Nature.* London: Allen Lane.

Bentall R (2009a) *Doctoring the Mind: Why Psychiatric Treatments Fail.* London: Penguin.

Bentall R (2009b) Formulating Zeppi. In Sturmey P (ed.) *Clinical Case Formulation: Varieties of Approaches.* Chichester: Wiley, pp. 119–131.

Bentall R (2016) Mental illness is a result of misery, yet still we stigmatise it. *The Guardian*, 26 February.

Bentall R and Pilgrim D (2016) There are no 'schizophrenia genes': Here's why. *The Conversation*, 8 April. https://theconversation.com/there-are-no-schizophrenia-genes-heres-why-57294 [accessed 24 May 2018].

Best B, Bonefeld W and O'Kane C (eds) (2018) *The Sage Handbook of Frankfurt School Critical Theory.* London: Sage.

Bhugra D et al. [40 co-authors]. (2017) The World Psychiatric Association-Lancet Psychiatry Commission on the future of psychiatry. *The Lancet*, 4(10), pp. 775–818.

Bickerdike L, Booth A, Wilson P.Farley K and Wright K (2017) Social prescribing: Less rhetoric and more reality. A systematic review of the evidence. *British Medical Journal*, 7(4). https://bmjopen.bmj.com/content/7/4/e013384 [accessed 19 May, 2019].

Birmingham University (2019) Brain wiring differences identified in children with conduct disorder. www.birmingham.ac.uk/news/latest/2019/04/brain-wiring-differences-in-children-with-conduct-disorder.aspx [accessed 20 May, 2019].

Blackmore S (2000) *The Meme Machine.* Oxford: Oxford University Press.

Blackmore S (2017) *Consciousness: A Very Short Introduction.* Oxford: Oxford University Press.

Bocock R, 1978, *Freud and Modern Society: The Making of Sociology*, Nelson.

Boseley S (2018) The drugs do work: Antidepressants are effective, study shows. *The Guardian*, 21 February.

Boseley S, Collyns D, Lamb K and Dhillon A (2018) How children around the world are exposed to cigarette advertising. *The Guardian*, 9 March.

Boyer P and Peterson M (2012) The naturalness of (many) social institutions: Evolved cognition as their foundation. *Journal of Institutional Economic*, 8(1), pp. 1–25.

Brown G W (1959) Experiences of discharged chronic schizophrenic patients in various types of living group. *Milbank Memorial Fund Quarterly*, 37(2), pp. 105–131.

Brune M (2008) *Textbook of Evolutionary Psychiatry.* Oxford: Oxford University Press.

Buller D (2012) Four fallacies of pop evolutionary psychology. *Scientific American, Special Editions*, 22(1s), pp. 44–51.

Bullmore E (2018a) This revolution in our understanding of depression will be life-transforming. *The Observer*, 29 April.

Bullmore E (2018b) *The Inflamed Mind: A Radical New Approach to Depression.* London: Short Books.

Buss D (2017) *Evolutionary Psychology: The New Science of the Mind*, 5th edn. Abingdon: Routledge.

Buss D, Kruger D and Kurzban R (2009) Evolutionary theory and psychology. Psychological science agenda [Science Briefs]. *American Psychological Association.* www.apa.org/science/about/psa/2009/05/scibrief.aspx#Povinelli,%20Penn,%20and%20Holyoak [accessed 22 January, 2019].

Cacioppo J and Berntson G (1992) Social psychological contributions to the decade of the brain: Doctrine of multilevel analysis. *American Psychologist*, 47(8), pp. 1019–1028.

Cacioppo J and Decety J (2011) Challenges and opportunities in social neuroscience. *Ann N Y Acad Sci*, 1224(1), pp. 162–173.

Cacioppo J and Patrick W (2009) *Loneliness: Human Nature and the Need for Social Connection.* London: W W Norton & Company.

Cadwalladr S (2013) Susannah Cahalan: 'What I remember most vividly are the fear and anger'. *The Guardian*, 13 January.

Cahalan S (2012) *Brain on Fire: My Month of Madness.* London: Penguin.

Cairney P and Oliver K (2017) Evidence-based policymaking is not like evidence-based medicine, so how far should you go to bridge the divide between evidence and policy? *Health Research Policy and Systems*, 15(35). https://health-policy-systems. biomedcentral.com/articles/10.1186/s12961-017-0192-x [accessed 21 January, 2019].

Campaign for Tobacco-Free Kids (2019) Tobacco and kids: Marketing. www.tobacco freekids.org/fact-sheets/tobaccos-toll-health-harms-and-cost/tobacco-and-kids-marketing [accessed 7 January, 2020].

Carey N (2012) *The Epigenetics Revolution: How Modern Biology is Rewriting our Understanding of Genetics, Disease and Inheritance.* London: Icon.

Chater N (2018) *The Mind Is Flat.* London: Allen Lane.

Chomsky N (2007) *Failed States: The Abuse of Power and the Assault on Democracy.* London: Penguin.

Cipriani A, Furukawa, T, Salanti G, Chaimani A, Atkinson L, Ogawa Y, Leucht L, Ruhe H, Turner E, Higgins J, Egger M, Takeshima N, Hayasaka Y, Imai H, Shinohara K, Tajika A, Ioannidis J, Geddes J (2018) Comparative efficacy and acceptability of 21 antidepressant drugs for the acute treatment of adults with major depressive disorder: a systematic review and network meta-analysis. *The Lancet*, 391(10128), pp. 1357–1366.

Clapp M, Aurora N, Herrera L, Bhatia M, Wilen E and Sarah Wakefield (2017) Gut microbiota's effect on mental health: The gut-brain axis. *Clinical Practice*, 7(4), p. 987. www.ncbi.nlm.nih.gov/pmc/articles/PMC5641835/ [accessed 29 November, 2018].

Cohen B (2016) *Psychiatric Hegemony: A Marxist Theory of Mental Illness.* London: Palgrave McMillan.

Comfort N (2018) Genetic determinism rides again: Nathaniel Comfort questions a psychologist's troubling claims about genes and behaviour. *Nature*, 561, pp. 461–463.

Connor S (2015) Many people have genes missing but are still fit and healthy. *The Guardian*, 1 October.

Council for Evidence-based Psychiatry (2018) Do antidepressants work? The new research proves nothing new. http://cepuk.org/2018/02/22/antidepressants-work-ne w-research-proves-nothing-new/ [accessed 24 February, 2018].

Cozolino L (2010) *The Neuroscience of Psychotherapy: Healing the Social Brain*, 2nd edn. London: W W Norton & Company.

Dalton V, Kolshush E and McLoughlin D (2014) Review: Epigenetics and depression: return of the repressed. *Journal of Affective Disorders*, 155(1), pp. 1–12.

Davis E (2017) *Post-Truth: Why We Have Reached Peak Bullshit and What We Can Do About It*. London: Little Brown.

Dawkins R (1976) *The Selfish Gene*. Oxford: Oxford University Press.

Dawkins R (2018) *Science in the Soul: Selected Writings of a Passionate Rationalist*. London: Black Swan.

Dempsey-Jones H (2018) Neuroscientists put the dubious theory of 'phrenology' through rigorous testing for the first time. *The Conversation*, 22 January.

Dennett D (2017) *From Bacteria to Bach and Back: The Evolution of Minds*. London: W W Norton & Company.

Department of Health [UK]. (2006) *Our Health, Our Care, Our Say: A New Direction for Community Services*. London: Department of Health [UK].

de Ridder J, Peels R and van Woudenberg R (eds) (2018) *Scientism: Prospects and Problems*. Oxford: Oxford University Press.

Dorling D (2015) *Inequality and the 1%*. London: Verso.

Doudna J and Charpentier E (2014) The new frontier of genome engineering with CRISPR-Cas9. *Science*, 346(6213), 28 November. http://science.sciencemag.org/ content/346/6213/1258096 [accessed 29 June 2018].

Doudna J and Sternberg S (2017) *A Crack in Creation: The New Power to Control Evolution*. London: Bodley Head.

Dunt I (2016) *Brexit: What the Hell Happens Now?* Tonbridge: Canbury.

Dupre J (2014) *Processes of Life: Essays in the Philosophy of Biology*. New York: Oxford University Press.

Eagleman D (2015) *The Brain: The Story of You*. Edinburgh: Canongate.

Edgerton R (1992) *Sick Societies: Challenging the Myth of Primitive Harmony*. New York: Free Press.

Eisenberg L and Kleinman A (eds) (1980) *The Relevance of Social Science for Medicine*. New York: Springer.

Ewbank M, Passamonti L, Hagan C, Goodyer I, Calder A and Fairchild G (2018) Psychopathic traits influence amygdala–anterior cingulate cortex connectivity during facial emotion processing. *Social Cognitive and Affective Neuroscience*, 13(5), pp. 525–534.

Fallon J (2014) *The Psychopath Inside: A Neuroscientist's Personal Journey into the Dark Side of the Brain*. London: Current.

Feyerabend P (1970) Against method: Outline of an anarchistic theory of knowledge. Minnesota Center for Philosophy of Science (University of Minnesota). http://mcps. umn.edu/assets/pdf/4.2.1_Feyerabend.pdf [accessed 15 January, 2019].

Feyerabend P (2011) *The Tyranny of Science*. Cambridge University Press: Polity.

Fitz N (2015) Economic inequality: It's far worse than you think. *Scientific American*, 31 March. www.scientificamerican.com/article/economic-inequality-it-s-far-worse-tha n-you-think/ [accessed 27 September, 2018].

Fitzgerald M (2015) Do psychiatry and neurology need a close partnership or a merger? *British Journal of Psychiatry*, 39(3), pp. 105–107.

Fond G, Macgregor A and Miot S (2013) Nanopsychiatry, the potential role of nanotechnologies in the future of psychiatry: A systematic review. *Eur Neuropsychopharmacol*, 23(9), pp. 1067–1071.

Foucault M (1961) *Folie et Déraison: Histoire de la folie à l'âge classique* [Madness and Civilization]. Paris: Librarie Plon.

Foucault M (1963) *Naissance de la Clinique* [Birth of the Clinic]. Paris: Universitaires de France.

Foucault M (1966) *Les mots et les choses: Une archéologie des science* [The Order of Things: An Archaeology of the Human Sciences]. Paris: Gillimard.

Foucault M (2006) *Psychiatric Power: Lectures at the Collège de France*. Basingstoke: Palgrave MacMillan.

Francis C (2012) *Epigenetics: How Environment Shapes Our Genes*. London: W W Norton & Company.

Fudge J, Powers J, Haber S and Caine E (1998) Considering the role of the amygdala in psychotic illness: A clinicopathological correlation. *Journal of Neuropsychiatry Clinical Neuroscience*, 10(4), pp. 383–394.

Fund for Peace (2018) *Fragile States Index 2018 – Annual Report*. Fund for Peace. http://fundforpeace.org/fsi/2018/04/24/fragile-states-index-2018-annual-report/ [accessed 4 February, 2019].

Gallagher J (2019) Cheap common drugs may help mental illness. *BBC*. www.bbc.co.uk/news/health-46809517 [accessed 9 January, 2019].

Gallop (2019) *Gallup 2019 Global Emotions Report*. www.gallup.com/analytics/248906/gallup-global-emotions-report-2019.aspx [accessed 21 May, 2019].

Gandal M, Haney J, Parikshak N, Leppa V, Ramaswami G, Hartl C, Schork AJ, Appadurai V, Buil A, Werge T, Liu C, White K, Horvath S and Geschwind D, CommonMind Consortium, PsychENCODE Consortium, iPSYCH-BROAD Working Group (2018), Shared Molecular Neuropathology Across Major Psychiatric Disorders Parallels Polygenic Overlap. *Science*, 359(6376), pp. 693–697.

Gargiulo P and Mesones-Arroyo H (eds) (2018) *Psychiatry and Neuroscience Update – Vol. II: A Translational Approach*. New York: Springer.

Gates B (2017) Bill Gates's 7 predictions for our future. World Economic Forum, 8 May. www.weforum.org/agenda/2017/05/bill-gates-is-pretty-good-at-predicting-the-future-this-is-what-he-thinks-will-happen-next1 [accessed 9 July, 2018].

Gates S, Nygård H, Strand H and Urdal H (2014) *Trends in Armed Conflict, 1946–2014*. Peace Research Institute Oslo. www.prio.org/utility/DownloadFile.ashx?id=8&type=publicationfile [accessed 4 February, 2019].

Geher G (2015) What is evolutionary psychology? 5 foundational concepts for understanding evolutionary psychology. *Psychology Today*, 18 August. www.psychologytoday.com/us/blog/darwins-subterranean-world/201508/what-is-evolutionary-psychology [accessed 22 January, 2019].

Genomics England (2018) The UK has sequenced 100,000 whole genomes in the NHS. www.genomicsengland.co.uk/the-uk-has-sequenced-100000-whole-genomes-in-the-nhs/ [accessed 8 December, 2018].

Gibson M and Lawson D (2015) Applying evol anthropol. *Evol Anthropol*, 24(1), pp. 3–14.

Goffman E (1961) *Asylums: Essays on the Social Situation of Mental Patients and Other Inmates*. New York: Anchor.

Goldacre B (2009) *Bad Science*. London: Harper Perennial.

Goldacre B (2012) *Bad Pharma: How Drug Companies Mislead Doctors and Harm Patients.* London: Fourth Estate.

Goldacre B (2015) *I Think You'll Find It's a Bit More Complicated Than That.* London: Allen Lane.

Gøtzsche P (2015) *Deadly Psychiatry and Organised Denial.* Copenhagen, Denmark: People's Press.

Gøtzsche P (2018) Cipriani review does not add anything. Council for Evidence-based Psychiatry. http://cepuk.org/2018/02/22/peter-gotzsche-cipriani-review-not-add-anything/. [accessed 24 February, 2018].

Gould S J (1997) Darwinian fundamentalism. *New York Review of Books*, 12 June. www.nybooks.com/articles/archives/1997/jun/12/darwinian-fundamentalism/?page=1. [accessed 12 December, 2018].

Grawe K (2005) *Neuropsychotherapy: How the Neurosciences Inform Effective Psychotherapy.* Abingdon: Routledge.

Greenfield S (2016) *Day in the Life of the Brain: The Neuroscience of Consciousness from Dawn Till Dusk*: London: Allen Lane.

Greenhill K (2011) *Weapons of Mass Migration: Forced Displacement, Coercion, and Foreign Policy.* New York: Cornell University Press.

Haas B and Reuters (2017) China's Shanghai sets population at 25 million to avoid 'big city disease'. *The Guardian*, 26 December.

Hacker P (2015) Philosophy and scientism: What cognitive neuroscience can and cannot explain. In Robinson D and Williams R (eds) *Scientism: The New Orthodoxy.* London: Bloomsbury, pp. 97–116.

Hallowell E (2018) *Because I Come from A Crazy Family: The Making of a Psychiatrist.* London: Bloomsbury.

Harari Y (2015) *Sapiens.* London: Vintage.

Harari Y (2017) *Homo Deus: A Brief History of Tomorrow.* London: Vintage.

Harden K (2018) Heredity is only half the story. www.spectator.co.uk/2018/10/heredity-is-only-half-the-story/ [accessed 10 December, 2018].

Hart D (2017) 'The Illusionist'. *The New Atlantis*, 53, pp. 109–121. www.thenewatlantis.com/publications/the-illusionist [accessed 1 November, 2018].

Hayes J, Lundin A, Wick S, Lewis G, Wong I, Osborn D and Dalman C (2019) Association of hydroxylmethyl glutaryl coenzyme a reductase inhibitors, l-type calcium channel antagonists, and biguanides with rates of psychiatric hospitalization and self-harm in individuals with serious mental illness. *JAMA Psychiatry*, 9 January. https://jamanetwork.com/journals/jamapsychiatry/fullarticle/2719703. [accessed 10th January, 2019].

Heinrich C, Bergami M, Gascón S, Lepier A, Viganò F, Dimou L, Sutor B, Berninger B and Götz M (2014) Sox2-mediated conversion of ng2 glia into induced neurons in the injured adult cerebral cortex. *Stem Cell Reports*, 3(6), pp. 1000–1014.

Helliwell J, Layard R and Sachs J (eds) (2019) *World Happiness Report (2019).* New York: Sustainable Development Solutions Network.

Helman C (2007) *Culture, Health and Illness*, 5th edn. London: Hodder Arnold.

Herriot P (2008) *Religious Fundamentalism: Global, Local and Personal.* Abingdon: Routledge.

Higgins E (2018) *The Neuroscience of Clinical Psychiatry*, 3rd edn. Philadelphia, PA: Lippincott Williams and Wilkins.

Hossain N, Byrne B, Campbell A, Harrison E, McKinley B and Shah P (2011) *The Impact of The Global Economic Downturn on Communities and Poverty in the UK.* York: Joseph Rowntree Trust.

Hunter M, Gillespie B and Yu-Pu Chen S (2019) Urban nature experiences reduce stress in the context of daily life based on salivary biomarkers. *Frontiers Psychology,* 4 April. www.frontiersin.org/articles/10.3389/fpsyg.2019.00722/full [accessed 11 April, 2019].

Insel T (2015) Psychiatry is reinventing itself thanks to advances in biology. *New Sci,* 3035, 19 August. www.newscientist.com/article/mg22730353-000-psychiatry-is-rein venting-itself-thanks-to-advances-in-biology/ [accessed 13 November 2015].

Insel T and Collins F (2003) Psychiatry in the genomics era. *Am J Psychiatry,* 160(4), pp. 616–620.

Institute for Economics and Peace (2017) *Global Terrorism Index 2017.* Sydney, Australia: Institute for Economics and Peace.

Institute for Policy Studies (2018) Inequality and health. https://inequality.org/facts/inequality-and-health/ [accessed 27 September, 2018].

International Neuropsychiatric Association. About the International Neuropsychiatric Association. www.inawebsite.org/about-ina [accessed 30 January, 2019].

James O (2016) *Not in Your Genes: The Real Reasons Children are Like Their Parents.* London: Vermillion.

Jasanoff A (2018) *The Biological Mind: How Brain, Body, and Environment Collabo- rate to Make Us Who We Are.* New York: Basic Books.

Jenkins P (2018) *Minding Our Future.* London: Universities UK Task Group on Stu- dent Mental Health Services, Universities UK.

Johnstone L (2014) *A Straight Talking Introduction to Psychiatric Diagnosis.* Ross-on- Wye: PCCS.

Johnstone L and Boyle M (2018) The power threat meaning framework: an alternative nondiagnostic conceptual system. *Humanistic Psychology,* 5 August. http://journals. sagepub.com/doi/abs/10.1177/0022167818793289?journalCode=jhpa [accessed 30 October, 2018].

Johnstone L and Dallos R (eds) (2013) *Formulation in Psychology and Psychotherapy,* 2nd edn. Abingdon: Routledge.

Jolly C (2016) A life in evol anthropol. *Annu Rev Anthropol,* 45, pp.1–15. www.annua lreviews.org/doi/10.1146/annurev-anthro-102215-095835 [accessed 16 January, 2019].

Jones J (1993) *Bad Blood: Tuskegee Syphilis Experiment.* New York: Free Press.

Jones N and Luhrmann T (2016) Providing culturally competent care: Understanding the context of psychosis. *Psychiatric Times,* 33(10), 31 October. www.psychiatrictimes.com/sp ecial-reports/providing-culturally-competent-care-understanding-context-psychosis [acce ssed 28 June 2018].

Kallert T, Mezzich J and Monahan J (eds) (2011) *Coercive Treatment in Psychiatry: Clinical, Legal and Ethical Aspects.* Chichester: Wiley-Blackwell.

Kaltwasser C, Taggart P, Espejo P and Ostiguy P (eds) (2017) *The Oxford Handbook of Populism.* Oxford: Oxford University.

Keane J (2018) Post-truth politics and why the antidote isn't simply 'fact-checking' and truth. *The Conversation,* 23 March. http://theconversation.com/post-truth-politics-and-why- the-antidote-isnt-simply-fact-checking-and-truth-87364 [accessed 27 September, 2018].

King's Fund (2019) What is social prescribing?www.kingsfund.org.uk/publications/ social-prescribing [accessed January 28, 2019].

Kirov G (2017) Electroconvulsive therapy does work – and it can be miraculous. *The Conversation*, 20 April. https://theconversation.com/electroconvulsive-therapy-does-work-and-it-can-be-miraculous-76381.

Kozubek J (2018) *Modern Prometheus: Editing the Human Genome with Crispr-Cas9*. Cambridge: Cambridge University Press.

Krishnamurti J (2017) *Krishnamurti: The Essential Collection. Common Ground*: Champaign, IL: University of Illinois Research Park.

Kuma K (2004) *From Post-Industrial to Post-Modern Society: New Theories of the Contemporary*. Chichester: Wiley-Blackwell.

Kynge J and Jonathan Wheatley (2015) Emerging markets: Redrawing the world map. *Financial Times*, 3 August.

Laing R D (1960) *The Divided Self: An Existential Study in Sanity and Madness*. London: Tavistock.

Lassale C, Batty G, Baghdadli B, Jacka F, Sánchez-Villegas A, Kivimäki M and Akbaraly T (2018) Healthy dietary indices and risk of depressive outcomes: A systematic review and meta-analysis of observational studies. *Nature, Molecular Psychiatry*, 26 September, pp. 1–22. www.nature.com/articles/s41380-018-0237-8 [accessed 26 September, 2018].

Launer J (2016) Epigenetics for Dummies. *Postgraduate Medical Journal (British Medical Journal)*, 92(1085), 183–184.

Lennox B, Palmer-Cooper E, Pollak T, Hainsworth J, Marks J, Jacobson L, Lang B, Fox H, Ferry B, Scoriels L, Crowley H, Jones P, Harrison P and Vincent A (2017) Prevalence and clinical characteristics of serum neuronal cell surface antibodies in first-episode psychosis: A case-control study. *The Lancet (Psychiatry)*, 4(1), pp. 42–48.

Lessenich S, Dörre K and Rosa R (2015) *Sociology, Capitalism, Critique*. London: Verso.

Lewis O and Steinmo S (2012) How institutions evolve: Evolutionary theory and institutional change. *Polity*, 44(3), pp 314–339.

Lewontin R (2001) *It Ain't Necessarily So: The Dream of the Human Genome and Other Illusions*. New York: New York Review of Books.

Lewontin R, Rose S and Kamin L (1984) *Not in Our Genes: Biology, Ideology, and Human Nature*. New York: Pantheon.

Lieberman J (2015) *Shrinks: The Untold Story of Psychiatry*. Weidenfeld & Nicolson.

Liu L and Zhu G (2018) Gut–brain axis and mood disorder. *Frontiers in Psychiatry*, 9, p. 223. www.frontiersin.org/articles/10.3389/fpsyt.2018.00223/full [accessed 29 November, 2018].

Luhrmann T and Marrow J (2016) *Our Most Troubling Madness: Case Studies in Schizophrenia across Cultures (Ethnographic Studies in Subjectivity)*. Oakland, CA: University of California.

Luxton D (ed.) (2015) *Artificial Intelligence in Behavioral and Mental Health*. Cambridge, Massachusetts: Elsevier Academic.

Lyons S (2018) Wall Street at 30: Is greed still good? *The Conversation*, 8 December. http://theconversation.com/wall-street-at-30-is-greed-still-good-87612 [accessed 4 February, 2019].

Major Depressive Disorder Working Group of the Psychiatric Genomics Consortium (2018) Genome-wide association analyses identify 44 risk variants and refine the genetic architecture of major depression. *Nature Genetics*, 50(5), pp. 668–681.

Marsh A (2017) *Good for Nothing: From Altruists to Psychopaths and Everyone in Between*. London: Robinson.

Marmot M (2016) *The Health Gap: The Challenge of an Unequal World*. London: Bloomsbury.

Maudsley Biol Res Centre (2018) Clinical disorders and health behaviours cluster. www.maudsleybrc.nihr.ac.uk/research/clinical-disorders-and-health-behaviours/ [accessed 31 January, 2019].

Mazower M (2018) Fascism revisited? A warning about the rise of populism. *Financial Times*, 11 April. www.ft.com/content/6d57a338-3be9-11e8-bcc8-cebcb81f1f90 [accessed 4 February, 2019].

McCarthy-Jones S (2017) The concept of schizophrenia is coming to an end – here's why. *The Conversation*, 24 August. https://theconversation.com/the-concept-of-schizophrenia-is-coming-to-an-end-heres-why-82775 [accessed 25 September, 2018].

McGuffin P and Murray R (eds) (2014) *The New Genetics of Mental Illness*. Oxford: Butterworth-Heinemann.

McIntyre L (2018) *Post-Truth*. Cambridge, MA: MIT.

McCormack J and Korownyk C (2018) Effectiveness of antidepressants. Lots of useful data but many important questions remain. *British Medical Journal*, 9 March. www.bmj.com/content/360/bmj.k1073 [accessed 13 January, 2019].

Megget K (2016) Crispr goes commercial. Royal Society of Chemistry. www.chemistryworld.com/news/crispr-goes-commercial/9359.article [accessed 20 August, 2018].

Mental Health Foundation (2015) *Dementia, Rights, and the Social Model of Disability: A New Direction for Policy and Practice?* London: Mental Health Foundation.

Midgely M (2011) *The Myths We Live By*. Abingdon: Routledge.

Midgely M (2014) *Are You an Illusion?* Abingdon: Routledge.

Mill J S (1869) *The Subjugation of Women*. London: Longmans, Green, Reader, and Dyer.

Mills C (2014) *Decolonizing Global Mental Health: The Psychiatrization of the Majority World*. Abingdon: Routledge.

Monbiot G (2016) Neoliberalism is creating loneliness. That's what's wrenching society apart. *The Guardian*, 12 October.

Moncrieff J (2013) *The Bitterest Pills: The Troubling Story of Antipsychotic Drugs*. London: Palgrave Macmillan.

Moncrieff J (2014) A Critique of genetic research on schizophrenia – expensive castles in the air. *Critical Psychiatry, Mad in America: Science, Psychiatry and Social Justice*, 1 September. www.madinamerica.com/2014/09/critique-genetic-research-schizophrenia-expensive-castles-air/ [accessed 11 July, 2018].

Moncrieff J and Middleton H (2015) Schizophrenia: A critical psychiatry perspective. *Current Opinion Psychiatry*, 28(3), pp. 264–268.

Morrall P (2008) *The Trouble with Therapy: Sociology and Psychotherapy*. Chichester: Open University Press/McGraw-Hill.

Morrall P (2017) *Madness: Ideas about Insanity*. Abingdon-on-Thames: Routledge.

Morrall P, Worton K and Antony D (2018) Why is murder fascinating and why does it matter to mental health professionals? *Mental Health Practice*, 23 April. https://journals.rcni.com/mental-health-practice/evidence-and-practice/why-is-murder-fascinating-and-why-does-it-matter-to-mental-health-professionals-mhp.2018.e1249/abs [accessed 4 February, 2019].

Morrison A, Renton J, Dunn J, Williams S and Bentall R (2003) *Cognitive Therapy for Psychosis: A Formulation-Based Approach*. Abingdon: Routledge.

Mosley I (ed.) (2000) *Dumbing Down: Culture, Politics and the Mass Media*. Exeter: Imprint Academic.

Mostafavi, H, Pickrell J and Przeworski M (2017) Evolutionary geneticists spot natural selection happening now in people. *The Conversation*, 12 September. http://theconversa tion.com/evolutionary-geneticists-spot-natural-selection-happening-now-in-people-83621 [accessed 5 December, 2018].

Mukherjee S (2017) *The Gene: An Intimate History*. London: Vintage.

Müller J (2017) *What is Populism?* London: Penguin.

Najjar S, Steiner J, Najjar A and Bechter K (2018) A clinical approach to new-onset psychosis associated with immune dysregulation: The concept of autoimmune psychosis. *Journal of Neuroinflammation*, 15(50). www.ncbi.nlm.nih.gov/pmc/articles/ PMC5809809/ [accessed 26 July, 2018].

National Aeronautics and Space Administration [NASA]. (2018) Long-term warming trend continued in 2017. NASA and Goddard Institute for Space Studies. www.giss. nasa.gov/research/news/20180118/. [accessed 27 September, 2018].

National Health Service England (2019) Social prescribing. www.england.nhs.uk/persona lisedcare/social-prescribing/ [accessed 28 January, 2019].

NHS Digital (2019) The Prescription Cost Analysis, England 2018. Leeds: NHS Digital.

Nobel Assembly at Karolinska Institute (2018) 2018 Nobel Prize in Physiology or Medicine – Press Release. www.nobelprize.org/uploads/2018/10/press-medicine2018. pdf [accessed 1 October, 2018].

O'Connor C and Weatherall J (2018) *The Misinformation Age: How False Beliefs Spread*. New Haven, CT: Yale University Press.

Office of National Statistics (UK) Suicides in the UK: 2017 Registrations. www.ons. gov.uk/peoplepopulationandcommunity/birthsdeathsandmarriages/deaths/bulletins/ suicidesintheunitedkingdom/2017registrations [accessed 10 October, 2018].

Palumbo P, Mariotti M, Iofrida C and Pellegrini S (2018) Genes and aggressive behavior: Epigenetic mechanisms underlying individual susceptibility to aversive environments. *Frontiers in Behav Neurosci*, 12, 117. www.ncbi.nlm.nih.gov/pmc/a rticles/PMC6008527/ [accessed 6 December, 2018].

Panksepp J and Panksepp JB (2000) The seven sins of evolutionary psychology. *Evolution and Cognition*, 6(2), pp. 108–131.

Parkhurst J (2017) *The Politics of Evidence*. Abingdon: Routledge.

Pies R (2016) The astonishing non-epidemic of mental illness. *Psychiatric Times*, 1 November. www.psychiatrictimes.com/blogs/astonishing-non-epidemic-mental-illness.

Pinker S (2018) *Enlightenment Now: The Case for Science, Reason, Humanism and Progress*. London: Allen Lane.

Plant J and Stephenson J (2009) *Beating Stress, Anxiety and Depression: Groundbreaking Ways to Help You Feel Better*. London: Little, Brown.

Plomin R (2018) *Blueprint: How DNA Makes Us Who We Are*. London: Allen Lane.

Psychiatric Genomics Consortium (2018) What is the PGC? www.med.unc.edu/pgc. [accessed 10 July, 2018].

Quine W (1951) Two dogmas of empiricism. *Philosophical Review*, 60(1), pp. 20–43.

Richerson P and Boyd R (2005) *Not by Genes Alone: How Culture Transformed Human Evolution*. Chicago, IL: University of Chicago Press.

Rieder R, Wisniewski P, Alderman B and Campbell S (2017) Microbes and mental health: A review. *Brain Behavior and Immunity*, 66, pp. 9–17.

Rissmiller D and Rissmiller J (2006) Open forum: Evolution of the antipsychiatry movement into mental health consumerism. *Psychiatric Services*, 57, pp. 863–866.

Rogers J, Gonzalez-Madruga K, Kohls G, Baker R, Clanton R, Pauli R, Birch P, Chowdhury A, Kirchner M, Andersson J, Smaragdi A, Puzzo I, Baumann S, Raschle N, Fehlbaum L, Menks W, Steppan M, Stadler C, Konrad K, Freitag C, Fairchild G and De Brito S (2019) White matter microstructure in youths with conduct disorder: effects of sex and variation in callous traits. *J Am Acad Child Adolesc Psychiatry*, S0890–8567(19), pp. 30251–30255.

Rose H and Rose S (2014) *Genes, Cells and Brains: The Promethean Promises of the New Biology*. London: Verso.

Rose H and Rose S (2016) *Can Neuroscience Change Our Minds?* Cambridge: Polity.

Rose N (1998) Controversies in meme theory. *Journal of Memetics. Evolutionary Models of Information Transmission*, 2. http://cfpm.org/jom-emit/1998/vol2/rose_n. html [accessed 21 April, 2015].

Rose N (2018) *Our Psychiatric Future: The Politics of Mental Health*. Cambridge: Polity.

Rose N and Abi-Rached J (2013) *Neuro: The New Brain Sciences and the Management of the Mind*. Princeton, NJ: Princeton University Press.

Rose N and McGuffin P (2005) Will science explain mental illness? *Prospect Magazine*, October, pp. 28–32.

Rosenhan, D L (1973) On being sane in insane places. *Science*, 179, pp. 250–258.

Royal Australian and New Zealand College of Psychiatrists (2019) Section of Neuropsychiatry. www.ranzcp.org/membership/faculties-sections/neuropsychiatry [accessed 14 January, 2019].

Royal College of Psychiatrists (2019) Faculty of Neuropsychiatry. www.rcpsych.ac. uk/members/your-faculties/neuropsychiatry [accessed 14 January, 2019].

Russo J and Sweeney A (eds) (2016) *Searching for a Rose Garden: Challenging Psychiatry, Fostering Mad Studies*. Ross-on-Wye: PCCS.

Sanjak J, Sidorenko J, Robinson M, Thornton K and Visscher P (2018) Evidence of directional and stabilizing selection in contemporary humans. *Proceedings of the National Academy of Sciences*, 115(1), pp. 151–156.

Scheff T (1966) *Being Mentally Ill: A Sociological Theory*. Chicago: Aldine.

Schildkrout B (2016) How to move beyond the diagnostic and statistical manual of mental disorders/international classification of diseases. *Journal of Nervous and Mental Disease*, 204(10), pp. 723–727.

Schildkrout B (2017) Neuroanatomy and the 21st century psychiatrist. *Psychiatric Times*, 34(3), 21 March. www.psychiatrictimes.com/neuropsychiatry/neuroanatom y-and-21st-century-psychiatrist/page/0/1?GUID=EBC79EE0-EC28-48F7-A99F%2029 CB7FE8DC6E&rememberme=1&ts=11042017 [accessed 28 June, 2018].

Schildkrout B and Frankel M (2016) Neuropsychiatry: Toward solving the mysteries that animate psychiatry. *Psychiatric Times*, 33(12), 15 December. www.psychiatrictimes.com/ neuropsychiatry/neuropsychiatry-toward-solving-mysteries-animate-psychiatry?GUID= EBC79EE0-EC28-48F7-A99F-29CB7FE8DC6E&rememberme=1&ts=29122016 [acce ssed 5 July, 2018].

Schizophrenia Working Group of the Psychiatric Genomics Consortium (2014) Biological insights from 108 schizophrenia-associated genetic loci. *Nature*, 511(7510), pp. 421–427.

Schizophrenia Working Group of the Psychiatric Genomics Consortium (2016) Schizophrenia risk from complex variation of complement component 4, *Nature*, 530 (7589), pp. 177–183.

Schulze T and Adorjan K (2018) From the genomic revolution to friendly data sharing and global partnerships. *Psychiatric Times*, 35(8), pp. 1–4. www.psychiatrictimes.com/genet ic-disorders/psychiatric-genetics-2018-genomic-revolution-friendly-data-sharing-and-glo bal-partnerships [accessed 13 December, 2018].

Schumann C, Bauman M and Amaral D (2011) Abnormal structure or function of the amygdala is a common component of neurodevelopmental disorders. *Neuropsychologia*, 49(4), pp. 745–759.

Scull A (1977) *Decarceration: Community Treatment and the Deviant - A Radical View*. Upper Saddle River, NJ: Prentice Hall.

Scull A (1979) *Museums of Madness: The Social Organisation of Insanity in Nineteenth-Century England*. London: Allen Lane.

Scull A (2005) 'Killing cures': An exchange. www.nybooks.com/articles/2005/11/03/ killing-cures-an-exchange/ [accessed 7 January, 2020].

Scull A (2007a) Scholarship of fools. The frail foundations of Foucault's monument. *The Time Literary Supplement*, March 23, pp. 3–4.

Scull A (2007b) Mind, brain, law and culture – Book reviews by Andrew Scull. *Brain*, 130, pp. 585–591.

Scull A (2011) *Madness: A Very Short Introduction*. Oxford: Oxford University Press.

Shackelford T and Weekes-Shackelford V (eds) (2012) *The Oxford Handbook of Evolutionary Perspectives on Violence, Homicide, and War*. New York: Oxford University Press.

Shorter E (1997) *A History of Psychiatry: From the Era of the Asylum to the Age of Prozac. A History of Psychiatry*. New York: Wiley.

Stier M, Schoene-Seifert B, Rüther M and Muders S (2014) The philosophy of psychiatry and biologism. *Frontiers in Psychology*, 5(1032). www.ncbi.nlm.nih.gov/pm c/articles/PMC4166893/ [accessed 12 December, 2018].

Stevens A and Price J (2000) *Evolutionary Psychiatry: A New Beginning*, 2nd edn. London: Routledge.

Stewart G (2019) Social prescribing. *British Medical Journal*, 28 March, 364(1285). www.bmj.com/content/364/bmj.l1285/rr [accessed May 19, 2019].

Strachey J (2001) *Complete Psychological Works of Sigmund Freud*. London: Vintage.

Sweeney E (2019) No-deal Brexit scenario would create serious traffic congestion and supply chain chaos. *The Conversation*, 8 January. https://theconversation.com/ no-deal-brexit-scenario-would-create-serious-traffic-congestion-and-supply-chain-ch aos-109480 [accessed 4 February, 2019].

Szasz T (1961) *The Myth of Mental Illness: Foundations of a Theory of Personal Conduct*. New York: Hoeber-Harper.

Szasz T (1970) *The Manufacture of Madness: A Comparative Study of the Inquisition and the Mental Health Movement*. New York: Harper and Row.

Szasz T (1977) *Psychiatric Slavery When Confinement and Coercion Masquerade as Cure*. New York: Free Press.

Szasz T (1994) 'Mental illness is still a myth'. *Society*, 31(4), pp. 34–39.

Szasz T (2009) Merger of Psychiatry, Neurology [letter to the editor]. *Psychiatric News of the American Psychiatric Association*. https://psychnews.psychiatryonline.org/doi/ 10.1176/pn.44.5.0025 [accessed 31 October, 2018].

Szasz T (2010) The illegitimacy of the 'psychiatric bible'. *The Freeman*, 60, pp.16–18.

Szasz T (2011) The myth of mental illness: 50 years later. *The Psychiatrist*, 35, pp. 179–182.

Szmolka I (ed.) (2017) *Political Change in the Middle East and North Africa: After the Arab Spring.* Edinburgh: Edinburgh University Press.

Tallis R (2004) *Why the Mind is Not a Computer: A Pocket Lexicon of Neuromythology,* 2nd edn. Exeter: Imprint Academic.

Tallis R (2016) *Aping Mankind:* Abingdon: Routledge.

Taylor S (2012) *Back to Sanity: Healing the Madness of Our Minds.* London: Hay House.

Therrien A (2018) Anti-depressants: Major study finds they work. 22 February. www.bbc.co.uk/news/health-43143889 [accessed 13 January, 2018].

Thorley C (2017) *Not By Degrees Improving Student Mental Health In The UK's Universities.* London: Institute for Public Policy Research.

Tretter F and, Albus M (2008) Pharmacopsychiatry. *Systems Biology and Psychiatry –Modeling Molecular and Cellular Networks of Mental Disorders,* 41(1), S2–S18. www.ncbi.nlm.nih.gov/pubmed/18756416 [accessed 2 November, 2018].

United Nations (2018) Global issues – Overview. www.un.org/en/sections/issues-depth/global-issues-overview/ [accessed 14 August, 2018].

University College London Hospitals (2019) Professor Eileen Joyce. www.uclh.nhs.uk/OurServices/Consultants/Pages/ProfEileenJoyce.aspx [accessed 14 January, 2019].

Verhaegue P (2014) *What About Me: The Struggle for Identity in a Market-based Society.* Melbourne, Australia: Scribe.

Wessely S (2016) A fuller picture of modern psychiatry. *The Guardian,* 26 February.

Wessely S and James O (2013) Do we need to change the way we are thinking about mental illness? *The Observer,* 12 May.

Whitaker R (2005) *Anatomy of an Epidemic: Magic Bullets, Psychiatric Drugs, and the Astonishing Rise of Mental Illness in America.* New York: Broadway.

Whitaker R (2010) *Mad in America: Bad Science, Bad Medicine, and the Enduring Mistreatment of the Mentally Ill,* revised edn. New York: Basic Books.

Whitaker R and Cosgrave L (2015) *Psychiatry Under the Influence: Institutional Corruption, Social Injury, and Prescriptions for Reform.* London: Palgrave MacMillan.

Wiggershaus R (2010) *The Frankfurt School: Its History, Theory and Political Significance.* Cambridge: Polity.

Wilkinson R and Pickett K (2010) *The Sprit Level: Why More Equal Societies Almost Always Do Better.* London: Penguin.

Wilkinson R and Pickett K (2017) Inequality and mental illness. *The Lancet,* 4(7), 25 May, pp. 512–513.

Williams R and Robinson D (eds) (2014) *Scientism: The New Orthodoxy.* London: Bloomsbury.

Wilmott P and Young M (1957) *Family and Kinship in East London.* Harmondsworth: Penguin.

Wilson C (2018) Almost every antidepressant headline you'll read today is wrong. www.newscientist.com/article/2161911-almost-every-antidepressant-headline-youll-read-today-is-wrong/ [accessed 20 May, 2019].

Wilson E O (1975) *Sociobiology: The New Synthesis.* Cambridge, MA: Harvard University Press.

Wolff M (2018) Fire *and Fury: Inside the Trump White House.* London: Abacus.

Wolin R (2006) *The Frankfurt School Revisited.* Abingdon: Routledge.

Woolf S and Aron L (2013) *U.S. Health in International Perspective: Shorter Lives, Poorer Health.* Washington DC: National Academies of Science, Engineering, and Medicine.

Wootton D (2018) Comfort history. *The Times Literary Supplement*, 14 February. www.the-tls.co.uk/articles/public/comfort-history-enlightenment-now/ [accessed 9 July, 2018].

World Federation of Societies of Biological Psychiatry (2019) About the World Federation of Societies of Biological Psychiatry. www.wfsbp.org/about/ [accessed 30 January, 2019].

World Health Organisation (WHO) (2013) *Mental Health Action Plan 2013–2020*. Geneva: World Health Organisation.

World Health Organisation (WHO) (2017) *Depression and other Common Mental Disorders: Global Health Estimates*. Geneva: World Health Organisation.

World Health Organisation (WHO) (2014) *Social Determinants of Mental Health*. Geneva: World Health Organisation and the Calouste Gulbenkian Foundation.

World Health Organisation (WHO) (2017) *Depression and Other Common Mental Disorders: Global Health Estimates*. Geneva: World Health Organisation.

World Health Organisation (WHO) (2018a) *The International Statistical Classification of Diseases and Related Health Problems 11 Revision [ICD-11]. Mental, Behavioural or Neurodevelopmental Disorders*. Geneva: World Health Organisation.

World Health Organisation (WHO) (2018b) *Health Topics*. Geneva: World Health Organisation www.who.int/health-topics/ [accessed 14 August, 2018].

World Health Organisation (WHO) (2018c) *Schizophrenia: Key Facts [Causation]*. Geneva: World Health Organisation. www.who.int/news-room/fact-sheets/detail/schizophrenia [accessed 28 September, 2018].

Žižek S (1989) *The Sublime Object of Ideology*. New York: Verso.

3 Violence

Violence and humanity, seemingly, are inseparable. Human history is replete with violent acts, intentions, and amusements. As sociologist Larry Ray (2018) notes, everyday life is permeated routinely with real and fantasy violence.

There have been, are, and maybe always will be, violent incidents or one sort or another. What changes are the quantities, intensities, the characteristics of the perpetrators, victims, situations, discernments, justifications, and the consequences. The consequences of violence on both humans and their communities varies from that of imperceptibility to that of devastation. All forms of violence entail some sort of psychological (emotional) suffering. Violence is a seemingly intractable problem in society which matters massively in the making and mending of madness.

> Violence has probably always been part of the human experience. Its impact can be seen, in various forms, in all parts of the world ... as a result of self-inflicted, interpersonal or collective violence.
>
> (Krug et al., 2002, p. 3)

The overall extent and concentrations of violence fluctuate wildly from the tens of millions of people killed during the years of the two world wars to the countless number of people tortured, assaulted, and abused every day across the world and throughout human history. Violence, however, remains a major public health problem globally (Alvarez and Bachman, 2016). A British Home Secretary described violent crime as akin to a 'virulent disease' (Javid, 2019).

Nelson Mandela, after serving twenty-seven years in prison having been implicated in the advocation and implementation of violent sabotage. Indeed, he had seen violence as inevitable and excusable in certain circumstances:

> [I]n the end, we had no alternative to armed and violent resistance..... At a certain point, one only fight fire with fire.
>
> (Mandela, 1994, p. 194)

Mandela claiming that violence can be excusable should not detract from his overriding and ensuring peaceful pronouncements and accomplishments. Conversely, Mandela's equivocation about violence (if only so when examined over a lifetime), does signpost that understanding this subject is not straightforward.

Violent deliberations

Deciphering past and present frequencies and patterns is a central deliberation in the study of violence (Hickey, 2003; United Nations Office on Drugs and Crime, 2014; Brookman and Maguire 2017; Ray, 2018). For example, in England and Wales, a study in which data was collected from Accident and Emergency hospital departments for 2018 suggest that levels of violence in England and Wales have fallen since 2002 although there is an increase in knife crime (Sivarajasingam et al., 2019). At that point in time, this result coincided with the government sanctioned Crime Survey of England and Wales, yet police data showed a rise in knife crime, gun crime and homicide, and a recent rate of increase in violence of 19% (Sivarajasingam et al., 2019). Another study published contemporaneously and covering the year 2017–2018, concluded that 69% of 'knife-enabled' homicides in London occurred in just sixty-seven (1.4%) of the city's near 5,000 local areas (Massey, et al., 2019). The Office for National Statistics (ONS), the UK's largest independent producer of official statistics but which works with the government's Statistics Authority, uses data from both the Crime Survey of England and Wales and the police. The ONS (2019a) deduces from police recorded crime that there been a long-term reduction in total violent crime recorded by the police in England and Wales, but that the level has flattened. However, according to ONS, these two sources of data do not concur because the police use recorded crime figures and the Crime Survey information from victims. This leads to different emphases regarding the style and impact of crime. For example, police records give more insight into the lower-volume, but higher-harm violence, compared with the Crime Survey, and the reverse follows (ONS, 2019a). Curiously, given its reliance at least in part on figures from the police, ONS states:

> An increase in the number of crimes recorded by the police does not necessarily mean the level of crime has increased. For many types of crime, police recorded crime statistics do not provide a reliable measure of levels or trends in crime.
>
> (ONS, 2019b)

Data from the police is unreliable, ONS explains tautologically, because it accounts only for crimes recorded by the police. Supplementary explanations offered by ONS for regarding police data as unreliable is more concerning than tautology given the potential for distortion over patterns of crime and the public's attitude to the police. ONS comments that recorded crime can be affected by changes in police activity and recording practices, and by the willingness of victims to report incidents.

The cognitive psychologist Steven Pinker (2011) argues that violence if, measured over millennia, has been in decline. Human society today for Pinker is probably the most peaceful it has ever been. Notwithstanding the recent rise in knife crime the risk of being murdered in London was massively more during the Middle Ages (Gardner 2008). Research by the United Nations Office on Drugs and Crime is, at the time of writing (2019), the most comprehensive study on homicide available (UNODC, 2014). According to that study fatal violence in much of Europe and Oceania, and in some South American countries such as Brazil, as well as Russia, South Africa, the United States, and England and Wales, stabilised or declined when measured over decades prior to 2014. Pinker holds in high esteem the work of sociologist Norbert Elias, describing him as: 'the most important thinker you have never heard of' (Pinker, 2011, p. 59).

Leaving aside Pinker's spurious claim that he is unknown, Elias's thinking about violence is interesting given his personal identity and social situation. Elias, a German Jew who had served in the army during the first world war, relocated first to Paris then London when Hitler came to power (Mennell, 2017). For Elias (1939), humanity has been on a steady trajectory towards a state of civilisation, a major characteristic of which is a marked reduction in violence. Elias argues that, apart from de-civilising blips which he attempted to address in his later writing, society has become pacified due to the growth in the formation and influence of the State, and subsequently the cultural inculcation of self-control. This is a remarkable proposition because of its imperceptiveness. After he published his civilising thesis what ensued was two world wars, multiple genocidal episodes, the butchery associated with Soviet gulags and the Chinese 'cultural revolution', the blitzing of large swathes of South-Asia by USA, and manufacturing of weapons of mass destruction (a version of which were to be use by the USA on the Japanese civilian population, twice). All of these 'blips' occurred during Elias' lifetime. All had been instigated by governments and demonstrate 'self-control' only in the sense of the individual enactors of this violence having enough control over their otherwise 'civilised' performance to terrify, maim, and massacre. It is more remarkable that Pinker commits himself to Elias' thesis.

But, as noted in the research which examined violence in London, vulnerability to victimhood from forms of severe physical violence such as wounding and murder have increased markedly in specific locales. These 'hot spots' exist in parts of South America, the USA, and Africa (UNODC, 2014). Incidents of mass homicides have also taken place in countries reputed to be free from the type of compound killings occurring in North America which receive international media attention. New Zealand's questionable reputation for peacefulness given its colonial history, was shattered in 2019 when a self-proclaimed 'white nationalist' opened fire on worshippers at mosques in Christchurch New Zealand killing 50 people and wounding another 50 using, amongst other firearms, two semi-automatic assault rifles (New Zealand Government, 2019). On 21 April 2019 bombs were used to attack churches and hotels in Sri Lanka. At least

250 were killed and hundreds more injured. This was the worst violence in Sri Lanka, suspected to have been by Islamic terrorists, since the 26-year-long civil war ended in 2009 (BBC News, 2019). Although Pinker highlights peace, it is not much of a mark of peaceability that at least 170 million people were murdered by governments during the twentieth century, and that even by the beginning of the twenty-first century 90 million people continued to be at risk from ethic and politically motivated slaughter (Wilkinson 2005).

The Institute for Economics and Peace (2018) conclusion is that since the end of the 2010s the world has become less peaceful. Furthermore, reductions in homicide rates in many Western countries has been brought about not necessarily by an historical trend towards passivity, but assuredly by improvements in medical knowledge, treatment, and speedy conveyance to specialist trauma facilities. These advances increase chances of surviving otherwise fatal assaults (Gash 2016). There is also sizeable underestimation of violent crime including when life is lost. International homicide statistics only collated periodically. Data are not available for large parts of Africa and some Asian countries. Deaths through warfare, civil strife, terrorism, and clandestine government or paramilitary assassinations not necessarily be registered as homicides or collated at all (UNODC, 2017). Human rights researcher John Sifton (2015) points to the continuation and exacerbation of extreme and lethal brutality occurring in a range of countries where there is armed conflict. He also draws attention to the existence of various levels of violence 'all around us', that is in everyday interactions between citizens and social institutions. The latter is noted by Mandela.

Mandela acknowledges that no part of human society is immune from violence but points to the twentieth century as the most violent in the history of humanity. New technologies for killing on an enormous scale had been invented in that century. The list of those technologies is extensive as has been their reach. It includes widely distributed rapid-fire guns, aerial-bombing, poisonous chemicals, and the atom bomb, and civilians became susceptible if not 'legitimate' targets. The point is also made by Mandela that such patent destruction can detract from the perpetual and pervasive violence occurring in the everyday lives of millions of people throughout the world:

> Less visible, but even more widespread, is the legacy of day-to-day, individual suffering. It is the pain of children who are abused by people who should protect them, women injured or humiliated by violent partners, elderly persons maltreated by their caregivers, youths who are bullied by other youths, and people of all ages who inflict violence on themselves.
>
> (Mandela quoted in Krug et al., 2002, p. 12)

Whilst wars and genocides end eventually, Mandela observes that everyday violence is passed on from one generation and community to another. Perpetration and victimisation find new sponsors and casualties unless there is a transformation in the social conditions in which they were formed originally.

Anthropologist Rahul Oka and his colleagues refute the argument, posited by Pinker, that modern day larger human groupings, are less violent than their forbearers living in small bands and tribes (Oka et al., 2017). Their research reaches the conclusion that people who lived in smaller societies were no more, or less, prone to violence than are those living in today's social settings. Ray (2018) comments that Pinker's thesis of a decline in violence is difficult to sell given the violent incivilities of the twentieth century, and Ray's observation that the civilisation idea is 'controversial' is a remarkable under-statement. Ray does document other criticisms of Pinker's position. These include his significant underestimation of the number of people slaughtered during the twentieth century, his 'confirmation' bias through the selective use of research, and for not grasping the difficulty of comparing medieval vio-lence with modern versions.

The matter of society and violence is also scrutinised by Fromm, and he reflects on the effect of the claimed 'civilisation' of human performance and culture. Fromm embraces Freud's idea about aggression:

> Freud, revising his earlier theory centred around the sexual drive, had already in the 1920s formulated a new theory in which passion to destroy ('death instinct') was considered equal in strength to the passion to love ('life instinct', 'sexuality').
>
> (Fromm, 1973, p. 1)

As did Freud (Bocock, 2002), Fromm also embraces the 'sociological imagi-nation' through which there is a recognition of the power of society to increase and decrease human instincts or to override completely biological partiality.

For Fromm (1964; 1973), there are variations in the background to violent performances in humans. The human psyche, he argues, contains the seeds which can geminate into expressed and enjoyed violence. What Fromm refers to as 'defensive violence', is rooted in fear and a predisposition for survival, and for this reason Fromm suggests that it is probably the most recurrent sort of violence. 'Defensive violence' can be a positive force, employed by an individual as an inherent reaction to real or imaginary threats to protect her/ himself or others (Buechler, 2017), that violence which is employed to protect life, freedom, dignity, property – one's own or that of others. But humans can, and do according to Fromm, employ 'destructive' violence which is not associated with the biological drive for survival, the death instinct, or any societal pressure to destroy or revel in mediated destruction. Although destructiveness may be generated from within the individual, at times in human history, highly malignant violence, argues Fromm, is assuredly pro-voked and sculpted by society.

When an economic system accentuates growth, profit, and the purchasing and the collecting of material possessions which have little if any essential utility, violence becomes, amplified, and admired. Violent actions and entertainments, ranging from the minute to the massive, the insouciant to the incessant, and the sadistic to the salacious, are embedded, promulgated, tolerated, and normalised in such societies. However, equivalent violence is also to found in societies in which the populace is subjugated to dictatorial rule, where the State determines all or most aspects of public and private life. Fromm's idea that both sorts of societies are insane rests for a large part on his assertion that the consequences of their violent cultures is the disempowerment and degradation of its human inhabitants. An extension of this view incorporates the debasement and degradation of animals and environments. However, Fromm implies a cause and effect reflexive relationship between violence and the enfeebling and perversion of human dignity. What Fromm suggests is that excessive indulgence of violence is a reaction to disenfranchisement and dehumanisation found in both over-controlling and commodified social systems. The upshot of a culture inculcated with illiberalism and indignity is increased incidences of mental disorder.

Factors in human social so-called progress which breed destructiveness include: the mechanisation of social and working life; the powerlessness of the individual to temper the clout of wealthy, politically and commercially influential, and the control apparatuses of the State; and the passivity and dispiritedness of the over-controlled and over-consuming citizen; unresolvable psychological dissonance due to the profound contradiction between professed societal values and the actuality of everyday personal experience. Conditions such as these create malignancy in the human psyche which yields quantities and intensities of violence not found, posits Fromm, in early humans

> [P]rehistorical man, living in bands as hunter and gatherer, was characterised by a minimum of destructiveness and an optimum of cooperation and sharing, and that only with the increasing productivity ad division of labor, the formation of large surplus, and the building of states with hierarchies and elites, large-scale destructiveness and cruelty came into existence and grew as civilisation and the role of power grew.
>
> (Fromm, 1973, p. 435)

In direct contradiction to Pinker's 'decline in violence' hypothesis, hunters and gathers were, argues Fromm, the least aggressive of human ancestors. Fromm avows firmly that as civilisation grew so did violence rather than the other way around.

Some causes of violence seem to be discernible because the 'fault' appears to lie purely with the perpetrator whether this is an individual, group, community, or society. Other causes are obscured because, as with most if not all personal and social issues, they are rooted deep in a convoluted mix of predispositions and precipitating biological, psychological, and societal predispositions and precipitations. Genes expressions, biochemical deficits overloads, personality traits, and situational dynamics, are entangled in what is probably an unfathomable contributory *mêlée*, with one aspect or another perhaps dominating but always contingent on its corporeal, dispositional, and cultural connections.

Medical practitioner and epidemiologist Etienne Krug along with collea-gues (Krug et al., 2002) accept that no single factor explains why some indi-viduals behave violently toward others or why violence is more prevalent in some communities than in others. What is offered by Krug is an 'ecological model' to try to bring some semblance of comprehension and thereby solu-tion to violence. The ecological model seeks to identify the personal, relationship, community, and societal factors, which may lead to violence. Regarding society, globalisation is accepted as having enlarged economies, created millions of jobs, and raised living standards, On the other, globalisa-tion has increased inequalities, destroyed social cohesion, provided freer access to alcohol, drug abuse, and firearms, all of which contribute to vio-lence. Krug's appreciation of the effects of globalisation contributes to other perspectives with sociological leanings. Ray (2018) records that Karl Marx, almost as an incidental to his theorising on historical social transformation, refers to violence as a 'cleansing force', and Michel Foucault inevitably links violence to power.

Apart from controversy over causation, the meaning of violence is sur-rounded by a variety of connotations and typologies attributed in different contexts, and by different people and organisations (Ray, 2018). All social and natural phenomena, including the topic of each chapter in this book, are subject to connotational caprice. A choice must be made to convey some sense about the subject in question. Krug divides violence into three cate-gories according to characteristics of the perpetrators (Krug et al., 2002). The first type, 'self-directed violence', refers to violence an individual inflicts upon her/himself. The second type, 'interpersonal violence', covers violence inflicted by another individual or by a small group, on another individual or small group. Violence instigated by larger groups such as states, organised political groups, militia groups, and terrorist organisations, is categorised as 'collective violence'.

The debates about meaning, whether violence is declining or rising, and causation, misses the mark in terms of personal suffering – that is the suffer-ing of the individual concerned and the suffering of society which cannot or will not stop all violence, or at the very least strive to limit its occurrence to a rarity rather than a regularity. Whether it is one or one million children or adult who is murdered, injured, abused, or neglected, whether it is one case or one million cases of physical or psychological abuse, whether it is inter-personal or self-inflicted, civil or external war, whether is configured as execrable or entertainment or it is significant in terms of the harm inflicted on those involved and society.

Violence is always a private trouble as well as a public issue no matter how high or low the levels or intensities. Whether it is 'only' one person battered by one other person, or it is the threat of humanicide from the premeditated exploding of nuclear bombs, incidental ushering of natural disasters because of human 'progress', or unceasing slaughtering *en masse* of other forms to support human life, violence endures. Violence has its upturns and downturns, its intensities, discernments opacities, and indifferencies, but it never disappears. Violence implies physical enactment with physical impacts, from bruises to genocide. However, violence can also comprise psychological instigations and impressions. That violence and humanity are so intertwined is sickening societal insanity. Violence is not only sickening, it is the foremost insanity of society because it is the source of so much suffering. This primary insanity can, however, either be visible or veiled.

Visible violence

Violence which causes death is *ipso facto* the most serious form although it may not cause the most suffering. Prolonged persecution of a victim or victims may induce more psychological angst physical agony than a swift execution unless the former proceeds the latter or the method of killing is messy. For example, severe suffering may occur in cases of prolonged periods in prison prior to the carrying out of a death sentence, and a subsequent botched dispatching of the prisoner (Sarat, 2014). Nonetheless, to-date there is no reversing of human life.[1] Therefore, when appraising violence as a societal insanity the statistics on state of killing are paramount. However, as already mentioned, those statistics are not sound and do not necessarily follow similar levels of increases and decreases to that of overall violence.

Officially there are 1.4 million deaths from all forms of violence globally each year, 90% of which occur in low and middle-income countries (World Health Organisation, 2019). Half a million of these deaths are classified officially as homicides, but the actual figure is considered much higher (UNODC 2014). Poverty and gun-ownership are strongly correlated with murder (Dorling 2005; UNODC 2014).

The ONS (2019b) reports that has been an increase in police recorded homicides in England and Wales of 6% in the year ending December 2018. The number of illegal killings for that year was 732. This is the highest since 2007, although it had reached to over 1,000 in 2003 from approximately 300 per year in the early 1960s. A knife or sharp instrument was used in 285 of these homicides, and this is the highest number since the official recording of methods of killing began in 1946. As in previous years, women were much more likely than men to be killed by partners or ex-partners, and men were more likely than women to be killed by friends or acquaintances. In contrast to the stated position of the police a few months earlier, a 2% decrease to the number of recorded gun crimes (ONS, 2019b). Violent crime, particularly homicide, increased in the USA during 2015 and 2016. Recorded incidents of violent crime in the USA for 2017 are nearly 1.3 million and for murder over 17,000. There was, however, a decrease in violent crime during the first half of 2018 (Federal Bureau of Investigation, 2019). In Australia, the number of homicide victims decreased from 453 victims in 2016 to 414 victims in 2017. The number of sexual assault victims, however, increased for the sixth consecutive year from 23,040 victims in 2016 to 24,957 victims in 2017, a rise of 8% (Australian Bureau of Statistics, 2018).

Although deaths caused by terrorism in many parts of the world are relatively rare, the number of deadly acts of terrorism globally has increased markedly in recent decades (Roser and Nagdy 2017). The number of fatalities from terrorism peaked in 2014, but from 2016 began to drop from nearly 24,000 in 2016 below 17,300 in 2017 (Institute for Economics and Peace, 2018). This was mainly because of reduced incidents in Iraq and Syria. Europe also experienced less fatalities. Afghanistan had more deaths from terrorism than any other country in 2017. In Europe there has been an increase in terrorist incidents, 282 during 2017, and the social, psychological and financial cost of terrorism remains considerable and widespread. The estimated economic impact globally of terrorism in 2017 was US$52 billion. But this figure is regarded as an underestimation (Institute for Economics and Peace, 2018). Estimations of psychological and societal are vague and separating causes from consequences is problematic. Furthermore, there is no single internationally accepted definition of terrorism or universally recognised typology. Collecting valid and reliable data on terrorist acts and aftermaths is much more difficult than those of homicide. Terrorists and governments with their respective agendas may wish to inflate, deflate, ignore, or invent events (Institute for Economics and Peace, 2018).

Violence globally accounts for nearly 1.4 million deaths per year (World Health Organisation, 2019). This corresponds to over 3,800 people killed every day. Violence is a significant public health, human rights, and human development problem. Most deaths due to violence occur in low- and middle-income countries. Countries with higher levels of economic inequality tend to have higher rates of death due to violence. Within countries, the highest death rates occur among people living in the poorest communities. Homicide and suicide are the major causes of death globally among men aged 15–44 years. For every young person killed by violence, an estimated 20–40 receive injuries serious enough for medical treatment to be sought (World Health Organisation, 2019). World Bank (2018) describe violence against women as a global pandemic. Physical harm, including sexual abuse and genital mutilation, affects one-in-three women. 200 million women have experienced female. An average of 137 women across the world are killed by a partner or family member every day. Mass shootings account for a small percentage of homicides. The USA in 2016 only 71 (0.5%) of homicides were the result from mass shootings. There were in that year 23,000 suicides, 50% of which were from guns (Small Arms Survey, 2019[2]).

Armed conflict is responsible for huger numbers of injuries and fatalities involving combatants and those covered by the euphemistic and morally misleading militaristic term 'collateral damage'. Those who take up arms, not always willingly, use them and have them used against them, and are knowingly exposed to harm. However, so can the innocent and unaware. Moreover, the injuring and killing of non-combatants may be an accidental consequence of conflict or a calculated risk acceptable to military leaders to deliberately undermine the morale of the enemy.

Examples of incidental and premeditated slaughtering of civilians include aerial bombing in numerous twentieth century wars, to the targeting' of specific individuals in the twenty-first[t] century by 'precision' missiles (Holland, 2004; Rosen, 2016). But incidental killing of civilians through aerial bombing is a twenty-first century conflict phenomenon. Amnesty International and the conflict research agency Airwars (2019) two-year investigation into civilian deaths in Raqqa, Syria, concludes that 1,600 civilian lives lost as a direct result of thousands of US, UK and French air strikes and tens of thousands of US artillery strikes in the Coalition's military campaign against the terrorist group Islamic State from June to October 2017. Many of the air bombardments were inaccurate and tens of thousands of artillery strikes were indiscriminate.

Terrorist tactics are frequently aiming to frighten and weaken populations whose way-of-life, religion, or politics they are contesting. Therefore, terrorism invoke collateral damage when it is the structure or culture of a community which is their ultimate target rather than those individuals who they maim and slay. Islamic State in Raqqa had over four years perpetrated war crimes and crimes against humanity, used civilians as human shields, mined exit routes, and shot at those trying to flee (Amnesty International, 2018).

Sociologist Zygmunt Bauman (2011) applies includes as collateral damage to the unintended consequences of social inequality. For Bauman, inequality (discussed in detail in Chapter 4) is connectable to higher rates of morbidity and mortality, along with a multitude of social problems. What Bauman is pointing out is that millions if not billions of people become 'collateral damage' in an age of globalised wealth, health, housing, and employment, differentiation, and who become submissive to consumerism, commodification, and 'profit-led' neoliberal ideals. Extending Bauman's argument, climate warming and the ensuing undermining of the environment and threat to human existence is collateral damage from industrialisation and post-industrial globalised society.

The research organisation 'Small Arms Survey' is staffed by an international team producing data on trends in non-fatal and fatal violence through the use of handguns, rifles, sub-machine guns, machine guns, grenade launchers, portable anti-aircraft guns, and missile launchers. According to the Small Arms Survey's data published in 2019, there are approximately 875 million small arms in circulation globally. These have been manufactured by more than 1,000 companies from nearly 100 countries (Small Arms Survey, 2019). Firearms (handguns, rifles, and machine-guns) are responsible for about 60% of world-wide deaths from all violence. In Central America, this figure rises to 77%. More deaths and injuries from armed violence occur in non-conflict and non-war settings.

Non-conflict armed violence includes homicides, suicides, and extrajudicial killings. The number of homicides in countries such as El Salvador, Jamaica, and South Africa, are more each year than deaths from many contemporary wars, and mostly they are carried out using firearms. The number of guns owned by civilians in the USA is estimated at 390 million, although countries such as Switzerland and Finland have more guns *per capita* because they have compulsory military service. New Zealand has one of the world's highest rates of gun ownership in the world, country with a population of fewer than 5 million people owning up to 1.5million firearms (Small Arms Survey, 2019; Lyons, 2019). At the time of writing, the New Zealand Government is intending to ban the type of rapid-fire weapons used in the 2019 Christchurch mass killings (Lyons, 2019).

A think-tank, the Institute for Economics and Peace, uses qualitative and quantitative indicators to produce its 'Global Peace Index'. Three thematic themes are covered in the Index: societal safety and security; domestic and international conflict; the degree of militarisation. In the 2018 version of the Global Peace Index which refers to the year 2017, the average level of global peacefulness has declined for the fourth consecutive year. Deterioration in peacefulness is to be found in 92 countries, with improvement in only 71. Moreover, the gap between the least and most peaceful countries is increasing. The Middle East and North Africa are the least peaceful regions, and the least peaceful countries include Syria, Iraq, Afghanistan, Colombia, South Sudan, Somalia, and Central African Republic, El Salvador, and Lesotho. Europe has also deteriorated in Peacefulness has also deteriorated in Europe because of increased political instability, terrorism, and fear of crime (Institute for Economics & Peace, 2018).

Veiled violence

The total sum of violence and entire amount of suffering caused by violence is incalculable. Instances of covert violence can be estimated and suffering from those occasions can be assessed. However, much of violence is covert, and therefore many if not most violent episodes are mostly unaccounted (Krug et al., 2002). Terrorist atrocities, armed conflict, civilian rioting, and many interpersonal murders, are witnessed by both participants and authorities involved in containment and arraignment. Television and internet news broadcasting supplies prompt and constant visual and narrational details of visible violence frequently accompanied by interviews with primary or secondary victims. Journalists, clinicians and academics also interview perpetrators and publish their findings. Easily accessible video-sharing websites such as YouTube reproduce myriad accounts of murder and mayhem. Much more violence than this openly observed violence occurs out-of-sight, but of course not to the perpetrators or the victims and possibly not wholly to the police, politicians, and at least elements of the public. To categorise any violence as invisible is questionable. Whether violence occurs in domestic situations, in the workplace, or in social institutions such as those ostensibly providing care for the physically disabled, the elderly, people with learning difficulties, or the mad, it is difficult to envisage the absence of knowledge or suspicion by friends, family, colleagues, or professionals. That said, violence in these settings may be obscured to outsiders because perpetrators may wish to frame their deeds having happened through other means than their own malevolence, and victims may wish or be forced to present their injuries as accidental or immaterial – that is if they haven't been killed. Invisible violence is perhaps better understood as ignored than unseen or veiled rather than apparent.

Bullying, for example, has been an ignored or veiled form of violence perhaps for most of human collective existence until being made more discernible and defined in recent times. A large study into bullying in schools conducted by the United Nations Educational, Scientific and Cultural Organisation (UNESCO, 2019) comprised quantitative and qualitative data from 144 countries. This research indicated that a significant minority of students had been psychologically and physically (either of which could be sexual) bullied by their peers at least once in the previous month. Bullying is reported as affecting both male and female students. Male students were victims of physical bullying more than girls, and girls were victims of psychological bullying than boys. Online social media and mobile-phones were increasingly used for psychological bullying. Particularly susceptible victims of bullying were those children who were regarded by their peers as different because of their personalities, appearance, nationality, or ethnicity.

Regarding difference, across the world women and girls of all ages with disabilities are singled out for bullying and other modes of violent discrimination (United Nations Development Program, 2015). Targeted especially are females with learning and psychological difficulties are the main targets of violence. Apart from peers, women and girls with disabilities are vulnerable to bullying by family members and non-family carers. A case study from Albania reveals the position faced by females with disabilities:

> A 25 year old woman with mental disabilities living in the rural area was being subjected to violence by her husband. She went to the social service offices to re-apply for her disability benefit. She had bruises in her face.... For the moment, the woman and her daughter are in a shelter for women victims of violence.
>
> (United Nations Development Program, 2015, p. 40)

Intimate partner violence is a pandemic private trouble and public issue throughout the world (Karakurt and Silver, 2013), lethal and non-lethal. In heterosexual relationships, violence by current or former spouses and lovers affects women more than men. Same-sex intimate partner physical violence is being disclosed more. What is also becoming more apparent is that psychological abuse between partners is pervasive. With the intended or unintentional outcome of controlling and dominating a partner, verbal attacks which humiliate, ridicule, and frighten may be the forerunner to, or combined with, physical abuse (Karakurt and Silver, 2013).

Children are generally especially vulnerable to both physical (including sexual) and psychological veiled violence. The violence children suffer can be designated as 'veiled' in most cases because the young are not as capable as older people of recognising and reporting harm done to them, and if the perpetrators are adults, they are capable of disguising their abuse and, if necessary, misleadingly presenting injuries and even fatalities.

Data from 190 counties examined by the United Nations International Children's Emergency Fund (UNICEF, 2014) indicates that many forms of violence are inflicted on children and that the violent infliction is commonplace. Across the world children are hit, molested sexually, bullied, and emotionally abused. Yet, the report reveals, much of the violence is not acknowledged because it is commonplace and thereby normalised. The physical violence children are subjected to ranges from torture, corporal punishment, and vicious bullying, to what may appear to be negligible bodily contact. Instances of physical violence against children include hitting with a hand, whip, cane, stick, belt, shoe, or kitchen utensil, kicking, shaking, pinching, biting, pulling hair, burning, scalding, and forced ingestion. Sexual violence is defined by UNICEF (2104) as any sexual activity imposed by an adult on a child against which contravenes criminal law. Such illegal sexual activities can include encouraging and forcing children into prostitution, to become 'sexual slaves', or underage marriage, to engage in sexualised talk, touching, and penetration. Technology is increasingly used to lure children into proscribed and exploitative sexual encounters (Internet Watch Foundation, 2018). Mobile phones and social media are utilised by sexual predators as well 'cyberbullies' (both of which may be older children) to locate and target young people (Parents Against Child Exploitation, 2019).

According to the British charity the National Society for the Prevention of Cruelty to Children (2019) psychological violence, particularly if long-term and in multiple forms including brutality and neglect, can have a profoundly undermining influence on mental well-being in later life. The charity supplies an extensive list of examples of psychological violence which includes: regular humiliation, criticism, blaming, scapegoating, and threatening; imposing unreachable standards regarding educational achievement and behaviour; exposure to domestic violence between adults, and to criminal acts such as the taking of illegal drugs; and failing to support social development by, for example, not allowing friendships. What can be added to that list is 'hazing', confining and isolating, abandonment, and neglecting the emotional, educational, and medical, needs together with not ensuring the child's physical safety (UNICEF, 2014). The repercussions for the victims and for society, according to the report have considerable detrimental consequences. This degree of pervasive veiled violence damages children and their communities and is recycled from one generation to the next. Everyday violence may be pervasive, but it is not inevitable (UNICEF, 2014).

Vicarious violence

As declared in the next section of this chapter, violence, whether visible or veiled, is damaging physically, psychologically, and socially. Despite the fear and harm it causes, verbal and non-verbal human performances of violence against other humans and life forms, at times in its most brutal and grotesque kind, attract a pervasive and perverse allure. Criminologist Elie Godsi (2004) notes that the extensive and pervasive fascination with violence covers the most ruthless of real deeds committed by humans on other humans, such as rape, the abuse of children, sadism, and killing, all increasingly displayed graphically. The more 'civilised' society is, the more the fascination with violent entertainment, and the more striking is that rise if the decline in violence proposal is accepted (Ray, 2018). Historian Richard Bessel (2015) remarks that violence is a 'modern obsession'. For Godsi, the consumption of violence has reached 'frenzied proportions'.

Real violence appears repeatedly in 24-hour news broadcasting from multiple media sources, many of which can be revisited at will. A mass of information and countless documentaries about murders, genocide and serial killing, along with the narratives of some killers, can be accessed easily via internet search engines and video websites. Along with the 'true crime' category of factual violence, fictional violence forms the focus of a host of television programmes, films, magazines and books. The well-established genres of 'crime fiction', 'Nordic noir', 'murder mystery' and 'thriller' feature made-up violence centrally in their plots. 'Murder mystery' holidays, weekend-breaks and dinners, where imagined killings are acted out, have become commonplace and are promoted as permissible and pleasurable (Morrall et al., 2018).

Media coverage of actual violent events is to be expected and can serve a positive purpose by exposing heinous acts carried out by individuals and governments, with the possible consequences of penance, punishment, and prevention. But what purpose may be served by a fascination with actual or abstract cruelty and carnage, and it that purpose positive or negative? Is this fascination either an adaptive or maladaptive atavistic legacy, an aberrational or unresolved stage of childhood in the psychoanalytic sense, or is an embedded and universal social norm or a transient social deviance which surfaces in certain cultures such as the present consumer society? That is, is the fascination with violence 'functional' (fascination serves a positive purpose for the individual and/or society) or 'dysfunction' (fascination has a negative effect on the individual and/or society). There are enough ideas and evidence to indicate that violence fascinates (Kottler 2011, Worsley, 2014; Sifton 2015; Bauer-Clapp 2016). But there is scant robust theorising or empirical research for the reasons why. There are, however, some fascinating viewpoints.

British essayist and self-confessed opium addict Thomas De Quincey offered a most imaginative idea. In 1827 De Quincy published an essay titled *Murder Considered as One of the Fine Arts.* De Quincey's proposition in the essay is that murder, and by implication other types of violence, because it is 'appreciated' by the public and connoisseurs of cultural artefacts, should be deemed 'art' (De Quincey, 1925). It then follows, argues De

Quincy that murderers should be respected as 'artists'. Literature, drama and newspapers, points out De Quincey, are drenched in murderous scenes and narratives, and therefore are integral to fictional or factual 'aesthetics' of storylines. For De Quincey each story has the aesthetic ingredients of shape, rhythm, shade, and feeling, designed to portray meaning. He extrapolates that each murder also contains these constituents. As for De Quincy's own artistic murderousness, he confesses that he has only ever killed a cat, his own which he had caught stealing food from his pantry. In the killing of the cat he does call upon Shakespeare, wielding the knife he envisages the death of Brutus. De Quincey was in this essay, ironically, intending to be entertaining rather than earnest.

Pubic voyeurism of violence has a long history (Gatrell, 1996). For example, the gladiatorial battles were staged exhibitions of interpersonal slaughter as well as the slaying of bigger version of De Quincey's quarry. This was for communal pleasure and for the demonstration of the Emperor's command over the life and death of the populace. Huge audiences turned up to watch executions of criminals, those with eschewed political positions, royal heritage at a time of republican fervour, or who were alleged to be wielders of witchcraft, in many European countries until the nineteenth century. In contemporary times Saudi Arabia continues to behead publicly those convicted of murder and a variety of non-lethal transgressions, with dozens killed during in one mass execution (Amnesty International, 2019). The terrorist group 'Islamic State' (*Daesh* in Arabic) has gained unprecedented levels of international attention and vehement disapprobation by placing choreographed executions into the public domain via the internet. These globalised spectacles of violence are intended to install fear in its adversaries but according to political scientist Simone Friis (2018), also to demonstrate Islamic State's capacity to erect an alternative political order. For Bessel (2015), the collectively observed death penalty, serves both as mass entertainment, or as a stark symbol of the power of the state (or would-be state in the case of Daesh) and often both.

English literature scholar Peter Conrad (2002) argues that the fascination with murder can be linked to sexuality. Conrad points to the cinematic work of Alfred Hitchcock, who blended lethal violence with sub-textual eroticism. This linkage, argues Conrad, is what made Hitchcock so successful as a film director and so popular amongst the public. Interesting, much of the violence, as with the sexuality, was implied and nuanced rather than laid bare and crudely exhibited as happens with much of current 'noir' cinematic and television entertainment. In noir films there is an acceptance and exploitation of the bondage between sex and violence. Journalist Simran Hans (2018) writing for the British Film Institute, observes that the bonding of sex and violence is also embodied in the book genre the 'erotic thriller': 'Sex and death are the lifeblood of the erotic thriller.... [T]his narrative mode borrows heavily from film noir' (Hans, 2018).

In these films and books, notes Hans, women are frequently brutalised to engender in the audience 'cheap' and 'vulgar' excitement. Nonetheless, discloses Hans, these 'sexy thrillers' are 'pretty enjoyable'.

An idea of Sigmund Freud (1920) is that aggression and sex are the most fundamental of human drives. The make-up the human psyche and consequential conscious and unconscious performance are an outcome of a negotiation between these drives and the needs of society. Sociologist Denis Duclos (1998) adopts Freud's approach to argue that there is a perpetual struggle within the psyche and society between barbarism and civilisation, and that this tension furnishes what he describes as a 'werewolf culture'. In this werewolf culture, individuals have been socialised to deny and resist their basic drives, and society through the regulatory apparatuses of the State endeavours to modify this inherent source of gratification. However, the drive to enjoy what is 'taboo', as with the nightly deadly pursuits of the werewolf, emerges as the shape of occasional bursts of actual violence but mostly through substitute acceptable socially acceptable pastimes such as the erotic thriller. The entertainment, sport, and travel industries exploit these latent and closet tendencies thereby amplifying and extending the 'night' element of the werewolf culture to the extent that society becomes riddled with symbols of violence.

Criminologist Scott Bonn (2014) argues that the public's fascination with, and the media accounts of, serial killing, is far in excess of the sum of actual murderous events, number of killers, and number of victims. Serial killers, suggests Bonn, have become socially ascribed 'celebrity monsters'. In that role they deliver an addictive emotional 'rush' and a conduit for the fears, anger, and lust, to their audiences. Hence, Bonn is also connecting erotic emotionality to vicious vicarious violence.

Henry Bacon (2015) is a scholar of film and television. He suggests that fictional violence in the media serves the psychological and societal function of making real violence fathomable. This approach implies that vicarious violence as found in films has a biological, psychological, and societal functionality. This stance is similar to the conclusions reached from a study by psychologist Jeffrey Kottler (2011). Kottler interviewed a host of people whose opinions had relevance to violence. These included psychologists, psychiatrists, criminologists, homicide detectives, murderers, victims of violent crime, researchers in the field of media, film directors and producers, and consumers of vicarious violence. What Kottler extracts from those interviews is that the emotional arousal obtained from violent entertainment may have benefits at both the level of the individual and for society. The evolutionary make-up of humans, argues Kottler, incorporates a biological predisposition for arousal when violence is observed or anticipated. This is the survival 'flight/fight' mechanism. Biological predisposition is, for Kottler, overlaid with cultural messages not intended to subdue but entice excitement regarding violence. The fascination with bloody brutality rather than instigating replication in the observer, denoting personal maladaptation or sordidness, and/or epitomising a degraded social system, according to Kottler, a fascination with violence allows humans to 'cleanse' themselves of their inherent viciousness. The positive consequence of this personal cleansing is a 'cleaner' society, that one less polluted by real violence. Kottler's perspective chimes with explanations influenced by Freud (1920) which regard the fascination with violence are sublimation. The fundamental human gratification which would otherwise be achieved through actual violence is gained, in most cases, from enjoying but not participating in the violence of others. To invoke other Freudian concepts, through violent entertainment the 'pleasure principle' is pandering to the 'death wish'. Sublimated and fanaticised killing, in particular, assuages fear of inevitable expiration.

Far from cleansing, Bessel (2015) contends that Western countries' preoccupation with violence is polluting society. Violence, factual and fictional, should not be accepted as an inevitable, and certainly not valuable, aspect of society or humanity. Bessel suggests that the public are not enjoying violence but increasingly find it abhorrent. The public have become more sensitive not sensitised to scenes of real and simulated violence, which has increased political and academic attention aimed at prevention. Bessel argues that the public's abhorrence was intensified by knowledge of the casualties and cruelties as for the second world war. Media technology had advanced appreciable at the time of that war, and was to develop further in subsequent conflicts, thereby enabling war correspondents and makers of documentaries to revel in graphic visual and descriptive detail almost every aspect of the war and associated suffering. As modern media technology has become more and more sophisticated, there has been an exponential growth in explicit imagery and narratives relating not only to conflicts, but murders and terrorist atrocities, rapes, war crimes, and mass graves. But rather than desensitising the public, the reaction to the prevalence of violent imagery and accounts has, in Western societies, become increasingly one of revolution. The sharp rise in living standards and life expectancy experienced throughout the West in the ensuing decades, adds Bessel, means life is more congenial and people are keener to avoid their lives being interrupted or ended by violence. There is an ethical trajectory in social attitudes heading towards not accepting or enjoying violence. That trajectory does, acknowledges Bessel, have intermittent deviations into real and vicarious dissoluteness. He accepts that despite being appalled, there remains substantial public amusement from violence, although much of the pleasure arises from the fictional variety. However, simulated violence for Bessel, is qualitatively different from real events, and it is the latter that prompts emotional discomfort.

Germaine Greer is an academic, writer, and broadcaster. She submits the paradox between male actual violence and female voyeurism. Men are twice as likely as women to be victims of homicide, and female corpses, frequently mutilated, far outnumber those of men, in television crime dramas and literature, and images of murdered women appear and reappear in the news on what Greer suggests is the 'slightest of pretexts'. Yet it is women, Greer points out, who are the majority of consumers in nearly all genres of entertainment in which violence including murder and rape feature as a core part of the plot:

> Strange as it must seem, the endless array of female cadavers laid out on slabs and dragged out of the undergrowth in crime drama on TV is designed to reel in a mainly female audience.... Female victimisation sells. What should disturb us is that it sells to women.
>
> (Greer, 2018)

Journalist Zoe Williams (2018), however, counters the implication of Greer's presentation of this gender paradox regarding violence. Women, argues Williams, are searching for the solving of the puzzle which coincides with descriptions and visualisations of murder and rape rather than craving either. They are also, Williams, continues, attempting to comprehend why they (women) are in the main the victims of violence, grateful that they are not so in these instances, and capable of separating fact from fantasy. Williams also asserts that women may, in this voyeuristic role, have become yet again victims of patriarchy when they are accused of inappropriate pleasure from scenes and reports of violence. Greer tone in questioning gender differences in voyeuristic violence could be interpreted as admonishing women for their prurient inclinations. The proposition by Williams that there is nothing improper about women's prurience could have what presumably is the unintended consequence of legitimising pleasure from surrogate sadistic sexual practices in which the victims by-and-large have not submitted to concomitant pain (and for some death) willingly.

The first series of the BBC 'spy-action thriller' 'Killing Eve' was televised 2018 (BBC iPlayer, 2019). It has received critical and commercial success in both the UK and USA, wining multiple awards including one for its leading actor who plays a psychopathic assassin. Chitra Ramaswamy, journalist for the liberal-left British newspaper *The Guardian*, delivers passionate praise for the programme: 'Picking apart the details of Killing Eve is probably the most fun you can have in 2018.... There's so much to love' (Ramaswamy, 2018).

Ramaswamy says that there is 'so much to love' about this drama, but her 'greatest pleasure' is gained from its anti-patriarchy pro-feminist comedic undertones. In the first episode of the first series the (female) assassin performs a series of explicit and gruesome killings of both men and women. None of the women slain in that first episode were depicted as deserving of their violent death.

Indulgence in violence entangles both men and women as perpetrators, victims, or patrons. An acquired fascination by or pleasure in violence has been termed 'appetitive aggression' (Elbert et al., 2017). Appetite aggression is thought to be acquired due experience or exposure to violence either as a child or adult. Previous experience of or exposure to violence sets the body to react by, for example, a release of biochemicals such as adrenaline, cortisol, and endorphins, when confronted with violent events in the present. The sense of urgency and euphoria that these biochemicals produce furnish not only a fear of, but a lust for, violence, a paradoxical mix of biological and psychological effects in a feedback loop. At the behest of the person's biology, horror is mixed with hunger for violence. This biological-psychological interaction offers one explanation for conducting 'visible' violence and for enjoying violence vicariously. It also can explain the 'cycle of violence' enwrapping and entrapping victims and perpetrators, passing from one generation to the next, and embedding in the cultural make-up of a society.

Today's society is global and so it would seem is an appetite for violence. Society is marked by an appetite for violence and makes-up the menu for violence. That is, the conditions for conducting veritable violence and consuming invented violence is concocted in and by society. Without societal connivance (in the sense of endorsement or tolerance by people in power and entrenchments in powerful institutions), the menu might not contain violent options.

Violent aftermaths

Pain and pleasure can undoubtedly be associated with violence. Similarly, the violent implementation can be visible or veiled, the proposition that violence brings pain is supportable patently but there is also an oblique equivalent. Moreover, gaining pleasure from violence, directly or indirectly, may not be socially defensible. Alongside personal suffering, there is also the suffering of society. Much of the physical damage from violence for individuals and society is obvious. Much psychological damage is indiscernible in the immediate and may surface only gradually or not until later in life. Much societal damage may never be recognised, or if recognised only partially (for example, the financial cost) and not necessarily as a serious sign of society's insanity.

There are conspicuous and concealed, physical, psychological, and social detrimental aftermaths of fatal and non-fatal interpersonal violence (Wilkinson and Pickett, 2010). The aftermath of violence on primary victims, the targets of violence, may death. Violence also creates and has aftermaths for secondary victims, the families, friends, and close associates of the primary victims Morrall 2006; Morrall et al., 2011; 2013). Furthermore, violence creates and has aftermaths for tertiary victims, the communities of primary and secondary victims, and where violence is rife and entrenched, their society. The ultimate tertiary victim, where the spread is worldwide and prolonged, is global society. Inter-state wars, civil wars and genocide, damage the fabric of whole societies, but so does self-inflicted and interpersonal violence Calculated, and collateral violence, kills and leaves as residue of enfeebled and ruined lives, and Individuals who survive violence are vulnerable to life-changing and potentially life-threatening physical and psychological disorders. The dread, distress, disease and degradation from whole-scale calculated and collateral violence, such as occurs during inter-state wars, civil wars and genocide, can destabilise the political and economic of States (Rothbart and Korostelina 2013, Syrian Centre for Policy Research 2017; Centers for Disease Control and Prevention, 2017).

Secondary victims of homicide describe the effects on them as 'devastating'[3] (Krug et al., 2002; World Health Organisation 2014; Citizens Against Homicide 2017). The impact of homicide on the victim's partner or close relative may result in a severe and distinct form of bereavement which can lead to a type of post-traumatic stress (Morrall 2006, Network of Victim Assistance 2016). Describes. The emotional aftermath of murder is described by the National Organisation of Parents of Murdered Children (2017) as 'grief like no other'. Homicide, especially if in high numbers, may provoke in society a collective sense of sadness and anxiety, and higher rates of physical morbidity and mortality and diagnosis of mental disorder (Wilkinson and Picket 2010; Amnesty International, 2017).

Violence correlates with increased rates of smoking, drug and alcohol addiction, cardiac disease, cancer, diabetes, chronic pain disorders, sexually transmitted diseases, unwanted pregnancies, severe depression and/or anxiety, self-harming including suicide, and post-traumatic stress disorder (Friborg et al., 2015; Alvarez and Bachman, 2016; United Kingdom Faculty of Public Health 2016; World Health Organisation, 2019;). Violence globally is among the leading causes of death for people aged 15–44 years (Krug et al., 2002).

Changes in the temperament and neurological composition of the brain has been documented in combatants and civilians caught-up in civil unrest, warfare, and terrorism (UNODC, 2014; World Health Organisation, 2014; Raine, 2014). The experience of partaking in or witnessing traumatic events such as armed conflict there is generally a 'stress' response, the body's 'flight or fight' defence against harm. Alongside other biochemicals, the hormone cortisol is released to prepare the affected person for what is taken as an emergency. The individual's blood pressure rises as does her/his heart rate, sweating increases, and in extreme situations bowel and bladder evacuation might also occur thus reducing weight to further enable flight or fight. Following, the violent event the primary victim or witness may suffer 'shock' physiologically and psychologically. Shock if unresolved physically (that is 'naturally') or through medical intervention can be life-threatening. Unresolved psychological shock may lead to prolonged anxiety, depression, and post-traumatic stress disorder (PTSD) (Mental Health Foundation, 2016). Symptoms of PTSD include: depression and anxiety; emotional numbness; recurrent 'flashbacks', that is re-experiencing the violent event; avoiding items of places associated with the event; panic attacks; lack of concentration on otherwise everyday activities; disturbed sleep; drug or alcohol misuse; outbursts of and anger. Treatment for PTSD is either psychotherapy (commonly cognitive behavioural), drug therapy for depression and anxiety, or these approaches combined (Mental Health Foundation, 2019a; 2019b). What is missing in the available treatment regimens for PTSD and other personal aftereffects from violence is therapy for society.

The early findings from a study which surveyed 16857 serving UK police officers and civilian staff involved in police operations indicated that nearly one in five had signs of PTSD (Miller and Burchell, 2019). Most of those who completed the survey were unaware that they had signs of PTSD, but two-thirds revealed that they had a 'mental health issue' which they attributed to their work. Examples of trauma experienced by the officers and staff were reviewing material relating to paedophile and terrorist activities, deaths from vehicle accidents, suicides, stabbings, and murders. An illustrative case is that of Police Officer Lee Jackson who in 2015 had responded to an instruction to attend a violent domestic dispute (Shaw, 2019). He recalls:

> It was a Friday night on my own.... I pulled up to stop some people arguing because it was starting to get a little bit more physical. I ended up being attacked – someone tried to gouge my eye out.
>
> (Jackson, quoted in Shaw, 2019)

Jackson's eye became infected which caused partial blindness temporarily. Soon after the violent attack on him he experienced nightly 'flashbacks' and deterioration in performance at work and in his personal relationships He was eventually diagnosed with PTSD for which he received six months of what is reported as 'one-to-one counselling' (Shaw, 2019).

Whilst exposure to and enduring violence should never be 'acceptable', police work is at times unavoidably traumatic. Police officers and their civilian colleagues are, however, adults and have choice about their situation. They elect to enter police work, can elect to leave that work, and can ask for help as did (eventually) Police Officer Jackson. Children are not in that position. Incidental, and certainly intentional, pain caused to children should be unacceptable in any society let alone one supposedly civilised. Across global society both physical and psychological violence where the victim is a child is common (UNICEF, 2014).

Analysis of composite data from a series of international surveys suggests that annually more than 1 billion children are victims of violence. The analysis of these surveys also links violence to increased risk in later life of criminality, drug abuse, serious physical disease and psychological distress (Centers for Disease Control and Prevention, 2017). The World Health Organisation (2019) concurs with these results, adding that children who are victims of violence have a higher risk of alcohol abuse, smoking, and unsafe sexual behaviour, and decades later are more vulnerable to heart disease and cancer.

The British Royal College of Psychiatrists (2017) recognises that children either as witnesses or victims, who are exposed to real violence can experience depression, anxiety, increased aggressiveness, and post-traumatic stress disorder. Children appear to be highly susceptible to PTSD. An epidemiological study of 2232 young people in England and Wales indicated that one in 13 had experienced PTSD by 18 years of age. Half of those who had experienced

PTSD had also experienced a major depressive episode and one in five had attempted suicide. The highest risk of developing PTSD is associated with physical or sexual assault and threats from adults, bullying by peers, and after accidents or illness (Lewis et al., 2019).

The British charity, the National Society for the Prevention of Cruelty to Children (NSPCC, 2019) affirms that the psychological abuse of children increases the risk of emotional instability and possibly mental disorder diagnoses at the time and in the future. An inability to feel, express, and regulate emotions appropriate to their situation which may result in impulsivity or aggression, lack confidence, self-harm, be unable to maintain relationships, be diagnosed with attention deficit or an eating disorder, depression, and anxiety. The NSPCC provides a long list of psychological abuses which could have emotionally injure children. Included in the list are: berating, belittling, condemning, insulting, mocking, embarrassing, shaming, humiliating, taunting, goading, deceiving, blackmailing, and moralising. In turn, suggests the NSPCC, the abused may become the abuser, using some of the same tactics. However, it is difficult to separate in this list of suggested psychological abuses those which may contribute negligibly or substantively to emotional disharmony in children. Berating a child for wrongdoing, attempting to install moral standards, or lying to a child about the existence of Santa Claus, may not be held without equivocation to be abusive.

Bullying does appear to have a significant negative effect on children's mental health, quality of life and academic achievement. Children who are frequently bullied are nearly three times more likely to feel like an outsider at school and more than twice as likely to miss school as those who are not bullied recurrently. They have worse educational outcomes than their peers and are also more likely to leave formal education after finishing secondary school (UNESCO, 2019).

But, that violence affects children emotionally is unequivocal. The most adverse aftermaths affecting the emotional well-being of children arise from violence. Children who report high levels of exposure to violence either as victim or witness report the highest levels of anger, anxiety, and reduced or absence of empathy and compassion for others (Flannery, 2018). Interpersonal violence has what UNICEF (2014) describes as a 'grave effect' on children to the extent of altering adversely their life-course in terms of education, employment, and financial security, and in worst cases it ends their lives. Children who grow up in a violent household or community have a greater tendency than those who don't to internalise and display what they have witnessed.

Children who are prey to armed conflict are amongst the most vulnerable to a host of physical harm and psychological distress. The Syrian internal armed conflicts ensued after the 'Arab Spring' protests in 2011, and which were in due course to involve external forces including the USA and Russia. Much of the material and social infrastructure in the then largest Syrian city, one of the oldest continuously occupied cities, was in ruins (Burns, 2017;

Maclean, 2017). Aleppo remains in 2019, the time of writing this book, a destroyed and dangerous city (*Aljazeera News*, 2019). Journalists Olivia Alabaster and Zouhir Al Shimale (2016), in their newspaper article titled 'Life Among Barrel Bombs for Aleppo's Children', quote 14-year-old Hala who witnessed her mother killed by a shell when it landed on their home:

> Whenever I remember this moment, my tears just fall by themselves.... I have been having nightmares, and I awake suddenly in the middle of the night and I just can't sleep again.... I feel very exhausted.

The article also contains comments from medical practitioners in the city. John Kahler is a paediatrician from the USA who notes how children have become distrustful, couldn't be comforted emotionally, are prone to tearfulness, temper tantrums, bed-wetting, and 'anxiety disorder'. Syrian epidemiologist Abdulkarim Ekzayez, with the charity Save the Children observes that there is a lot of children affected detrimentally psychologically and socially, who will not play with their peers, do not laugh, and show signs of anxiety.

Children's vulnerability to psychological abuse may arise from witnessing factual or fake violence on television, and in videogames, and social media[4] (Wayne, 2016; Dmitrieva 2017). The abuse occurs because of 'vicarious traumatisation'. Blame for this trauma lies with adults (specifically parents, politicians, and media operatives) for allowing if not encouraging children to witness digitalised violence.

According to the American Academy of Child and Adolescent Psychiatry (2014) children living in the USA watch an average of four hours of television daily, and hundreds of studies examining the effects of this level of television viewing is emotional abuse. These studies indicate that extensive viewing of television violence by children causes greater aggressiveness, but the same effect may come from watching one programme in which there is particularly violent content. In one study of violence in US television shows, 60% of a sample containing approximately 10,000 programs over one week included acts of violence (Kunkel 2007). Over 50% of the violence in these shows involved one or more killings. The study observed that millions of children in the US were watching television on average for about 20 hours per week and were exposed to much of its violent content. Where the violence is real or portrayed as realistic, repeated, or is unpunished, then there is an increased likelihood of the child emulating what has been viewed. As with witnessing violence face-to-face, and more so from enduring violence, the aftermath may be delayed until later life.

Daniel Flannery (2018), researcher in violence prevention also argues that children's exposure to violence in the media does undermine their psychological well-being by, for example, amplifying fearfulness. Most children (92%) use the internet daily with a constant use for nearly a quarter (24%), and this suggests Flannery, leads to exposure to possible immediate, intense, and repeated minor and major forms of violence. The internet provides unfettered access to images of actual violence and thereby potential modelling for copycat acts (Gansner, 2017). Flannery and others (Gentile, 2014; Hollingdale and Greitemeyer, 2014, Beresin, 2015) refer to evidence suggesting that playing computer-generated games can desensitise children to violence and increase the risk of committing violence as well as being diagnosed with mental disorder. There is evidence that the neurological circuitry and structures of children and adults may be affected by exposure to fake or real violence experienced in actual events or in the media (Bacon, 2015, Eagleman, 2015, Hummer, 2015).

For novelist Teddy Wayne (2016) 'doom-and-gloom news' is available constantly on mobilephones and the internet allowing the intricate details of horrendous harshness and unfettered anguish to be documented consciously and internalised unconsciously. The day-to-day experience of face-to-face violence in medieval times and the gruesomeness of mass twentieth century arm-to-arm warfare is hardly comparable with viewing killings and cruelty vicariously, nomatter if real. But, media portrayal of violence until relatively recently has been confined to print and then the occasional television broadcast most of which had limited audiences compared with today's pandemic of portrayals of factual and fake blood, guts, corpses, savagery, and hardheartedness.

The claim that observing violence in digitalised media is a sound predicator of acts of violence, including murder and school shootings, is contentious (Ferguson, 2015; Bushman and Anderson, 2015; Ray, 2018). However, the daily diet of death, destruction, and maliciousness on television not only makes the world appear miserable but furnishes a view of others as potential terrorisers if not executioners and may have an insidious effect on self-appraisal and perpetuation which is insidious rather than linkable directly to acts of violence (Gerbner, 1996). With reference to children, display and digestion of actual and fictional violence in the media adds to a 'culture of violence' within which they grow up (Kunkel 2007).

What is also contentious is the cost of violence. Economist John Keynes's (1936) idea is that paying people to dig holes and fill them in again has an economic value to society. Wages paid for hole digging can stimulate growth when they are used to buy products and services thereby expanding the economy. The same argument can apply to violence including the most destructive variety, war (Institute for Economics and Peace, 2011; Pham, 2017). For example, armament and entertainment industries require violence, tangible and imaginary, to sell their goods. Health, criminal justice, and security services employ staff and operate specialist facilities. But, the evidence to the contrary is sizable. Indeed, the direct and indirect monetary loss to economies due to violence is gauged as monumental. The direct costs refer to the immediate consequences of violence on the victims, perpetrators and public systems including health, social, and judicial services. The indirect costs of violence refer to lost productivity, psychological distress on individuals, and the amplification of fearfulness about the safety, trustworthiness, and solidity of society. Globally, the economic impact of violence against children alone is estimated at hundreds of billions of dollars per year (Centers for Disease Control and Prevention, 2017). Gender-based violence is not only devastating for survivors of violence and their families, but also entails significant economic costs. Violence against women is estimated to cost more than double what most governments spend on education. (World Bank, 2018). Child abuse and neglect in the USA along affects over 1 million children every year (Gelles and Perlman, 2012). For 2017 the overall global economic impact of violence is calculated as $14.76 trillion (Institute for Economics and Peace, 2018).

What is not contentious is that violence, personal madness, and societal insanity, are entwined.

Summary

Ray (2018) posits that if violent tendencies are inherent in humans it does not follow that they will be expressed, and even in its expression it will be shaped by the society in which it arises. So far humanity has never ceased to express violence although society has manifestly moulded the features of violent episodes, its quantities, potency, and perpetrator-victim composition.

Violence is always a private trouble as well as public issue. The position of Pinker (2011) and Elias (1939) is that humanity is walking a path which leads to a civilised state. Although the route is littered with atavistic detritus, humans are on the whole shedding their barbaric predilections.

Fromm (1955) has a completely different position. For Fromm, 'civilisation' is the main problem, and one which doesn't cure but causes the personal problem of violence along with a myriad of other dehumanising performances attendant on what Pinker and Elias want to consider as the humanising setting of today's consumer-orientated globalised society. Applying Fromm's perspective not only is this kind of society insane, but to claim that such a society is civilised is an insanity. Visible, veiled, and vicarious violence is a hard-and-fast fixture of 'civilised' societies, as is the diagnosis of mental disorder. Take the example of apartheid, the defining social structure in South Africa for over four decades during the twentieth century, an institutionalised racial divide against which Mandela was willing to challenge with violence. The repercussions from apartheid are stark:

> Apartheid has negatively affected the lives of all South African children but its effects have been particularly devastating for black children. The consequences of poverty, racism and violence have resulted in psychological disorders, and a generation of maladjusted children may be the result.
>
> (Hickson and Kriegler, 1991, p. 141)

These effects of violence and from other incivilities are likely to reoccur in the generations that follow those that have been caught-up in the dozens of 21st century armed conflicts, only one example of which is the Syrian civil war.

It matters morally when murder manifests as a recreational spectacle. Core to civilised society, argues Elias (1939) is empathy, based on an individual's respect for the rights of others and restricting his or her own desires. But personal control over violent tendencies was paramount and respecting the prerogatives of fellow citizens did not extend to accepting violence – not the perpetration of violence nor the vicarious 'enjoyment' of violence. Fatal and non-fatal violence damages the physical and mental well-being of individuals and the well-being of society. Finding murder/violence fascinating may have similar detrimental effects.

There is a widening of the health and wealth gap both within countries and internationally (Wilkinson and Pickett, 2010; Fitz, 2015; Dorling, 2015; Marmot, 2016; Institute for Policy Studies, 2018). Income inequality along with raw penury are key to determining whether a part of the world or region in a country has a high risk of fatal and non-fatal violence (United Nations Office on Drugs and Crime, 2014). Inequality also connects with madness, and it is this public issue and private trouble which forms the next chapter.

Notes

1 In 2019 researchers from Yale University reported on how they had reactivated cells in the brains of pigs hours after death (Vrselja et al., 2019).
2 This is a composite reference with the specific points made in this chapter are taken from the subsections of the 'Small Arms Survey Focus Areas'.
3 To-date, there appears to be no published research establishing the meaning of reported 'devastation' claimed by secondary victims. There is anecdotal evidence of negative outcomes for secondary victims, few of which seem to concur with the strict definition of that term.
4 A detailed exploration of social media appears in Chapter 6.

References

Alabaster O and Shimale Z (2016) Life among barrel bombs for Aleppo's children: The psychological trauma of being trapped in a war zone will last long after the conflict ends, doctors say. *Aljazeera*, 1 August. www.aljazeera.com/news/2016/07/life-barrel-bombs-aleppo-children-160731130545021.html [accessed 1 April. 2019].
Aljazeera News (2019) Rockets kill 11 in Syria's northern city of Aleppo. www.aljazeera.com/news/2019/04/rockets-kill-11-syria-northern-city-aleppo-reports-190415064940091.html [accessed 8 May, 2019].
Alvarez A and Bachman R (2016) *Violence: The Enduring Problem*, 3rd edn. Singapore: Sage.
American Academy of Child and Adolescent Psychiatry (2014) TV violence and children. www.aacap.org/aacap/families_and_youth/facts_for_families/fff-guide/children-and-tv-violence-013.aspx [accessed 29 March, 2019].
Amnesty International (2018) Syria: 'Deadly labyrinth' traps civilians trying to flee Raqqa battle against Islamic State. www.amnesty.org/en/latest/news/2017/08/syria-deadly-labyrinth-traps-civilians-trying-to-flee-raqqa/ [accessed 25 April, 2019].

Amnesty International (2019) Saudi Arabia: 37 killed in 'chilling' execution spree [press release, 23 April]. www.amnesty.org.uk/press-releases/saudi-arabia-37-killed-chilling-execution-spree [accessed 29 April, 2019].

Amnesty International/Airwars (2019) Rhetoric versus reality in the war in Raqqa. https://raqqa.amnesty.org/ [accessed 25 April, 2019].

Atwan A (2015) *Islamic State: The Digital Caliphate*. Oakland, CA: University of California Press.

Australian Bureau of Statistics (2018) *Victims of Crime, Australia*. Australian Bureau of Statistics, 28 June. www.abs.gov.au/ausstats/abs@.nsf/Lookup/by%20Subject/4510.0~2017~Main%20Features~Vicitms%20of%20Crime,%20Australia~3 [accessed 9 April, 2019].

BBCiPlayer (2019) *Killing Eve*. www.bbc.co.uk/iplayer/episodes/p06jy6bc/killing-eve [accessed 16 May, 2019].

BBC News (2019) Sri Lanka attacks: What we know about the Easter bombings. *BBC News*, 25 April. www.bbc.co.uk/news/world-asia-48010697 [accessed 25 April, 2019].

Bacon H (2015) *The Fascination of Film Violence*. New York: Palgrave MacMillan.

Bauer-Clapp H (2016) Heritage of violence: Editor's introduction. *Journal of Landscapes of Violence*, 4(1), pp. 1–4. https://scholarworks.umass.edu/lov/vol1/iss1/8/ [accessed 29 March, 2019].

Bauman Z (2011) *Collateral Damage: Social Inequalities in a Global Age*. Cambridge: Polity.

Beresin E (2015) The impact of media violence on children and adolescents: Opportunities for clinical interventions. www.aacap.org/aacap/Medical_Students_and_Residents/Mentorship_Matters/DevelopMentor/The_Impact_of_Media_Violence_on_Children_and_Adolescents_Opportunities_for_Clinical_Interventions.aspx [accessed 8 February 2018].

Bessel R (2015) *Violence: A Modern Obsession*. London: Simon & Schuster.

Bocock R (2002) *Sigmund Freud*, 2nd edn. London: Routledge.

Bonn S (2014) *Why We Love Serial Killers: The Curious Appeal of the World's Most Savage Murderers*. New York: Skyhorse.

Brookman F and Maguire M (eds) (2017) *The Handbook of Homicide*. Chichester: Wiley.

Buechler S (2017) Erich Fromm's concept of reactive violence. *International Forum of Psychoanalysis* [*Violence, Terror and Terrorism Today: Psychoanalytic Perspectives, Part I*], 26(3), pp. 193–197.

Burns R (2017) *Aleppo: A History*. Abingdon-on-Thames: Routledge.

Bushman B and Anderson C (2015) Understanding causality in the effects of media violence. *American Behavioral Scientist*, 59(14), pp. 1807–1821.

Care Quality Commission (2017) *Review of Children and Young People's Mental Health Services (Phase 1 Report)*. London: Care Quality Commission.

Centers for Disease Control and Prevention (2017) Towards a violence-free generation. www.cdc.gov/violenceprevention/pdf/vacs-one-page.pdf [accessed 13 February, 2018].

Citizens Against Homicide (2017) About CAH. www.citizensagainsthomicide.org/about-cah [accessed 8 February 2018].

Cockerham W (2016) *Sociology of Mental Disorder*. New York: Routledge.

Conrad P (2002) *The Hitchcock Murders*. London: Faber and Faber.

De Quincey T (1925; original 1827) *On Murder Considered as One of the Fine Arts*. London: Allan & Co.

Dmitrieva K (2017) *Why Are We Fascinated with Violence? An Investigation of Mass Media's Role in Depicting Violence as Entertainment*. University of Rhode Island,

Paper 574. http://digitalcommons.uri.edu/srhonorsprog/574/?utm_source=digitalcomm ons.uri.edu%2Fsrhonorsprog%2F574&utm_medium=PDF&utm_campaign=PDFCo verPages [accessed 6 March, 2018).

Dorling D (2005) Prime suspect: Murder in Britain. In Dorling D, Gordon D, Hillyard P et al., *Criminal Obsessions: Why Harm Matters More Than Crime*. London: Crime and Society Foundation.

Dorling D (2015) *Inequality and the 1%*. London: Verso.

Duclos D (1998) *The Werewolf Complex: America's Fascination with Violence*. London: Berg.

Eagleman D (2015) *The Brain: The Story of You*. Edinburgh: Canongate.

Elbert T, Moran J and Schauer M (2017) Lust for violence: Appetitive aggression as a fundamental part of human nature. *Neuroforum*, 23(2), pp. A77–A84. www.degruy ter.com/downloadpdf/j/nf.2017.23.issue-2/nf-2016-A056/nf-2016-A056.pdf [accessed 15 March, 2019].

Elias N (1939) *Über den Prozeß der Zivilisation. Soziogenetische und psychogenetische Untersuchungen* [two volumes]. Basel, Switzerland: Haus zum Falken.

Federal Bureau of Investigation (2019) *Preliminary Semiannual Uniform Crime Report, January–June, 2018*. https://ucr.fbi.gov/crime-in-the-u.s/2018/preliminary-report/home [accessed 4 April, 2019].

Ferguson C (2015) Does media violence predict societal violence? It depends on what you look at and when. *Journal of Communication*, 65(1), pp. E1–E22. https://academic.oup. com/joc/article-abstract/65/1/E1/4082340?redirectedFrom=fulltext [accessed 10 May 2019].

Fitz N (2015) Economic inequality: It's far worse than you think. *Scientific American*, 31 March. www.scientificamerican.com/article/economic-inequality-it-s-far-worse-than-you-think/ [accessed 27 September, 2018].

Flannery D (2018) Here's how witnessing violence harms children's mental health. *The Conversation*, 16 February. http://theconversation.com/heres-how-witnessing-violence-ha rms-childrens-mental-health-91971 [accessed 29 March, 2019].

Freud S (1920) *Jenseits des Lustprinzips* [Beyond the Pleasure Principle]. In Strachey, J. (ed.) (2001) *The Standard Edition of the Complete Psychological Works of Sigmund Freud*. London: Vintage.

Friborg O, Emaus N, Rosenvinge J, Bilden U, Olsen J and Pettersen G (2015) Violence affects physical and mental health differently: The general population based Tromsø study. *PLoS ONE*, 10(8), e0136588. https://journals.plos.org/plosone/article?id=10. 1371/journal.pone.0136588 [accessed 18 March, 2019].

Friis S (2018) 'Behead, burn, crucify, crush': Theorizing the Islamic State's public displays of violence. *European Journal for International Relations*, 24(2), pp. 243–267.

Fromm E (1955) *The Sane Society*. New York: Rinehart.

Fromm E (1964) *The Heart of Man: Its Genius for Good and Evil*. New York: Harper & Row.

Fromm E (1973) *The Anatomy of Human Destructiveness*. New York: Holt, Rinehart & Winston.

Gansner M (2017) 'The internet made me do it'—Social media and potential for violence in adolescents. *Psychiatric Times*, 34(8). www.psychiatrictimes.com/couch-crisis/-inter net-made-me-do-itsocial-media-and-potential-violence-adolescents [accessed 29 March, 2019].

Gardner D (2008) *Risk: The Science and Politics of Fear*. London: Virgin.

Gash T (2016) *Criminal: The Truth About Why People Do Bad Things*. London: Allen Lane.

Gatrell V (1996) *The Hanging Tree: Execution and the English People 1770–1868*. Oxford: Oxford University Press.

Gelles J and Perlman S (2012) *Estimated Annual Cost of Child Abuse and Neglect*. Chicago, IL: Prevent Child Abuse America. www.preventchildabuse.org/images/research/pcaa_cost_report_2012_gelles_perlman.pdf [accessed 4 May, 2019].

Gentile D (2014) *Media Violence and Children*. Santa Barbara, CA: Praeger,

Gerbner G (1996) *The Hidden Side of Television Violence*. London: Routledge.

Godsi E (2004) *Violence and Society: Making Sense of Madness and Badness*. Ross-on-Wye: PCCS Books.

Greer G (2018) Shows like The Bridge repeatedly depict violence against women – so why are we watching? *Radio Times*, 5 May. www.radiotimes.com/news/tv/2018-05-05/tv-violence-women-the-bridge-germaine-greer/.

Hans S (2018) 10 great erotic thrillers: Base instincts and fatal attractions abound in these 10 unmissably sexy thrillers. www.bfi.org.uk/news-opinion/news-bfi/lists/10-great-erotic-thrillers [accessed 29tApril, 2019].

Hickey E (2003) *Encyclopedia of Murder and Violent Crime*. London: Sage.

Hickson J and Kriegler S (1991) Childshock: The effects of apartheid on the mental health of South Africa's children. *International Journal for the Advancement of Counselling*, 14(2), pp. 141–154.

Holland J (2004) Military objective and collateral damage: Their relationship and dynamics. *Yearbook of International Humanitarian Law*, 7, pp. 35–78.

Hollingdale J and Greitemeyer T (2014) The effect of online violent video games on levels of aggression. https://journals.plos.org/plosone/article?id=10.1371/journal.pone.0111790 [accessed 11 March, 2019].

Hummer T (2015) Media violence effects on brain development: What neuroimaging has revealed and what lies ahead. *American Behavioral Scientist*, 59(14), pp. 1790–1806.

Institute for Economics and Peace (2011) *Economic Consequences of War on the U.S. Economy*. Sydney: Institute for Economics and Peace. http://economicsandpeace.org/wp-content/uploads/2015/06/The-Economic-Consequences-of-War-on-US-Economy_0.pdf [accessed 12t May, 2019].

Institute for Economics and Peace (2016) *Global Peace Index 2016*. Sydney: Institute for Economics and Peace.

Institute for Economics and Peace (2018) *Global Terrorism Index 2018*. Sydney: Institute for Economics and Peace.

Institute for Policy Studies (2018) Inequality and health. https://inequality.org/facts/inequality-and-health/ [accessed 27 September, 2018].

Internet Watch Foundation (2018) *Trends in Online Child Sexual Exploitation: Examining the Distribution of Captures of Live-streamed Child Sexual Abuse*. Cambridge: Internet Watch Foundation/Microsoft.

Javid S (2019) Home Secretary speech on protecting young people's futures. Home Office, 15 April. www.gov.uk/government/speeches/home-secretary-speech-on-protecting-young-peoples-futures [accessed 16 April, 2019].

Joint Commissioning Panel for Mental Health (2013) *Guidance for Commissioners of Child and Adolescent Mental Health Services [England]*. London: Joint Commissioning Panel for Mental Health.

Karakurt G and Silver K (2013) Emotional abuse in intimate relationships: The role of gender and age. *Violence and Victims*, 28(5), pp. 804–821.

Keynes J (1936) *The General Theory of Employment, Interest, and Money by John Maynard Keynes*. London: Macmillan.

Kottler J (2011) *The Lust for Blood: Why We Are Fascinated by Death, Murder, Horror, and Violence*. New York: Prometheus.

Krug E, Dahlberg L, Mercy J, Zwi A and Lozano R (eds) (2002) *World Report on Violence and Health*. Geneva: World Health Organization.

Kunkel D (2007) *The Impact of Media Violence on Children*. Testimony before the U.S. Senate Committee on Commerce, Science, and Transportation. Washington, DC. www.gpo.gov/fdsys/pkg/CHRG-110shrg76392/html/CHRG-110shrg76392.htm [accessed 14 February, 2018].

Lewis S, Arseneault L, Caspi A, Fisher H, Matthews T, Moffitt T, Odgers C, Stahl D, Teng J and Danese A (2019) The epidemiology of trauma and post-traumatic stress disorder in a representative cohort of young people in England and Wales. *The Lancet*, 6(3), pp. 247–356.

Lyons K (2019) Christchurch attacks: New Zealand brings in sweeping gun-law changes. *The Guardian*, 21 March.

Maclean R (2017) 'Everything we built for 20 years, gone in a blink' – life in the ruins of Aleppo. *The Guardian*, 28 March.

Mandela N (1994) *Long Walk to Freedom*. London: Little, Brown and Company.

Marmot M (2016) *The Health Gap: The Challenge of an Unequal World*. London: Bloomsbury.

Massey J, Sherman L and Coupe T (2019) Forecasting knife homicide risk from prior knife assaults in 4835 local areas of London, 2016–2018. *Cambridge Journal of Evidence-Based Policing*, 3, pp. 1–20.

Mennell S (2017) About Norbert Elias. http://norbert-elias.com/en/about-norbert-elias/ [accessed 27 April, 2019].

Mental Health Foundation (2016) *The Impact of Traumatic Events on Mental Health*. London: Mental Health Foundation.

Mental Health Foundation (2019a) Post-traumatic stress disorder (PTSD)www.mentalhealth.org.uk/a-to-z/p/post-traumatic-stress-disorder-ptsd [accessed 18 March, 2019].

Mental Health Foundation (2019b) Depression. www.mentalhealth.org.uk/a-to-z/d/depression [accessed 18 March 2019].

Miller J and Burchell B (2019) Police Care UK/University of Cambridge. www.cam.ac.uk/policeptsd [accessed 9 May 2019].

Morrall P (2006) *Murder and Society*. Chichester: Wiley

Morrall P (2008) *The Trouble with Therapy: Sociology and Psychotherapy*. Buckingham: Open University Press/McGraw-Hill.

Morrall P (2010) *Sociology and Health: An Introduction*. London: Routledge.

Morrall P (2017) *Madness: Ideas about Insanity*. Abingdon-on-Thames: Routledge.

Morrall P, Hazelton M and Shackleton W (2011) Homicide and health: The suffering of secondary victims and the role of the mental health nurse. *Mental Health Practice*, 15(3), pp. 14–19.

Morrall P, Hazelton M and Shackleton W (2013) Psychotherapy and social responsibility: homicide. *Psychotherapy and Politics International*, 11(2), pp. 102–113.

Morrall P, Worton K and Antony D (2018) Why is murder fascinating and why does it matter to mental health professionals? *Mental Health Practice*, 21(7), pp. 34–39.

National Organization of Parents of Murdered Children (2017) Grief – The human experience. www.pomc.com/grief.html [accessed 8 February, 2018].

National Society for the Prevention of Cruelty to Children (NSPCC) (2019) Emotional abuse: What is emotional abuse? www.nspcc.org.uk/preventing-abuse/child-abuse-and-neglect/emotional-abuse/what-is-emotional-abuse/ [accessed 29 March, 2019].

Network of Victim Assistance (2016) Homicide. www.novabucks.org/otherinformation/homicide [accessed 8 February 2018].

New Zealand Government (2019) New Zealand history: Crime timeline. https://nzhistory.govt.nz/culture/nz-crimetimeline [accessed 17th April, 2019].

Office for National Statistics (ONS) (2019a) The nature of violent crime in England and Wales: Year ending March 2018. Office for National Statistics, 7 February [corrected version]. www.ons.gov.uk/peoplepopulationandcommunity/crimeandjustice/articles/thenatureofviolentcrimeinenglandandwales/yearendingmarch2018#main-points [accessed 4 April, 2019].

Office for National Statistics (ONS) (2019b) Crime in England and Wales: Year ending December 2018. www.ons.gov.uk/peoplepopulationandcommunity/crimeandjustice/bulletins/crimeinenglandandwales/yearendingdecember2018#main-points [accessed 26 April, 2019].

Oka R, Kissel M, Golitko M, Sheridan S, Kim N and Fuentes A (2017) Population is the primary driver of war group size and conflict casualties. *Proceedings of the National Academy of Sciences*, 114(52), pp. E11101–E11110.

Parents Against Child Exploitation (2019) https://paceuk.info/for-parents/advice-centre/understanding-online-risks/ [accessed 25 April, 2019].

Pham P (2017) Is war good for economies? *Forbes*, 6 November. www.forbes.com/sites/peterpham/2017/11/06/is-war-good-for-economies/#5bfbd8f64d9d [accessed 12 May, 2019].

Pinker S (2011) *The Better Angels of Our Nature: Why Violence Has Declined*. New York: Viking.

Raine A (2014) *The Anatomy of Violence*: London: Penguin.

Ramaswamy C (2018) From fridging to nagging husbands: How Killing Eve upturns sexist clichés. *The Guardian*, 12 October.

Ray L (2018) *Violence and Society*, 2nd edn. London: Sage.

Rosen F (2016) *Collateral Damage: A Candid History of a Peculiar Form of Death*. London: C Hurst & Co.

Roser M and Nagdy M (2017) Terrorism. www.ourworldindata.org/terrorism [accessed 8 February, 2018].

Rothbart D and Korostelina K (2013) *Why They Die: Civilian Devastation in Violent Conflict*. Ann Arbor MI: University of Michigan Press.

Royal College of Nursing (2017) *Child and Adolescent Mental Health Key Facts*. London: RCN.

Royal College of Psychiatrists (2017) Mental health and growing up factsheet. www.rcpsych.ac.uk/healthadvice/parentsandyoungpeople/parentscarers/domesticviolence.aspx [accessed 8 February, 2018].

Sarat A (2014) *Gruesome Spectacles: Botched Executions and America's Death Penalty*. Redwood City, CA: Stanford University.

Schraer R (2019) Christchurch shootings: How mass killings have changed gun laws. *BBC News*, 18 March. www.bbc.co.uk/news/world-47612116 [accessed 20 March, 2019].

Shaw D (2019) PTSD 'at crisis levels' among police officers. *BBC News*, 9 May. www.bbc.co.uk/news/uk-48201088 [accessed 9 May, 2019].

Sifton J (2015) *Violence All Around*. Cambridge, MA: Harvard University.

Sivarajasingam V, Page N, Green G, Moore S and Shepherd J (2019) *Violence in England and Wales in 2018: An Accident and Emergency Perspective.* Cardiff: Violence Research Group, Crime and Security Research Institute, Cardiff University.

Small Arms Survey (2019) Small arms survey focus areas. www.smallarmssurvey.org/home.html [accessed 21st April, 2019].

Syrian Center for Policy Research (2017) Social degradation in Syria report. www.scpr-syria.org [accessed 8 February 2018].

Tasman A (2016) Hot topics of 2016: In and around psychiatry: Violence. *Psychiatric Times*, 20 December. www.psychiatrictimes.com/cultural-psychiatry/hot-topics-2016-and-around-psychiatry/page/0/1 [accessed 1 April, 2019].

United Kingdom Faculty of Public Health (2016) The role of public health in the prevention of violence: A statement from the United Kingdom Faculty of Public Health. www.fph.org.uk/media/1381/the-role-of-public-health-in-the-prevention-of-violence.pdf [accessed 8 May, 2018].

United Nations Development Program (2015) Invisible violence: An overview on violence against women and girls with disabilities in Albania. Tirana, Albania. www.al.undp.org/content/dam/albania/docs/misc/disabilities.pdf [accessed 29 March, 2019].

United NationsEducational, Scientific and Cultural Organization (UNESCO) (2019) *Behind the Numbers: Ending School Violence and Bullying.* Paris: UNESCO.

United Nations International Children's Emergency Fund (UNICEF) (2014) *Hidden in Plain Sight: A Statistical Analysis of Violence Against Children.* New York: UNICEF.

United Nations Office on Drugs and Crime (UNODC) (2014) *Global Study on Homicide 2013: Trends, Contexts, Data.* Vienna: United Nations.

Vrselja Z, Daniele S, Silbereis J, Talpo F, Morozov Y, Sousa A, Tanaka B, Skarica M, Pletikos M, Kaur N, Zhuang Z, Liu Z, Alkawadri R, Sinusas A, Latham S, Waxman S and Sestan N (2019) Restoration of brain circulation and cellular functions hours post-mortem. *Nature*, 568, pp. 336–343.

Wayne T (2016) The trauma of violent news on the internet. *The New York Times*, 10 September.

Wen L and Goodwin K (2016) Violence is a public health issue. *Journal of Public Health Management and Practice.* 22(6), pp. 503–505.

Wilkinson I (2005) *Suffering: A Sociological Introduction.* Cambridge: Polity.

Wilkinson R and Pickett K (2010) *The Spirit Level: Why Equality is Better for Everyone.* London: Penguin.

Williams Z (2018) Are women responsible for all the extreme sexual violence on screen? *The Guardian*, 1 May.

World Bank (2018) Gender-based violence: Violence against women and girls. World Bank, 5 October. www.worldbank.org/en/topic/socialdevelopment/brief/violence-against-women-and-girls. [accessed 11 March, 2019].

World Health Organization (2014) *Global Status Report on Violence Prevention.* Switzerland: World Health Organization.

World Health Organisation (2019) Ten facts about violence prevention. www.who.int/features/factfiles/violence/en [accessed 11 March, 2019].

Worsley L (2014) *A Very British Murder: The Curious Story of How Crime was Turned into Art.* London: BBC Books.

4 Inequality

Inequality is a key indicator of insane society. The contention that the public issue of inequality is linkable to the private trouble of madness is compelling.

There is much agreement across academic and professional disciplines and from policy makers that inequalities and the diagnosis of mental disorder (and physical ill-health) are linked. Furthermore, there is a general acceptance that the link is strong, and whilst 'proof' is problematic, it is probably causal. Confirmation and indictment of wealth inequality arises not only from left and liberal think-tanks, parties, and individual campaigners. It also come from agencies (organisations) and agents (individuals) with the opposite political stance and those of governments.

Public Health England (2018) is an executive agency of the UK's Department of Health and Social Care. The agency is unequivocal about the close association between a diagnosis of mental disorder and factors in society. For example, in England psychotic disorder is diagnosed at a rate of nine times higher in people in the lowest fifth household income compared to those in the highest fifth. It recognises that these differences are connectable to the reduction in quality of life, contracting serious physical diseases, and a shortened lifespan. 'Death' inequality is the subject of the second section in this chapter. Unravelling the specific causative iniquities is accepted by Public Health England as complex, and involve factors such as poverty, inadequate education, poor housing or homelessness, unemployment, underemployment or reprehensible work settings, deficient diet. It declares these inequalities as 'unfair' and 'avoidable', and recommends improvements in which people live and work, and the building of stronger communities and social connections by reducing social isolation and increasing social cohesion. Such advocations are both laudable and lamentable.

What is missing from much of the analysis of this linkage, however, is an awareness or admission of the fundamental causes of inequality and concomitant fundamental solutions. Public Health England and most other agents and agencies commenting on inequality do not address the rudimentary reasons for the dispropionate distribution of wealth, death, and madness which lie in the insane structural make-up of society, that is the asymmetrical allocation of power. A discussion on that insanity forms the third part of this chapter.

An association between social circumstances such as impoverishment and iniquitous wealth and diagnosed mental disorder (and physical ill-health) is supported by a profusion of empirical evidence. A selection of the evidence connecting societal faults to psychological distress is presented in this chapter. What is also presented is a section of ideas which expound on these connections. Some of these ideas, including that from Fromm, attempt to provide answers to the fundamental cause of such a distinct and pervasive societal insanity. The use and abuse of power needs to be considered as one causal connector.

The societal situation for which there is an abundance of evidence is that of 'wealth' inequalities, and that is the topic for the first section in the chapter. Wealth, however, covers several circumstances which have differing effects. Connecting one societal situation with one or more positive or negative psychological states is also problematic.

Take happiness and death. There is the foremost difficulty of forming a standard measurement across countries and social categories. Can the 'quotient' of happiness of a female responsible for four children who lives in basic and unstable conditions in a Democratic Republic of Congo village be compared with the luxurious condition which the billionaire-boss of a multinational corporation inhabits? Is the happiness quotient of President Donald Trump equatable with that of an unemployed construction worker in South Carolina? Wealth inequality is a major factor for happiness, but more-so is well-being inequality (Helliwell et al., 2019). However, there is no exponential rise in happiness levels as national wealth increases (Monbiot, 2017). Inequalities that arise from wealth and other social situations influence both morbidity and mortality levels. The influence is dramatic, and the drama is played out in countries which are overall are very wealthy and in those which are not. If there are wide divides between those people who possess most of whatever wealth is available and the rest of the population, then there will marked divides in lifespan. There is a similar gulf between wealthy and non-wealthy countries.

Power is apparent or can be unearthed in the clinical and academic literature connecting inequality and vulnerability to a diagnosis of mental disorder. It is the inequality in the distribution and discharge of power which is key to the inequality in the diagnostic distribution of mental disorder. Neoliberal capitalistic globalisation is marked by marked disparities in wealth, poverty, mental disorder diagnoses, and power.

Poverty is distinct from inequality. Both inequality and poverty have detrimental effects. The detrimental effects of poverty and inequality can be severe in terms of physical and psychological debility and premature death. There has been an increase in the material standard of living globally, mainly because of rising incomes in the emerging economies, especially of India and China. Most of the world's population are not living in dire poverty. However, an unequal distribution of wealth (and power) remains extreme and the extremities are widening.

Unequal wealth

A forum of countries committed to democracy and the market economy, the Organisation for Economic Co-operation and Development (OECD) was established in 1961. Membership consists of 36 countries with industrialising ('emerging'), industrialised, or post-industrial economies. The member countries are: Australia, Austria, Belgium, Canada, Chile, Czech Republic, Denmark, Estonia, Finland, France, Germany, Greece, Hungary, Iceland, Ireland, Israel, Italy, Japan, Korea, Latvia, Lithuania, Luxembourg, Mexico, the Netherlands, New Zealand, Norway, Poland, Portugal, Slovak Republic, Slovenia, Spain, Sweden, Switzerland, Turkey, the United Kingdom, and the United States. The OECD also 'works closely' with several non-member countries from Asia, Africa, Latin America and the Caribbean. Its purpose is to act as a forum for the governments of its members and associates to 'promote free market policies and trade'. It attempts to produce international policy regulations on taxation, the movement of goods and capital, the prevention of bribery, and corrupt practices on the internet (OECD, 2018a).

What 'free market policies and trade' appear to have generated so far is immense and imbedded inequality, which for the OECD has reached a 'tipping point'. That is, inequality and its aftermaths maybe insolvable. No matter that 'insanity is repeating the same mistakes and expecting different results',[1] the OECD (2018b) argues emphatically for more 'free market' and more 'trade' to rectify inequality and resolve its repercussions. No matter that the average income of the richest 10% of the population in OECD countries is approximately nine times that of the poorest 10%. No matter that social mobility in OECD countries has 'stalled'. No matter that there is an inequality 'crisis' throughout the OECD area of influence which is having 'severe social, economic and political consequences'. No matter that all of these acknowledge atrophying constituents of its avowed economic system on the physical and psychological health of its member's populations, the organisation's solution is more of the same:

> [T]here doesn't have to be a trade-off between growth and equality. On the contrary, the opening up of opportunity can spur stronger economic performance and improve living standards across the board.
>
> (OECD, 2018b)

The 'Gini Index' or 'Gini Coefficient' is one of the main measures of inequality used by the OECD (2018b). It is a statistical measure of income distribution or, less commonly, wealth distribution. Income is defined as household disposable annual income comprising earnings from employment and investments minus personal taxes. South Africa, Costa Rica, Mexico, Chile, Turkey, the USA, Lithuania, United Kingdom, New Zealand, and Israel were the top ten most unequal countries during the period 2014–2107. Some of the world's poorest countries (Central African Republic) have some of the world's highest Gini coefficients (61.3), while some of the wealthiest (Denmark) have some of the lowest (28.8). Yet the relationship between income inequality and GDP per capita is not one of perfect negative correlation, and the relationship has varied over time (OECD, 2018b).

The World Inequality Lab is an agency comprised of about twenty researchers based at the Paris School of Economics. Its members cooperate with an international network of researchers and produces a World Inequality Report every two years. Data sources are combined using national accounts, survey data, fiscal data, and wealth rankings. In the 2018 the World Inequality Report (Alvaredo et al., 2018) income inequality is noted to vary hugely across world regions. It is lowest in Europe and highest in the middle east. Furthermore, it notes that inequality within global regions varies greatly. In 2016 the share of total national income accounted for by just that nation's top 10% earners (top 10% income share) was 37% in Europe, 41% in China, 46% in Russia, 47% in USA-Canada, and in sub-Saharan Arica, Brazil, and India. in the middle east, the world's most unequal region according, the top attained 61% of national income. The report also makes the point that in recent decades, income inequality has increased in nearly all countries, but this has happened at different speeds. Since 1980, income inequality has increased rapidly in North America, China, India, and Russia, but moderately in Europe. At the global level, inequality has risen sharply since 1980 despite strong growth in China and India which includes considerable income growth in the poorest half of their populations.

The charity Oxfam has its origins in the founding by Quakers and academics of an agency in Britain attempting to tackle food shortage during the 1940s. Subsequently, agencies across the world formed a coalition of charities focusing on poverty and other social injustices under the umbrella organisation Oxfam International (2019a).

Using data from the transnational financial services agency, Credit Suisse, in 2016 Oxfam International, reported that global inequality had reached a point of crisis. the richest 1% now have more wealth than the rest of the world combined. Oxfam International also reported that the poorest people in the world live in areas most vulnerable to the damaging effects of climate change. However, it is the wealthy not the poorest poor who are responsible for most of the pollutants which are causing global warming (Oxfam International, 2016).

Three years later Oxfam International (2019b) reports that the crisis in inequality had not abated, and in some respects had worsened. Whilst the wealthy had become wealthier, nearly half of the world's population had to live on less than US$5.50 a day. Moreover, the growing gap inequality gap, it is argued by Oxfam International, is damaging economies and fuelling public anger across the globe. It also finds that Women and girls are hardest hit by rising economic inequality. While corporations and the super-rich enjoy low tax bills, millions of girls are denied a decent education and women are dying for lack of maternity care. Since the 2007/8 financial crisis the number of billionaires has almost doubled, wealthy individuals and corporations are paying lower rates of tax than they have in decades, whilst spending on public services has reduced. Every day ten thousand people die because they lack access to affordable healthcare. In developing countries, a child from a poor family is twice as likely to die before the age of five than a child from a rich family.

Inequality within rich countries also provides stark contrasts in how people live. Philip Alston is a lawyer and campaigner for human rights. He also serves as United Nations 'special rapporteur' whose brief covers human rights and poverty. Alston's official statement after a visit to the UK in 2018 is damming.

> [S]o many people are living in poverty.... [I]mmense growth in foodbanks and the queues waiting outside them, the people sleeping rough in the streets.... 14 million people, a fifth of the population, live in poverty. Four million of these are more than 50% below the poverty line, and 1.5 million are destitute.
>
> (Alston, 2018)

Alston records that civil society in the UK has been undermined by alterations in welfare provision, the closing, selling-off, easing-out, and underfunding of public facilities such as libraries, community, youth and recreational centres, swimming pools, and parks. Insecure, arduous, and inadequately paid work, and the unavailability of affordable homes. He describes as the 'sense of deep despair' which for him arises from impoverishment and for some near or definite destitution, along with unprecedented levels of loneliness has led the Government to appoint a Minister for Suicide Prevention in England, announced on World Mental Health Day in 2018.

Social geographer Danny Dorling (2018) observes that the gap between the very rich and the rest is wider in Britain than in any other large European country, and well into the twenty-first century it is the most unequal it has been since shortly after the First World War. The USA, however, is more unequal than any European nation, and the inequality gap is widening in many Western nations (Herbert, 2018).

Dorling warns that such inequality is a 'ticking timebomb' which could trigger major social unrest. However, for Dorling inequality in Britain, and by implication this is so for other similarly rich countries, has reached its peak. As happened after that war and again the Second World War, inequality can decrease. There are indications that this is happening and for reasons which parallel those which altered inequality following the two world wars. The threat and actuality of societal disorder which has surrounded the UK voting to leave the European Union and the rise of radical and popularists discourses, along with palpable unfairness, is evidence that a period of great change may be about to start. Dorling accepts that he may be wrong.

Indeed, Dorling in an earlier publication than his 'Peak Inequality' book suggests that inequality continues to impose a damaging influence on some people's lives –and deaths. Life expectancy, Dorling and his colleague, social scientist Stuart Gietel-Basten (2017a) highlight government figures released in 2017 that average life expectancy in the UK is reducing after over a hundred years of increase. Both men and women are dying one year younger than did they did in previous years. This will result in one million people dying earlier over the subsequent forty years period, and for Dorling and Gietel-Basten (2017b) inequality and poverty are largely to blame for the social and health morbidities that lead to increased mortality. The following year life expectancy in the UK did not improve, and any future increase is predicted to be only be gradual (Office for National Statistics, 2018a).

The USA, the richest country in the world but the most unequal amongst major developed countries. Average lifespan for people residing in Hawaii is nearly seven years longer than for those in Mississippi. Already with a low life expectancy compared with other major developed countries and is experiencing a similar decline in the last few years to that of the UK (National Center for Health Statistics, 2018).

Another major consideration relating to early deaths as a consequence of inequality and poverty is air pollution. Research by the World Health Organisation (2018) indicates that nine out ten people in the world are berating contaminated air. Pollutants realised into the air from, for example, manufacturing, vehicles including diesel ships, and domestic appliances especially fossil-fuel stoves, kill seven million mainly poor people annually (WHO, 2018). Ambient contamination penetrates the respiratory and cardiovascular systems which can lead to stroke, heart disease, lung cancer, chronic obstructive pulmonary diseases, and pneumonia.

Mental inequality

That inequality is associated mental disorder diagnoses is well established. There is also support from a series of sources that this is association is not merely correlational but causal. Put bluntly, it is becoming an unavoidable and manifest verity, as far as any social scientific or natural scientific 'fact' can be established as proof infinitum, that material differences make the diagnosis of mental disorder more probable for those who are most disadvantaged.

According to Public Health England (2018) inequality affects people diagnosed with severe mental illness far more than the rest of the population. Consequently, their life expectancy is up to twenty years less than the average, and this gap is widening.

In a special report for the journal *Psychiatric Times* a team of psychiatrists (Simon et al., 2018) are unequivocal that there is evidence of a strong for a causal relationship between poverty and mental health. Whilst both economic inequality and poverty lead to higher rates in the diagnosis of mental disorder, they can and do act independently. Focusing on poverty, they affirm that children born into poverty and who continue to live in poor conditions are more likely to fail at school because their intellect and attention is underdeveloped, commit criminal offences, be diagnosed as anxious or depressed, and receive a diagnosis of mental disorder later in life. Suicide if also more common in adulthood for those brought up in poverty. These psychiatrists do not leave biology behind. For them there is a complex compound of biological and social mechanisms linking poverty to psychological distress, including stressful life experiences which lead to neurochemical and neurocircuitry malfunctioning. Financial difficulties due to impoverishment – but also family discord and emotional detachment, parental psychological distress (especially a diagnosis of depression), neglect of physical and intellectual needs, and exposure to abuse – all interfere with the working of the brain and it related biological systems. They observe, however, that few psychiatrists receive adequate training in assessing the effects of poverty on their patients and how to incorporate mitigating treatments.

Similar to Simon et al. (2018), neuroscientist Joe Herbert (2018) is clear that poverty has deleterious effects. Herbert lists these effects as feeling lonely, defeated, inferior, isolated, lonely. These feelings, argues Herbert, are accentuated when poorer people live in an unequal society because added to the psychological harm from poverty is the harm from comparison. Again, biology is linked to social circumstances with Herbert pointing to the 'stress' of poverty and inequality causing a rise in the release of the 'fight or flight' hormone cortisol. Cortisol, amongst other tasks in the body, responds to such stressors. The release of high levels of cortisol regularly or continuously may result in damage to physical health, especially disorders of the circulatory system, as well increase the possibility of a diagnosis of anxiety and depression. Herbert is cautious about causation. He points out that the evidence of associating poverty and inequality with mental disorder diagnoses does not prove causation, but the prospect for so doing is strong.

A meta-analysis of research examining income inequality, diagnoses of mental disorder, and resilience (the ability to cope with life's misfortunes), Wagner Ribeiro and colleagues concluded that greater inequality is associated with higher rates of mental illness particularly of depression and anxiety disorders, and if the association is causal then. They remark that many of the studies they reviewed point to small effects, and there is inconsistency in the quality and homogeneity of the extant research, and the influence of biology must also be considered. However, they speculate If this association is causal and growing income inequality does lead to an increase in the prevalence of mental health problems, then its reduction could improve markedly the well-being of a country's population.

In a study of French-speaking urban areas of Montreal in Canada over three decades, growing up in poverty was found to connect with increases in the diagnoses psychotic disorder (Hastings et al., 2019). The World Health Organisation (2014) also conceives that mental disorder is likely to be diagnosed for people living in deleterious social and physical environments. Deficient nutrition, polluted or inadequate supply of water, and economic disparity are linkable to anxiety, depression, schizophrenia, and alcohol and drug dependency. Regarding water, data from a joint project by World Health Organization and the United Nations Children's Fund (WHO/UNCF, 2019) reveal that globally 1 in 4 health care facilities lacks basic water services and 1 in 5 had no sanitation service. These unhygienic health care facilities are responsible for the care up to two billion of the world's population.

Epidemiologists Richard Wilkinson and Kate Pickett in their book *The Spirit Level* (2010) argue that societies with greater inequality also had a range of more pronounced social problems. Inequality is associable with higher rates of violence, murder, higher rates of imprisonment, drug abuse, imprisonment, obesity, teenage pregnancies, infant mortality, lower maternal survival, educational attainment employment opportunities, and increases in physical disorder in diagnoses of mental disorder. Moreover, they contend that businesses with sizeable salary differences are far less efficient, that is less productive and therefore less profitable than those with narrow remunerative ratios. Also, the cohesion of communities and trust between people was weaker in unequal societies. People, suggest Wilkinson and Pickett, simply get along with each much better in more equal societies. For them the overall consequence of considerable inequality was considerable 'social stress'.

Wilkinson and Pickett are emphatic that the correlations between income inequality and these social problems is not only association but causal. Inequality for Wilkinson and Pickett causes social stress and social stress damages people and society. What the key to that causality they submit is social status. Inequality causes serious social problems and social stress and status competition is the intervening causative factor. For example, when inequality is excessive and embedded in a society in which material wealth and the display and consumption of material commodities is valued highly then interpersonal competitiveness and insecurity rises accordingly. People with low status because they are at the low end of a highly unequal society is much more likely to suffer from low self-worth and therefore the above (socially created) problems.

However, journalist and libertarian Christopher Snowdon (2010) condemns Wilkinson and Pickett's 'Spirit Level' thesis as delusional and partial for confusing correlation with causation.. Sociologist Peter Saunders, another libertarian, declares much of the evidence presented in that book as weak, selective, superficial, and replete with 'spurious correlations' and 'wonky statistics' used to connect inequality to, for example, childhood trauma, homicide rates and suicide rates. Their theory therefore is invalid.

In their book *The Inner Level* Wilkinson and Pickett (2018) and in previous publications (for example, Pickett and Wilkinson, 2015; 2017) focus on the psychological stress of inequality. Appraising a multitude of statistical data, they argue that people suffer from high levels of 'social anxiety' (that is, 'social stress' or 'shyness') in contemporary society which is founded on neoliberal capitalist economic. A distinguishing feature of neoliberal capitalism is inequality. Following their review of hundreds of research studies Wilkinson and Pickett conclude that the relationship between inequality and an exacerbation of social anxiety as well as a conspicuous upturn in the diagnosis of other mental disorders, is causal.

Inequality increases what Wilkinson and Pickett refer to as 'social evaluative threat' or 'status anxiety'. Individuals are constantly comparing themselves to others and evaluating their self-worth based on those comparisons. Those with less income and fewer high-grade material possessions feel less worthy than those who are believed to be wealthier or whose wealth is paraded. CEOs of many large transnational corporations, comment Wilkinson and Pickett, receive salaries hundreds of times greater than the lowest paid employees in the same company. Self-perceptions of personal worth are commensurate with these salaries.

A culture of narcissism develops where there is high social anxiety and evaluative threat. But Wilkinson and Pickett identify it as a defense mechanism in those with low self-worth and those who are rich but who presumably have high self-worth. They also suggest that a culture which places high value on individualism, greed, 'turbo-consumerism', 'logos', and low value on cooperation, 'psychopathic tendencies' are more manifest. However, they resolve that most people are not narcissists or psychopaths. For them 'epidemics' of mental disorder, especially depression and anxiety, but also schizophrenia, are real. Both children and adults are affected. They also highlight that globally there are each year one million suicides.

Wilkinson and Picket are in no doubt that there are much higher rates of mental disorder and suicide in rich but unequal countries compared to poor but more equal societies. They contend that the evidence of association is overwhelming and persuasively indicative of a one-way origin. For example, they also acknowledge the role of biology but argue that brain imaging shows that an individual's position in the social hierarchy alters neurological structures and processes, not the other way around.

They do, however, overplay their hand and have a 'blunderbuss' explanatory taxonomy of inequality evils which is difficult to credit without qualification and pruning. They also throw into the mix biological and psychological evolutionary theoretical and epigenetic snippets to explain why humans perform the way they do today. But then they assert human performance is a 'learned way of life'. That is, culture determines more than biology how humans think, feel, and behave. For Snowdon (2018) *The Inner Level* is as partial and defectively researched as he claims was *The Spirit Level*. Snowdon also attacks this thesis for its many tangential, opaque, and irrelevant data and theory offerings. He accuses them of presenting an incoherent narrative in which folk wisdom, anecdote, hunches, and 'wild extrapolations' from scientific studies are mixed.

Inequality, argue Wilkinson and Picket, undermines economic growth. Inequality leads to economic stagnation and instability, and (slightly) reduces innovation. Companies with a bigger pay ratios amongst their employees are also less efficient. But they also state 'growth [economic] has largely finished its work' (2018, p. 215). A new economy is needed to deal with climate change. A post-capitalist 'new society', one with 'more democratic and egalitarian model of business' such as cooperatives. Confusingly, they maintain that cooperativeness is higher in countries that are more equal, and a 'new society' with more democratic and egalitarian model of business such as cooperatives can help to create a 'post capitalist' world. Cooperatives can and do participate in capitalism. Cooperatives can't at the same time be a cause and consequence of a new society. Moreover, they do not elaborate sufficiently on what a novel political economic model for this new society. There is no sophisticated political and economic theory to replace the theories which have underpinned capitalism, communism, neo-conservatism, and communitarianism, or any of their derivatives.

A meta-analysis of research conducted concluded that rates of mental illness were higher in societies with larger income differences. The UK and the US are at the top of the graph on both mental illness and income inequality. If a country is materially well off, as measured by the gross-domestic-product per person, this is not linkable to diagnoses such as anxiety and depression. Material wellbeing protects individuals from rather than abandoning them to psychological distress.

Unequal power

Difference in the siting and circulation of power in society is the root of much wealth inequality and poverty. Thereby, power inequity is rooted in the making of madness.

Criminologist Scott Bonn (2017) uses the concept of the 'power elite' from the work of sociologist C. Wright Mills who he describes as visionary. Sixty years previously, Mills (1956) had described a 'power elite' as a small group of wealthy individuals made up of corporate owners, chief executives, senior military officers, and politicians, and who have substantial influence over social policy. This description for Bonn stands today. The power elite pursue their own interests without due respect to the morality of their decisions, manipulating society mostly in secrecy. The power elite is not made up of a homogenous group of people and is not entirely a closed order. Although most come from similar social backgrounds, there are social outsiders accepted especially those who have made fortunes or become prevalent politically, and regularly, there are new entrants (and presumably some leave, perhaps when they lose their fortunes or their political clout). What binds them are the values and practices associated with the accumulation and protection of wealth, and the social networks to which they belong. Furthermore, the power elite reproduce themselves by passing on to future generations their wealth, and introducing their offspring to the same social networks, schools and universities, and employment opportunities that they had enjoyed.

Power and privilege, argue Oxfam International (2016), is used to skew the economic system to increase the financial benefits of those people who already occupy the rich section of global society or heading towards that social stratum, to the detriment of those who are already impoverished or in danger of falling into that category. But it is not only the poor who are disadvantaged by the skewing of power but the rest of population who aren't rich. Power has been used to construct global network of tax havens which allow the rich to hide their wealth, avoid taxation, and utilise it nefariously to maximise profit.

Concentrated power and wealth have resulted in the share of a country's income going to ordinary workers falling whilst the share going to owners of and senior executives running large corporations, along with and their political associates, has increased significantly. In countries which have increased their gross national product over previous decades, workers are losing more and more of their share from growth. This has occurred in almost all rich countries and in most developing countries (Oxfam International, 2016). One again, paradox arises.

It is Monbiot's observation that inequality within the workplace furnishes an unequal impact on the environment that provides this example of irony.

> The most lucrative, prestigious jobs tend to cause the greatest harm [corporate chief executives]. The most useful workers [care workers] tend to be paid the least and treated the worst.
>
> (Monbiot, 2017, p. 184)

Not only is there huge power and remunerative differentials at work (and in society overall), but the actions of the corporate elite in maximising their company's profit and in spending their inflated salaries causes a huge difference in the amount of damage done to the physical environment.

Powerful political allies of the rich, who themselves benefit either in their careers or financial by so doing, have implemented polices to favour the rich. Cronyism between politicians and the rich over the last thirty years has allowed the long-standing ability of the powerfully rich to protect and then further their power and to become 'supercharged'. Reduction of corporate and capital gains tax, deregulation of rules on business operations, the lack of regulation on tax avoidance, intensified regulation of trade unions, and the privatisation of former State-owned assets and services, austerity measures for public spending, along with tax havens, have contributed to the fruitful enactment of power. Power has and continues to pay-off through cronyism, and the ways in which it does can be considered as corrupt (Oxfam International, 2019b).

A plethora of research, records political scientist Bo Rothstein (2018), again underscores the negative impact of wealth inequality. These include higher levels of violence and lower levels of satisfaction with life. What Rothstein focuses on is the reduction of trust in society. There are, suggests Rothstein, two types of trust. Social trust refers to the extent to which individuals believe and rely on other individuals. Institutional trust refers to which society's organisations such as political parties, the police and judiciary, and the media, can be believed and relied upon. What is paramount in terms of overall trust, posits Rothstein, is that the public sphere is not regarded as corrupt – which it is inevitably when there is a marked disparity in wealth.

It is, states Oxfam International (2019b), 'market fundamentalism' that drives this process of embedding power and wealth inequity into what has become a globalised economic system. That system is sustained by a hoard of well-paid professional advisers from the trades of finance and banking, financial law, accounting, and investment. The intellectual legitimacy for market fundamentalism is derives from the philosophy of 'neoliberalism' (Biebricher, 2019). Dorling (2018) blames the Prime Ministership of Margaret Thatcher and that of Tony Blair for inequality rising in Britain because they either explicitly or in effect drove a neoliberal economic policy.

Economist Angus Deaton (2019) believes that inequality as it is today is threatening 'democratic capitalism' in much of the developed world. He is supportive of capitalism because it has, he maintains, lifted billions of people out of deprivation, provided employment for much of the world's population, and a cornucopia of goods and services. But what it hasn't provided is equality. He associates that deficiency in contemporary capitalism with a decrease in lifespan, in some of the richest countries, an increase in suicide, and drug and alcohol abuse and the diseases they generate. These lethal consequences of capitalism arise from an intensification in the misery of everyday life which again results from how this economic system has 'matured' – that is, become neoliberal.

Oxfam International's answer to neoliberalism is what it describes is a 'human economy'. This alternative system is characterised first by a righting of the wrongs which favour the rich over the rest (for example: get rid of tax havens; re-establishing the legitimacy of workers to strike; boosting public spending on health and education). A human economy, founded on justice and inclusion, would furnish economic prosperity (Oxfam International, 2019b). Inequality has been cited, suggests Oxfam International, as an important element in the election of Donald Trump as President of the USA, the election in the Philippines of Rodrigo Roa Duterte, and the UK electorate voting to leave the European Union. What Oxfam is recommending is a renovation, not the transformation, of society. It is not promoting of even perceiving an alternative to economic prosperity.

Neoliberal economic prosperity has allowed the accumulation of enormous assets by a few people. Oxfam International (2009b) lists some of the richest people in the world:

1   Bill Gates, founder of Microsoft, has a fortune amounting to $75 billion;
2   Amancio Ortega, founder of one of the world's largest fashion firms Inditex, $67 billion;
3   Warren Buffett, Chief Executive and largest shareholder in the multi-national conglomerate Berkshire Hathaway, 60.8 billion;
4   Carlos Slim Helu owner of the retail, industrial, and construction conglomerate Grupo Carso, $50 billion;
5   Jeff Bezos, founder, chairman and chief executive of Amazon, $45.2 billion;
6   Mark Zuckerberg: American chairman, chief executive officer, and co-founder of Facebook, $44.6 billion.

Regarding salaries, John Hammergren of the USA medical supply company McKesson was the highest earner in 2018. His salary came to $131.2 million (*Forbes*, 2019). The annual salary of the Chief Executive Officer of the British Oxfam in 2018 for that year was £130,308 (Oxfam GB, 2019). In the same year the median average UK salary was £29,588 (Office of National Statistics, 2018b).

Economist and Nobel laureate Joseph Stiglitz (2012) argues that the exercise of political power by the rich over legislative and regulatory processes has conditioned the economic system to advantage the powerful at the expense of the rest. However, Stiglitz also argues that a free and competitive market benefits society, and then contradicts himself by stating that the only way it can function effectively and remain beneficial to society, is through 'government regulation and oversight'. For Stiglitz, inequality is especially destructive to society as it stifles economic growth by not using what he designates as its 'most valuable asset' – by which he means people.

Sam Dumitriu, an advocate of 'personal and economic freedom' and Head of Research at the think-tank the British 'free market' Adam Smith Institute claims that reports on inequality by agencies such as Oxfam are misleading. For Dumitriu, the world's poorest have received a massive pay rise because of neoliberalism except in those countries in which it hasn't been implemented. Therefore, what is needed is not less but more neoliberalism: '[I]n a free market individuals can only amass wealth by fulfilling the wants and needs of others. Work and trade does pay out for everyone involved' (Dumitriu quoted in Kilcoyne 2018).

Dumitriu uses the examples of the governments of China India and Vietnam, who have, he contends, raised the living standards of the poorest in their respective countries and they have done this by embracing the ideals of neoliberalism. These ideals include, reducing government interference in trade and commerce, enforcing property rights, and encouraging competitiveness. He also makes the point that rather concentrating on the wealth of the rich are doing, what organisation like Oxfam should be doing is caring about is the welfare of the poor.

The Brookings Institution is a USA think-tank comprising hundreds of what it refers to as 'scholars' who research public policies nationally and globally. It makes a similar point to that of Dumitriu by the claiming that half of the world's population by 2018 could be classified as middle class (Kharas and Hamel, 2018).

> For the first time since agriculture-based civilization began 10,000 years ago, the majority of humankind is no longer poor or vulnerable to falling into poverty. [J]ust over 50 percent of the world's population, or some 3.8 billion people, live in households with enough discretionary expenditure to be considered 'middle class' or 'rich'.

However, the Brookings report goes on to state that roughly the same proportion of the world's population are classifiable as poor or could easily become impoverished. Hence there are, for Brookings there seems to be two 'majorities', the rich and the poor.

Kenan Malik (2018), writer and academic with a background in neurobiology and the history of science, points out that Brookings are defining 'middle class' as 'not poor'. By implication, Malik argues, Bookings appear to be conflating middle class with 'ordinary folk' rather than a specific element of the social strata between working class and upper class. By using 'class' and 'discretionary expenditure' in their analysis Brookings have added confusion about global changes in wealth distribution and the cultural aspects and working conditions relating to differences in income. Many in Brookings' 'middle class', and more in the ones who have yet to enter that class, are forced to labour in demeaning circumstances, with minimal wages and limited rights. This is no less so in those countries cited by Brookings as having tipped over into middle-classness.

What Brookings also neglects, no matter the size of what it claims to be the middle-class, is an appreciation of how inequality in power remains flagrantly reified. Apart from the conspicuousness of enormous wealth which is not readily observable in the day-to-day lives of the poor (and in those Brookings considers 'middle class'), it is apparent perpetually in digital news, documentary, and popular entertainment, as well communicated through social media.

But, the most devastating reification of power differentials enacted through the neoliberal political programme is early death. For Dorling and Gietel-Basten (2017) there is no inherent biological reason for the reversal life expectancy in the UK. The ultimate culprit for them is likely to be societal in the form of the social policy of austerity introduced in 2010 by the British Government which, they contend, reduced welfare and health services for the elderly. A million early deaths in the UK could, they suggest, could be avoided if the knowledge about inequality furnished by social scientists and epidemiologists was utilised by the politically powerful.

Psychologist and psychoanalyst Paul Verhaeghe (2014) argues that neoliberalism has brought out the worst in people. Market fundamentalism for him is marked by increased inequality, 'universal egotism', and a rise in mental disorder. He also suggests that the workplace has become Kafkaesque. Conditions for millions of employed people are nightmarish because bureaucratic control and scrutiny, monitoring, measuring, auditing, and bullying have become standard. Neoliberalism is extracting the most it can from workers for the benefit of the bosses and shareholders of business.

For psychiatrist Jonathan Burns (Burns et al., 2014; Burns 2015) the continuous stress of living in highly disparate social circumstances increases the risk of schizophrenia. Burns argues it is indisputable that a relationship between inequality, poverty, and mental disorder exists. What causes inequality and poverty, and thereby susceptibility to a diagnosis of schizophrenia, is neoliberalism. Neoliberal (market-oriented) political doctrines lead to both increased income inequality and reduced social cohesion. Sociologist David Coburn (2000; 2004) also regards neoliberal polices such deliberately undermining welfare provision, with their legacy of inequality, as culpable in the reduced cohesion of society. Burns (Burns et al., 2014; Burns, 2015) affirms that income inequality must be included as a significant factor in researching the complex causes of schizophrenia.

Energetic power

Philosopher Roger Foster (2017) attempts to unify Marxist and Foucauldian ideas about the 'success' of neoliberalism by introducing Fromm's idea of 'social character. Fromm (1941; 1955; 1962; 1965) positions an idea about how social and economic arrangements such as capitalism and communism become inculcated culturally and personally. He regards both Foucauldian notion of 'governmentality' (Burchell et al., 1991) and Marxist notion of hegemony (Gramsci, 1971) as inadequate to explain the enculturation and internalisation of such systems. Foucault and Marx imply a dissemination of ideological control from the centralised elites down to masses. For Foucault this is achieved through a multitude of micro-processes and institutions which, taken together, push people towards performances consanguine to the interests of the powerful. For Marx it is more heavy-handed indoctrination delivered by a centralised elite via specific institutions of ideological and physical control – the media, education, religion, the police and the judiciary.

The masses, under a neoliberal system, have become accepting of competition, individual responsibility, and consumerism to the point that these tenets have become a way of life that is experienced as natural and legitimate. These tenets are virtually the opposite of those under a communist (or socialist) regime and at variance with those of other configurations of capitalism. Fromm attempts to answer the conundrum of how both become tolerated, if not savoured, by their respective populations. Foster's adoption of Fromm's concept of 'social character' is his attempt to answer the conundrum of how the neoliberal version of capitalism is considered in the main 'sane' by a global population despite its blatant discriminations, disasters, and disorderliness. Notwithstanding financial crises, global warming, and the accumulation of immense riches by a minority, it remains 'common sense' for most people.

For Foster (2017), the concept of social character is useful because it illustrates how the everyday experiences of individuals become fused with the tenets of the overarching social and economic system. Fromm, points out Foster, did not agree that people were simply empty vessels into which the elites could pour their self-serving missives. Nor for Fromm, points out Foster, are they knowingly arranging and absorbing into a whole the disparate communications from divergent sources which somehow coincide with the contingencies of free-market capitalism. There is a dynamic occurring involving individuals and societal structures and processes which is active and fluid, from which socialised human performance is created, and which fits with the dominant social and economic set-up.

Social character is not the set of opinions and preferences which make-up an individual's disposition, but the deep elements in the self which drive human performance, and which are beyond the drive to satisfy basic needs related to survival. These deep elements are the consequence of the interplay between social prescription and personal preference. However, personal preference has been shaped by the promise of personal pleasure and fulfilment and social success being possible by indulging the doctrines of the social and economic system in question. Moreover, neoliberalism has shifted the allegiance of a global population from other systems by and large through amplifying internal controls rather than engaging external threats. Self-responsibility along with individual rights are reciprocal principles reinforcing personal ownership and social legitimacy of neoliberalism and are basics of neoliberalism's version of social character (Foster, 2017).

However, there is madness inherent in fusing the personal with the socio-economic. Fromm fuses his psychoanalytic notion of 'psychic energy' with his more sociological understanding of how power operates in society. Unlike in classic Freudian thought, psychic energy does not originate from internal drives. Fromm's notion of psychic energy is not libidinous in character but societal. It is human vitality born from her/his social circumstances. 'Psychic energy' could be understood as 'cognitive dissonance' (Festinger, 1957). That is, holding two or more contradictory beliefs, values, or attitudes which then may lead to muddled thinking and inconsistent behaviours, can give rise to severe psychological discomfort, and changes in brain functioning (Gumley, et al., 1999). If severe, cognitive dissonance may also furnish the ascription of mental disorder, or considered to be a symptom of psychosis (Buckley, 2015).

For Fromm some social circumstances extinguish, stifle, or elicit psychic turmoil. Fromm refers to the possible occurrence of what he calls 'socially patterned defects'. These defects are the outcome of any unresolved tension between basic human needs and/or those which fit other social and economic systems and the requirements of the one attempting to assert its dominance, in this case neoliberalism. Inequality has its losers and some of them may still experience their disadvantage as exactly that no matter how powerful the messages about this being natural. People may, for Fromm, suffer socially engineered psychological disturbance, that is pathological psychic energy. Apparent epidemics of anxiety and depression may represent the outcome of an imperfect fusion between the needs of the populace and the needs of neoliberalism. Should these such features as inequality be experienced by more and more people as psychologically disturbing then the pressure will build for social transformation.

Just as neoliberalism encouraged and harnessed the (pathological) psychic energy experienced in previous societal circumstances to dominate how global society operates politically and economically, psychic energy can be encouraged and harnessed by a competitor. Political activists Jeremy Heimans and Henry Timms (2018) write about 'new power' which has come about because the networked age has revolutionised interpersonal and international communication, and how people engage with institutions and organisations. New power, suggest Heimans and Timms, is typified by collaboration, participation, and transparency, and devolvement of power to ordinary citizens. Mostly this new power comes about through the services and movements connected to digital communications, in particular the fluidity and spread of novel ideas and political and human rights campaigns in social media. 'Old-power' is typified by State, political, judicial, business, media, and educational institutions with rigid formal structures, and centralised and 'top-down' control. 'Hyper-connectivity' has empowered communities and minority groups as well as offering the majority a more democratic voice to, for example, fight inequality. However, the same technology is manipulatable by those already with (old) power and those who have grabbed big slices of new power. The use of algorithms by the internet commercial sector, and proscriptions on internet use by governments, undermine the benefits of new power.

Summary

Fromm's Marxist-orientated perspective, rather than his Foucault-Marx variant, shows that the globalisation of Western-inspired capitalism with the proliferation of international and intranational inequality is unambiguously a powerful example of social insanity. Western-inspired capitalism has become the dominant economic system and one which has concentrated power and possessions in an outstandingly privileged minority. Material disadvantage correlates with, and is probably causative of, madness in its medicalised forms of mental disorder such as anxiety and depression but may well also include psychotic disorders such as schizophrenia.

Both wealth inequality and poverty are linkable to the distribution of power in society. Being rich is the, most significant resource in exercising power in political arenas. Above and beyond factors such as educational attainment, inherited or achieved social status, entrepreneurial spirit, and military might (all of which may be connected to wealth either as precursors or corollaries), sizable incomes and/or considerable assets are used to gain political power.

A global power elite containing the very wealthy, leaders of big business, politicians, military chiefs, and media moguls, stands above all other social classes. Its power is pervasive, insidious, and advertently or inadvertently habitually nefarious. On the other hand, being in absolute poverty, whereby basic resources for survival are absent or precarious, or relatively poor, whereby the resources you own or to which you have access are noticeable few compared to others within the local, national, and global milieu, generates disempowerment.

In what way can this be a sane way to run the world? To recalibrate a phrase used by Alston (2018), wealth inequality, poverty, and the distribution of power is a political choice. So is social sanity.

Selfishness, the topic for the next chapter, is another questionable societal trait, as well as a dubious personal attribute. No matter its debatable standing, selfishness is rampaging through global society, at times expressed excessively as narcissism, and accompanied by its materialistic bedfellows of consumerism. It will be contended in Chapter 5 that selfishness, narcissism, and consumerism are an outstandingly malignant personal trouble and a virulently malign social issue.

Note

1 Origin of this quotation is unknown although it has been attributed to a range of sources including Narcotics Anonymous, Albert Einstein, and Benjamin Franklin.

References

Alston P (2018) *Statement on Visit to the United Kingdom, by Professor Philip Alston, United Nations Special Rapporteur on Extreme Poverty and Human Rights.* Office of the High Commissioner for Human Rights, 16 November. https://ohchr.org/EN/NewsEvents/Pages/DisplayNews.aspx?LangID=E&NewsID=23881 [accessed 18 November, 2018].

Alvaredo F, Chancel L, Piketty T, Saez E and Zucman G (2018) *World Inequality Report 2018.* Paris: World Inequality Lab.

Biebricher T (2019) *The Political Theory of Neoliberalism.* Stanford, CA: Stanford University Press.

Bonn S (2017) Beware of the power elite in society: A warning from the grave. *Psychology Today*, 7th August. www.psychologytoday.com/gb/blog/wicked-deeds/201708/beware-the-power-elite-in-society-0 [accessed 10 February, 2019].

Buckley T (2015) What happens to the brain during cognitive dissonance? *Scientific America*, 26(6), p. 72. www.scientificamerican.com/article/what-happens-to-the-brain-during-cognitive-dissonance1/ [accessed 5 March, 2019].

Burchell G, Gordon C and Miller P (eds) (1991) *The Foucault Effect: Studies in Governmentality.* Chicago, IL: University of Chicago Press.

Burns J (2015) Poverty, inequality and a political economy of mental health. *Epidemiological Psychiatric Science*, 24(2), pp.107–113.

Burns J, Tomita M and Kapadia A (2014) Income inequality and schizophrenia: Increased schizophrenia incidence in countries with high levels of income inequality. *International Journal of Social Psychiatry*, 60(2), pp. 185–196.

Coburn D (2000) Income inequality, social cohesion and the health status of populations: The role of neo-liberalism. *Social Science and Medicine* 51(1), pp. 135–146.

Coburn D (2004) Beyond the income inequality hypothesis: Class, neo-liberalism, and health inequalities. *Social Science and Medicine*, 58(1), pp. 41–56.

Cockerham W (2013) *Sociology of Mental Disorder*, 9th edn. New York: Routledge.

Deaton A (2019) A speech given by Sir Angus Deaton at the launch of the IFS Deaton Review, 14 May, 2019. www.ifs.org.uk/inequality/expert-comment/inequality-and-the-future-of-capitalism/ [accessed 25 July, 2019].

Dorling D (2018) *Peak Inequality.* Bristol: Policy Press.

Dorling D and Gietel-Basten S (2017a) Life expectancy in Britain has fallen so much that a million years of life could disappear by 2058 – why? *The Conversation*, 29 November.

http://theconversation.com/life-expectancy-in-britain-has-fallen-so-much-that-a-million-years-of-life-could-disappear-by-2058-why-88063 [accessed 27 February, 2019].

Dorling D and Gietel-Basten S (2017b) *Why Demography Matters.* Cambridge: Polity.

Festinger T (1957) *A Theory of Cognitive Dissonance.* Stanford, CA: Stanford University Press.

Forbes (2019) Ten highest paid CEOs. www.forbes.com/pictures/eggh45jef/john-hamm ergren-of-mckesson/#71da4aa26ead [accessed 3 March, 2019].

Foster R (2017) Social character: Erich Fromm and the ideological glue of neoliberalism. *Critical Horizons* 18(1), pp. 1–18.

Fromm E (1955) *The Sane Society.* New York: Rinehart.

Fromm E (1962) *Beyond the Chains of Illusion.* New York: Simon and Shuster.

Fromm E (1941) *Escape from Freedom.* New York: Farrar & Rinehart.

Fromm E (1965) *Man for Himself: An Inquiry into the Psychology of Ethics.* New York: Premier.

Gramsci A (1971) *Selections from the Prison Notebooks.* New York: International Publishers.

Gumley A, White C and Power K (1999) An interacting cognitive subsystems model of relapse and the course of psychosis. *Clinical Psychology and Psychotherapy,* 6, pp. 261–278.

Hastings P, Serbin L, Bukowski L, Helm J, Stack D, Dickson D, Ledingham J and Schwartzman A (2019) Predicting psychosis-spectrum diagnoses in adulthood from social behaviors and neighborhood contexts in childhood. *Development and Psychopathology,* 31(4), pp. 1–15.

Heimans J and Timms H (2018) *New Power: How It's Changing The 21st Century – And Why You Need to Know.* London: MacMillan.

Helliwell J, Huang H and Wang S (2019) Changing world happiness. In Helliwell J, Layard R and Sachs J (eds) *World Happiness Report (2019) World Happiness Report.* New York: Sustainable Development Solutions Network, pp. 10–46.

Herbert J (2018) The scandal of inequality and its effect on mental health: Financial inequality seems to be a major risk for mental illness. *Psychology Today,* 17 November, www.psychologytoday.com/gb/blog/hormones-and-the-brain/201811/the-scandal-inequality-and-its-effect-mental-health [accessed 11 February, 2019].

Kharas H and Hamel K (2018) A global tipping point: Half the world is now middle class or wealthier. The Brookings Institution, 27 September. www.brookings.edu/blog/future-development/2018/09/27/a-global-tipping-point-half-the-world-is-now-m iddle-class-or-wealthier/ [accessed 19 February, 2019].

Kilcoyne M (2018) *Oxfam's Inequality Mistake.* 22 January, Adam Smith Institute. www.adamsmith.org/news/oxfam-mistake-inequality-figures [accessed 19 February, 2019].

Lund C (2015) Poverty, inequality and mental health in low–and middle-income countries: Time to expand the research and policy agendas. *Epidemiology and Psychiatric Sciences,* 24(2), pp. 97–99.

Malik K (2018) As global poverty declines, we should beware the new class wars. *The Observer,* 7 October.

Mills C W (1956) *The Power Elite.* New York: Oxford University Press.

Monbiot G (2017) *How Did We Get Into This Mess?: Politics, Equality, Nature.* London: Verso.

Monbiot G (2018) *Out of the Wreckage. A New Politics for An Age of Crisis.* London: Verso.

National Center for Health Statistics [USA]. (2018) *Health, United States, 2017: With Special Feature on Mortality.* Hyattsville, MA: National Center for Health Statistics.

Office for National Statistics (ONS) (2018a) National life tables, UK: 2015 to 2017. Office for National Statistics, 25 September. www.ons.gov.uk/peoplepopula tionandcommunity/birthsdeathsandmarriages/lifeexpectancies/bulletins/nationallif etablesunitedkingdom/2015to2017#main-points [accessed 27 February, 2019].

Office forNational Statistics (ONS) (2018b) Employee earning in the UK: 2018. Press release, 25 October. www.ons.gov.uk/employmentandlabourmarket/peopleinwork/ea rningsandworkinghours/bulletins/annualsurveyofhoursandearnings/2018 [accessed 22 February, 2019].

Organisation for Economic Co-operation and Development (OECD) (2018a) About the OECD. www.oecd.org/about/ [accessed 13 February, 2019].

Organisation for Economic Co-operation and Development (OECD) (2018b) Income inequality. https://data.oecd.org/inequality/income-inequality.htm [accessed 6 February, 2019].

OxfamGB (2019) *Oxfam Annual Report & Accounts 2017/18 Trustees Annual Report.* Oxford: Oxfam.

OxfamInternational (2016) *An Economy for the 1%: How Privilege and Power in the Economy Drive Extreme Inequality and How this can be Stopped* [Oxfam Briefing Paper 210]. Nairobi, Kenya: Oxfam International.

OxfamInternational (2019a) History of Oxfam International. www.oxfam.org/en/coun tries/history-oxfam-international [accessed 18 February, 2019].

Oxfam International (2019b) *Public Good or Private Wealth?* Nairobi, Kenya: Oxfam International.

Patel V and Kleinman A (2003) Poverty and common mental disorders in developing countries. *Bulletin of the World Health Organisation*, 81(8), pp. 609–615.

Pickett K and Wilkinson R (2010) Inequality: An underacknowledged source of mental illness and distress. *Br J Psychiatry*, 197(6), pp. 426–428.

Pickett K and Wilkinson R (2015) Income inequality and health: A causal review. *Social Science & Medicine*, 128, pp. 316–326.

Platt L (2019) *Understanding Inequalities Stratification and Difference*, 2nd edn. Cambridge: Polity.

Public Health England (2018) Health matters: Reducing health inequalities in mental illness. www.gov.uk/government/publications/health-matters-reducing-health-inequalitie s-in-mental-illness/health-matters-reducing-health-inequalities-in-mental-illness [accessed 11 February, 2019].

Ribeiro W, Bauer A, Andrade M, York-Smith M, Pan P, Pingani L, Knapp M, Coutinho E and Evans-Lacko S (2017) Income inequality and mental illness-related morbidity and resilience: A systematic review and meta-analysis. *The Lancet*, 4(7), pp. 554–562.

Rogers A and Pilgrim D (2014) *A Sociology of Mental Health and Illness.* Maidenhead: McGraw-Hill.

Rothstein B (2018) How the trust trap perpetuates inequality: Corruption, distrust and inequality reinforce one another in a destructive loop. *Scientific America*, 1 November. www.scientificamerican.com/article/how-the-trust-trap-perpetuates-ine quality/ [accessed 9 February, 2018].

Saunders, P. (2010) *Beware False Prophets: Equality, the Good Society and The Spirit Level.* London: Policy Exchange.

Simon K, Beder M and Manseau M (2018) Addressing poverty and mental illness. *Psychiatric Times*. www.psychiatrictimes.com/special-reports/addressing-poverty-and-mental-illness [accessed 11 February, 2019].

Snowdon C (2010) The spirit level delusion: Fact-checking the left's new theory of everything. Washington, DC: Democracy Institute.

Snowdon C (2018) The inequality syndrome: The inner level is as myopic and poorly researched as its predecessor, the spirit level. *Spiked Magazine*, 23 July. www.spiked-online.com/2018/07/23/the-inequality-syndrome/#.W37JwX4nbuQ [accessed 2 March 2019].

Stiglitz J (2012) *The Price of Inequality*. London: W. W. Norton & Company.

Verhaeghe P (2014) *What About Me?: The Struggle for Identity in a Market-Based Society*. London: Scribe.

Wilkinson I (2005) *Suffering: A Sociological Introduction*. Cambridge. Polity.

Wilkinson R and Pickett K (2010) *The Spirit Level: Why Equality is Better for Everyone*. London: Penguin.

Wilkinson R and Pickett K (2017) Inequality and mental illness. *The Lancet*, 4(70), pp. 512–513.

Wilkinson R and Pickett K (2018) *The Inner Level: How More Equal Societies Reduce Stress, Restore Sanity and Improve Everyone's Wellbeing*. London: Allen Lane.

World Health Organisation (WHO) (2018) 9 out of 10 people worldwide breathe polluted air, but more countries are taking action. New Release, 2 May. www.who.int/news-room/detail/02-05-2018-9-out-of-10-people-worldwide-breathe-polluted-air-but-more-countries-are-taking-action [accessed 2 May 2018].

World Health Organization/United Nations Children's Fund (WHO/UNCF) (2019) *WASH in Health Care Facilities: Global Baseline Report 2019*. Geneva: World Health Organization and the United Nations Children's Fund.

5   Selfishness

As has been revealed in previous chapters, there is, as with most if not all personal and societal subjects, including every personal madness and societal insanity covered in the book, complexity. That complexity frequently includes paradox. The subject in this chapter, selfishness, is no exception.

Journalist and novelist William Storr (2017) plots the antecedents for individualism, ego-centrism, self-love, and self-promotion, back to ancient Greek society. Hiatuses have occurred in the overall historical trajectory towards a society based mainly on selfishness by intrusion of less self-regarding religious and political beliefs, social turmoil in which self-preservation not promotion of the self is of primary concern, and the more communitarian values of 'traditional' cultures. Storr, however, considers these qualities to have been re-affirmed in the USA, particularly through the neoliberal brand of capitalism. Selfishness has accompanied the spread of this unfettered profit-driven and deregulated economic mode globally from the 1970s onwards. Globalisation, and its concomitant capitalist system, endorses the 'autarkic' human. The self-sufficient, self-motivated, self-directing, autonomous, 'me-first' individual is an essential component of contemporary capitalism.

Paradoxically, an autarkic society implies a closed economic system whereas the ideal typification of global capitalism, underpinned by neoliberal values, is openness. A further paradox, and one which is palpable in everyday experience, is human inter-reliance whereby routinely and necessarily, individuals cooperate with other individuals at work, at home, and in leisure activities (Beck and Beck-Gernsheim, 2001). Atomisation and corporation would, therefore, appear to co-exist with mutual obligation and do so alongside increased digitalisation of daily life, the spread of networks and institutions worldwide, the normalisation of narcissism, as well as marked variations in levels of social trust (Ortiz-Ospina and Roser, 2016). Selfishness can only be considered a societal insanity, therefore, if that paradox is socially sanctified, societally suitable, and without sequelae. There are, however, several severe side-effects from selfishness for the self and society.

Writer and broadcaster Ruth Whippman (2016) points to one such side-effect arising from the paradoxical mix of individual self-sufficiency and globalised capitalistic interconnectivity. British-born Whippman comments on how, in her adopted home of the USA, there is an obsession amongst the middle-classes with personal happiness. But, she adds, this obsessiveness is making people miserable.

Moreover, the societal backdrop for what would appear to be individualistic desire is a self-help industry Whippman calculates to be worth more than $11 billion. The trade of this industry is pushing products advertised as motivating, achieving, soothing, actualising, spiritualising, and empowering. Achieving happiness through such personal endeavours has become, argues Whippman, has become a mark of social success. Whippman adds that serenity as a supreme aspiration had been only a middle-class mantra but is being adopted even by the poor.

The biggest difference between the habits of the middle-class populations in Britain and the USA, argues Whitman, is the latter is obsessed with attaining happiness or at least contentment and doing so through personal effort. Happiness-achieving strategies include mindfulness, self-help literature, internet courses, motivational trainers, yoga, meditation, spiritual direction, and problem-orientated or profound psychotherapy. People are training themselves to react to tribulations and possibilities with 'yes and' rather than 'no but', reframing failures as 'learning opportunities', and generally to be psychologically positive about whatever life presents including the inevitability of death. For Whitman, happiness in the USA has become the ultimate personal trophy, a sign of high social status which outranks occupational and financial success. She suggests that even that family and sexual relationships are foregone if they intrude on either the individual's road to or state of happiness. The self-help happiness doctrine is seeping through society, encouraging even the poorest that her/his individual hard-work will bring the reward of supreme serenity.

Striving for serenity, however, is not only questionable functionally and morally as a human goal, it is riven with incongruity. Happiness may never be attained, it may remain a goal and in so doing overlap with other self-defeating and inescapable emotional spirals such as worrying about worrying and feeling miserable about feeling miserable. These spirals become locked into an autonomic biological and psychological feedback loop making those involved vulnerable to a diagnosis of mental disorder entailing medical strategies which may only contain angst and misery rather than impel bliss. Moreover, the attainment of happiness through personal effort fits with capitalist ideology, especially, notes Whippman, the extreme version found in the USA. Individuals striving for personal perfection diverts attention from the imperfections in society which may be the source of personal deficiencies. The strain of battling for happiness in society in which unhappiness is systemically attuned is, suggests Whippman, a recipe for anxiety. Whippman provides examples of the systemic miseries in the USA: long working hours, little or no paid holidays, insecure employment, high rents, and inadequate health care coverage. Failing to be happy attracts 'victim-blaming' self-admonishment and negative reactions from others. The 'rat-race' to succeed in sublimity, as with all rat-races, has many more losers than winners, and this race has built-in impediments for all participants. No wonder, muses Whippman, the USA has such high levels of both despondency and discontent. Unhappiness and anxiety are different sides of the same contradictory cultural coin.

Narcissism

Seeking of happiness for oneself has a personal and societal cost. An orientation to satisfying the self means that commitments to society, community, and the family, are de facto secondary and perhaps altogether neglected. Time and effort spent by individuals on flattering their egos, pursuing personalised nirvanas, and profligate eroticism, undermine authentic affiliation to others and cultural mutualisation.

Full-blown devotion to achieving happiness is a severe form of selfishness and full-blown selfishness has been categorised as a mental disorder by psychiatrists since the mid-twentieth century (Morrall, 2017). An amplified sense of self-importance, hyperbolic self-promotion, profuse attention-seeking, and having little or no interest in others apart from feigning curiosity to gain further attention and/or to gain in one way or another for one's self, are symptoms of a 'narcissistic personality disorder'. Diagnosis hinges, however, on a symptom which narcissistic personality disorder has in common with personality disorder *per se*, that is the absence of empathy (Baron-Cohen, 2012).

Moving the focus from the narcissistic performance of the individual to that of society, historian and social critic Christopher Lasch (1979) suggests that a 'culture of narcissism' had begun in the nineteenth century and increased in intensity towards the latter part of the twentieth century. Lasch does not draw a link between the arrival of neoliberal tenets and the growth of narcissism but the timing corresponds.

Narcissism for Lasch is endemic and extolled in Western culture. Lasch was writing about narcissism in the 1970s. Had he been writing today he might judge that the lauding of narcissism has become global. Notwithstanding its partial (but still emphatic) geographical spread supposed by Lasch, he argued that it was not normal. Lasch had been influenced by Freud's idea about narcissism. Narcissism for Freud (1914) was necessary for the individual's understanding of his/her notion of 'self'. Introspection and auto-admiration are for Freud part of a process of development which would be followed by the socialisation of the individual to contain the ego's otherwise excesses. The psyche, for Freud and Lasch, becomes marred because of unrestrained egotism. For both Freud and Lasch there is also the marring of society if egos are uninhibited. A neither individual (adult) narcissism or a culture of narcissism can therefore be regarded as normal.

As did Lasch, psychologists Jean Twenge and Keith Campbell (2009) acknowledge that pathological narcissism in the individual (which could attract a diagnosis of narcissistic personality disorder) is not identical to the normalisation of narcissism furnished by a narcissistic culture. However, for Twenge and Campbell there is an intertwining of pathological narcissism in individuals and cultural narcissism. One feeds off and into the other. The cultural normalisation of narcissism conjoined with an escalation in the number of 'normal' narcissists, and the diagnosis of narcissistic pathology in other individuals, is difficult to disentangle and trying may be pointless. Where social approval is conferred on selfishness, and admiration is amplified if the selfish are socially successful, then this is 'normal' even if the individual concerned might have otherwise earned a diagnosis of pathology. Two characteristics of narcissists culturally conducive personality, her/his high level of grandiosity and absence of empathy, can be functional to core social intuitions. They may assist personal and organisational success in politics, business, and banking. Narcissists may have a competitive edge when attempting to achieve corporate and civic senior office (Ronson, 2012).

Contrarily, Twenge and Campbell go on to argue that a culture in which narcissism has become epidemic is itself pathological. When elevated selfishness gains reverence, remuneration, and influence, then for them the whole of the social system has become dysfunctional. What Twenge and Campbell are inferring is that a society in which the culture is narcissistic is not civilised. That is, humanity is not well served by selfishness just as it is not by violence and inequality (as well as the subjects of subsequent chapter, 'insecurity', and 'stupidity').

Taking a similar approach to that of Lasch, and Twenge and Campbell, journalist Rod Liddle (2009) looks beyond the individual to explain the prevalence of narcissism. However, he differs from their academic style, adopting a polemical approach peppered with rancour. Liddle is particularly rancorous towards the selfishness of celebrities. Celebrity in contemporary (globalised) society is admired and pursued because it implies outstanding individualistic success. But Liddle considers celebrities contemptible for their pre-eminent narcissism and unremitting self-indulgence, and for the attention-seeking public airing of trivial and shallow opinions, and the confessing of sins, virtues, and disorders. Liddle makes the connection between the narcissistic disclosures of celebrities with what Twenge (2014) describes as the 'me generation'. According to Twenge, the 'me generation' was born during 1955–1985 in Western countries, just at the time when the culture of narcissism and the cult of celebrity had begun to blossom. The absurdity of the celebration of celebrity and of celebrity's selfishness is that despite it fitting with other cultural norms, notably individualism and materialism, and the enormous effort employed to gain celebrity status and the attention afforded thereafter, happiness remains elusive. That is, neither the glorification of nor the revelling in celebrity assuages personal anguish or societal sanguinity.

Celebrity is admired and pursued as it ostensibly denotes full 'self' actualisation, a salutation to outstanding individual accomplishment. However, much of modern celebrity is not the outcome of unprecedented personal triumph but a means of achieving social success. Successfully selling 'the self' to the masses can bestow exalted esteem, sizeable financial remuneration, and concentrated if capricious public attention. No matter how fatuous or ignominious, the celebrity advertises and unleashes her/his thoughts via the written word, media broadcasts, and social media, on an insatiable and worldwide populace. The celebrity's self is fed by its own fame or infamy in a self-sustaining series of corpulent conceits. Celebrity is the epitome of narcissism, and narcissism epitomises celebrity. The consumption of celebrity epitomises the centrality of selfishness in contemporary society. The self-serving narratives of celebrities, even if exposing pathology, exemplify and augment 'normal' narcissism.

Liddle points out that people in the West live longer (although as been discussed already in the book this trend is reversing in some countries). Their material circumstances have improved markedly. People possess vast numbers of commodities. A wide range of leisure pursuits and holidays are accessible and affordable for most. These tremendous improvements in longevity and lifestyle, which have occurred over a relatively short period in the history of humans and their civilisations. Yet despite these apparent civilised advances, for Liddle humans are now characterisable by a disposition of dolefulness and querulousness which implies societal atavism, and for these supposed superior primates, regression into consummate selfishness. Liddle sums up the temperament of current humans as 'selfish whining monkeys'.

Twenge's 'me generation' and Liddle's 'whining monkeys' show no sign of dissolution. For clinical psychologist Leon Seltzer (2016), self-absorption, self-preoccupation, self-centredness, self-obsessiveness, self-interest, and egoism have become embedded in the human psyche. People are mainly preoccupied with their own affairs not the troubles of the world or even those of their neighbours. Little effort is made to understand the thoughts, feelings, and actions of others unless they impinge on personal affairs. Everyday speech can denote an individual's lack of attention to the needs or specialness of other people. The tendency to use self-referential terms (I, me, myself) to exclusion of references to others (you, us, we, they) is indicative of self-absorption.

Seltzer makes the point that is essential for individuals to pay attention to their own needs. It is, in Seltzer's view, morally acceptable and normal to fix on personal satisfaction and certainly on survival. But when serving the self becomes a fixation then this is unethical and abnormal. The abnormality concerns the undermining of psychological stability. Seltzer uses the phrase 'toxic self-absorption' to describe the state of over-indulgent grandiosity whereby the subjective assessment of one's 'self' stresses specialness. Toxic self-absorption is, suggests Seltzer, what underlines many maladies of the psyche. Some of these maladies are primary symptoms of medicalised madness. Reducing selfishness, posits Seltzer, should be the primary treatment for such maladies.

Seltzer is highlighting the high cost of selfishness to individuals. Not only may selfishness become toxic and susceptible to a diagnosis of mental disorder, but social relationships and physical health suffer. According to Seltzer, the toxicity of self-absorption can hinder or destroy personal connections, and even lead to early death. There is also a cost of selfishness to society. That cost is exceptionally significant when selfishness is implanted in political power.

More than 70,000 mental health practitioners, dozens of psychiatrists, and an assortment of former colleagues, have described one man in terms which epitomise extreme selfishness. Their opinions collectively of this person is that he is: impulsive, recklessness, paranoid, a bully, racist, not having a grip on reality with a poor understanding of consequences, not able to control his anger, lacking in empathy, irresponsible, emotionally stunted, belligerent, buffoonish, misogynistic, needing to constantly demonstrate his power, at times sounding cognitively impaired, dangerous, hedonistic, narcissistic, seriously mentally ill with little hope of improvement (Lee, 2017, 2018; Gartner, 2017; Sword and Zimbardo, 2017; Wolff, 2018; Newman, 2018; Comey, 2018). That man is the President of United States of America, Donald J Trump.

Trump, a business tycoon and reality television presenter, was elected as President in 2018. Former USA First Lady Barbara Bush is reported in a biography of her to be excoriating: the biographer records that Bush regards Trump as a symbol of 'greed and selfishness' (Page, 2019). Storr views his political ascendency as symptomatic of USA society presently, and what for him are values which lead to success in that setting:

> Trump … a definitive creature of the neoliberal, self-esteem, celebrity era. A sumptuously narcissistic self-publicist.
>
> (Storr, 2018, p. 240)

Economist Joseph Stiglitz (2019) concurs with Storr's view, describing Trump's election as President to be a celebration of 'unbridled selfishness and self-absorption'. On the other hand, Stiglich regards Trump's performance as disruptive rather than conducive to the present pivotal institutions in the USA. What Trump has done since gaining the presidency, argues Stiglitz, is to attack these institutions and thereby threaten the stability and prosperity of the USA, and by implication that of the global political and economic order. For Stiglitz, democracy is also jeopardised by Trump's politically motivated interfering with court and legislative procedures, his disparaging of the media, inattention to factualness. Stiglitz submits that there has been no moral leadership from Trump or any of his administration. This administration, continues Stiglitz, resembles a degree of dystopia that previously writers of science fiction could only have imagined.

Stiglitz's claim that it is the selfish who seem to win in this world leads to him implying that and this has dire implications for the way in which humans survive, and possibly for the very survival of humanity That is, if selfishness, particularly in its accentuated form, remains at the forefront of human performance, then an immoral free-for-all may ensue which may finish humanity not help it to endure.

Research by the Pew Center (2017) supports Storr's and Stiglitz's opinions. In its survey of nearly 2,000 adults in the USA, it found that most considered the descriptor of Trump's personality as 'selfish'. There was also only a minority who supported his policies.

There are other presidents of political selfishness than Trump. Boris Johnson became Britain's Prime Minister in July 2019 when Theresa May stood down. As with Trump, much has been written in the media about Johnson's personality. Johnson is a journalist turned politician. He served as Mayor of London from 2008 to 2016. Johnson then served as Britain's Foreign Secretary from 2016 to 2018. USA journalist Madeleine Kearns (2018) records that Johnson has been described by his own daughter as a 'selfish bastard'. During Johnson's period as Foreign Secretary fellow journalist Martin Fletcher was to describe him thus:

> [C]haotic, mendacious, philandering, egotistical, disloyal and thoroughly untrustworthy charlatan driven by ambition and self-interest.
>
> (Fletcher, 2017)

Another British journalist, Brian Reade, writing a few months before Johnson became Prime Minister, has an opinion of Johnson which is no more complementary than Fletcher's:

> Boris Johnson is a shallow, narcissistic, womanising liar
>
> (Reade, 2019)

Reade notes that a previous political ally of Johnson's, Michael Gove (who at that time was Secretary of State for Environment, Food and Rural Affairs) pronounced that he (Johnson) was selfish, and so ambitious that he would 'shaft' anyone impeding his aspirations. Reade (2019) notes that Trump is supportive of Johnson's political ambitions.

It is worth noting that Johnson has been described positively by others including members of his own political party (who voted him to lead their party). In a survey by YouGov (2019) of nearly 10,000 British adults, condemnatory views about Johnson where tempered by acclamations. The latter referred to his humour, intelligence, charisma, and his popularity even when this is in the mould of notoriety. However, for British journalist to write so disparagingly about anyone is risky financially and for the future of her/his career unless there is supportive, preferably solid, evidence for the expressed judgements. The reason for extra diligence by British authors, including journalists, is that laws on deformation are stricter in certainly under England and Welsh law than in the USA. The burden of proof in the USA rests with the person who brings a claim of libel, where in Britain the author must prove that what has been written is not libellous.

There is a further tempering to the admonishing tone about selfishness per se with the argument that it is self-evidently an effective strategy to achieve celebrity, political, and/or corporate success. Furthermore, it may be important, perhaps necessary attribute. Excessive modesty about one's aptitudes and undue deference to the status and outlooks of others may be self-defeating. That is, there may 'good selfishness' (Book of Life, 2019). If an individual always underplays her/his skills and is derisive about her/his opinions then this may lead to a lessening of personal achievement or a perceived lack of valuableness to fulfil the needs of employers, friends and family. Accurate self-assessment and salient pronouncements about competencies, as well incapacities, may be more self-motivational and of utility to others than either overdone selfishness or selflessness.

Essayist Kristin Dombek (2016) writes about the paradox of narcissism. There has been much publicity about how narcissists are found in all walks of life, to the point whereby narcissism, like anxiety and depression, is deemed to have reached epidemic proportions. This publicity has arisen from academic work, for example, Twenge and Campbell's (2009) and Lasch (1979). Moreover, their personality deficits are widely known. It is commonly understood that narcissists do not possess empathy and that this quality is otherwise a normal and necessary trait for humans to co-exist. But for Dombek there is a paradox in this recognition and consequent fear of the narcissistic partner, neighbour, boss, and politician. What is behind this apparent recognition (and definite fearfulness) is an attempt to resolve a psychological dissonant state within the identifier.

The idea of narcissism, argues Dombek, serves as a metaphorical depot for all the anxieties of the non-narcissist wrestles with as elements of everyday modern life. Narcissists, therefore, become scapegoats for the fears of 'normal' people about existence in a world in which new and ever-changing technologies and increasing demands on improving performance abound, including being happy. There is, for Dombek, pathological narcissism which is dysfunctional to the person concerned, for those with whom she/he associates, and for society. Pathological narcissism, however, is too often conflated with mere and possibly mild egotism. For Dombek, the fear that narcissists abound, and that their deficiency in empathy is dangerous, is contradictory. This is because the perception of the narcissists as lacking in empathy reveals a lack of empathy in the perceiver. Labelling some people as egoistical, and thereby untrustworthy, is an ego-defence-mechanism and one not to be trusted.

Consumerism

Being besotted with buying is a rampant reification of selfishness which borders on a narcissistic disorder for some individuals and is central to the cultural narcissism inherent in contemporary globalised capitalism. Can consumerism be defended similarly to selfishness? Every life form consumes to survive. Survival requires the acquiring of food, water, oxygen, and materials for shelter and protection or equivalent alternatives. Furthermore, humans have, ever since they began to collect or make adornments for their cave dwellings and cosseted ethereal experiences, always been consumers of entities not strictly necessary for survival. If the desire for accumulating such extras is realised, then a degree of extra satisfaction in that form merely continuing to exist is likely to be achieved. Consumerism may, however, be an ego-defence-mechanism, or at the very least an attempt to resolve some sort of sparsity of the psyche. For capitalism, consumerism is not only good but essential. The capitalist economic mode cannot exist without the symbiosis of production and consumption, no matter that this relationship is hardly ever in a state of equilibrium. The interdependence between production and consumption is always unwieldy and frequently chaotic. Underproduction and overproduction of food, industrial and armament hardware, household wares, property, and supplies for health care, leisure activities, and non-material happenings (for example, yoga, life-coaching, and spiritual practices) coexist with high demand and low demand for these products.

As with selfishness, negative rather than supportive testimonials abound. Consumerism as it is today, that is excessive and mainly material, is attacked from a range of standpoints.

For example, Pope Francis on Christmas Eve 2018 publicly condemned inequality and poverty but also denounced consumerism in specifically in developed countries. He reproached the populations of rich countries for living a life of materialism and recommended a much simpler way of living akin to that adhered to by Jesus.

> In our day, for many people, life's meaning is found in possessing, in having an excess of material objects. An insatiable greed marks all human history, even today, when, paradoxically, a few dine luxuriantly while all too many go without the daily bread needed to survive.
>
> (Pope Francis, quoted by Pullella, 2018)

Francis is not the only Pope to have commented on consumerism on Christmas Eve. Pope Benedict, Francis's predecessor, in 2011 urged his congregation, and because it was reported in the media his comment became available to consumers globally, to stop being enticed by the commodification of Christmas (*BBC News*, 2011).

The implication of rebukes by these two Popes is that it is immoral to indulge in excessive consumerism and it is up to individuals to desist. He is not recommending a structural revamping society. He is not the only Pope to reprimand not only Catholics but now the vast majority people in global society. Very few people in the world do not 'excessively' consume. Televisions, mobile-phones (cell phones), motor vehicles, computers with access to the internet, garments with logos, and 'junk' food, are no longer unusual the poorest of countries (Hill, 2011; Worldwatch Institute, 2015).

From another standpoint, that of a traveller, materialism has run amok. The long-distance motorcyclist and travel-writer Ted Simon went around the world for a second time at the age of 70 having first accomplished that feat some thirty years previously. On the second journey he travelled nearly 60,000 miles visited 47 countries. His account of what he experienced was not 'progress':

> It seemed to me impossible to say anything upbeat and optimistic about the changes I had seen. Even if people were materially better off than they had been, they didn't know it, and were not happier because of it. On the contrary, the little they had convinced them that they needed much more.
>
> (Simon, 2008, p. 420)

His point about acquisition is that desire for more becomes habitual, and the compulsion to acquire more and more and this doesn't sustain or increase contentment but drives discontent. Furthermore, Simon concludes from his comparing what he saw change from his first world motorcycling expedition with his second that as more is acquired, then the societal and physical environment suffers. Writing after the second journey he reports that 'unsustainable growth' had resulted in the disappearance or dilution of whole cultures, sets of customs, swathes of animals, and ecological systems.

Psychologist Oliver James (2007; 2008) claims that 'selfish capitalism' has spread a virulent variety of materialism which has infected society with what he terms infection he terms 'affluenza'. People suffering from this infection strive to get meaning from accumulating and parading commodities they have bought. Frank Lipman (2009), a practitioner of integrative medicine, argues materialism is having an enormous impact on the pace of life. Long hours are spent commuting to work and then long hours and longer years working to try to increase earnings to buy more things. Relaxation in leisure-time may not be possible because it is likely to be spent in the confines of busy cities or crowded holiday resorts. Time spent buying both essentials and frivolities is made more fevered because of the superfluity of choices including whether to choose to buy from the maelstrom of the internet or from hectic high-streets. Lipman concludes that People, he claims, have become 'spent'.

Communist Antonio Gramsci was imprisoned by the Italian Fascists in the 1920s. During his 11 years in prison he was to write copiously on a range of topics which become known as *The Prison Notebooks* (Gramsci, 1971). His topics included Italian history, the role of intellectuals and education in society, Machiavelli, the organisation of working practices along the lines of 'Fordism' and 'Taylorism', feminism, the connection between science, religion, and common sense, Marxism, and about revolutionary social transformation.

One of the ideas contained in Gramsci's notebooks is that of 'hegemony'. 'Hegemony' refers to how the powerful in society manipulate the rest of the population into believing what they (the powerful) want them to believe so that they can gain and retain their privileged position. For the most part, argues Gramsci the masses are influenced not through overt measures such as threats of or actual violence and incarceration, but through indoctrination.

The powerful attain and retain power through ideological control. The public become convinced that a set of beliefs have political, economic, moral, and legal authenticity.

Messages of legitimacy are delivered through the media, government policy, and educational and employment practices, and most effectively by the non-verbal, verbal, subliminal, and discernible reactions especially of significant others. But much 'accepted wisdom' is dispensed during the perpetual encounters with others who are not necessarily discerned as significant but do have significant influence on 'normalising' behaviour, emotions, and thoughts. To step out-of-line is likely to incite condemnation and possibly ostracisation. The likelihood of the latter is, according to human rights lawyer Dexter Dias (2017), is a very effective method of social control because if enacted then it can lead social death accompanied by an experience of pain akin to severe physical trauma. Selfishness is exemplified by excessive consumption but performing selfishly by excessively consuming, if Gramsci's idea of hegemony is adopted, is the consequence of ideological indoctrination that whereby the self is sanctified through accumulation.

Historian Frank Trentmann (2016) observes that the refashioning of human identity into one by which consuming is dominated has affected public services. Public transport, health care, indispensable utilities such as the supply of water, lighting, and heating, even when not privatised are set up as supermarkets. Trentmann opines that the neoliberal champions of unfettered capitalism consider this shift in how humans live their lives to be a positive development as increases prosperity and underscores democratic values especially the freedom to choose.

The thesis of sociologist Ritzer (1993) is that society has become 'MacDonaldized'. By the MacDonalization of society Ritzer means, as did Marx that the driving force in personal relationships and societal processes, institutions, and demarcations is the economy. But Ritzer calls upon Max Weber's (1930) idea of 'rationalization' whereby as human civilisation progresses traditional (irrational) values are replaced by reasoned ideals. Current capitalism is, Ritzer's proposition continues, founded on 'rational consumerism'. Efficiency, calculability, predictability, technology, homogenisation, rules, and regulations affect every aspect of human and organisational activity. At the centre of these activities is the consumer who is making logical and beneficial choices. But, for Weber and Ritzer, the consuming rational citizen there is a danger of becoming dehumanised as is exemplified in the tedious, trivial, underpaid, over-supervised, and frequently unhealthy work for both employees and customers found first in fast-food outlets but extending rapidly across many areas of the economy.

Adopting an approach which is indebted to ideas emanating from the 'Frankfurt School' of critical theorists, journalist Stuart Jeffries (2016; 2017) records that having the freedom to choose from an array of products, essentially serving the same purpose, does not generate contentment but misery. Moreover, having a multitude of makes of baked-beans or versions of the same motor-vehicle from which to choose is not freedom but coercion because it generates an angst-ridden obsessiveness over which is the right choice. There is a compulsion to buy but the process of buying is mediated through advertising, the manipulations of retail psychology, and the over-arching ideological indoctrination of capitalism. The mantra that there may be a better toothbrush, a better heating boiler, or motorcycle to buy than the one already owned is inculcated into the culture of contemporary society. Buying a better one with a concomitant much improved price becomes not only a choice but a necessity because the previous one has an in-built limited life-span or if broken cannot be mended or to do so is too expensive. There is an economic cost but psychological reward for buying the new product as it assuages the disappointment from the ownership of something seemingly defective. But, this pay-off is akin to the short surge from an intake of sugar. Disappointment, sadness, and obsessiveness soon take over and another replacement sought.

Much of the theorising by the Frankfurt School owes a debt to Marx (Jeffries, 2017). The obsessive compulsion to acquire goods (along with services in today's world) which are not necessary was described by Marx as 'commodity fetishism'. The fetishisation of commodities occurs when, for example, a tin of beans is bought because its brand implies higher value than its contents warrant. Beans are nutritional, and nutrition is necessary to sustain life. But, if all beans are nutritionally similar, then buying a brand because of its extravagant label and embellished media advertising (and possibly because the manipulative positioning, of the product in the shop) is probably succumbing to commodity fetishism rather than utilising conscious and uncontaminated choice. What's more, the individual becomes identified by the commodities she/he obtains. The acquirer is acquiring an identity which reflects her/his acquisitions, and seemingly so doing intentionally. The sellers of the fetishised brand of beans benefit financially, particularly as their product is likely to have a higher profit margin. Jeffries suggests the powerful overall in society benefit from commodity fetishism. When this fetishism is widespread (and not merely about bean buying), social change, potentially revolution, is mitigated, and those in power remain so.

Apart from beans, sexuality serves as a good case to support the contention that consumerism is out of control. Sex has been substantially commodified. The 'mainstreaming' and normalisation of sexual exhibitionism, paraphernalia, and information transpired in the late twentieth century (Attwood, 2009). This process was aided by the introduction of mass electronic communication systems, and mass travel. 'Sex texting' and 'sex-selfies' are now not an unusual element of adolescent culture. Social media and dating sites specifically tailored to sexual encountering are widely and easily accessed. Childhood is sexualised through the refashioning of adult fashion for young consumers. Whilst there are laws protecting children from physical sexual contact (above all with adults) they are vulnerable to exposure to sexualised internet content, advertising, television programmes and videos, and susceptible to enticement from pimps and paedophiles. Erotic titillation has gone hardcore to be point that there has been a 'pornification' of human consciousness and society (Schulz, 2009; Paul, 2006).

The commodification of sex has also been abetted by the continuation and expansion of liberalised social attitudes towards what previously would formerly have been tagged as private, shameful, deviant, or criminal. There has been a separation of sexual identify, gender, and chromosomal disposition, and sexual conduct has become fluid. But liberalised attitudes towards sex and sexual identity historically has not been, and still is not universal (Compsto, 2006: Young et al., 2015). The main religions of Christianity, Islam, and Judaism, have and still do have an ambivalent or hostile approach to sex which for sex therapist Marty Klein is more fitting for the people living in the Dark Ages or for nomads:

> [T]oday ... educated people actually believe that God cares about which orifice, which time of the month, which sperm, which embryo, which partner.... God has more important things to worry about -global warming, a nuclear North Korea, the HIV epidemic orphaning millions of African children, how to feed China & India.
>
> (Klein, 2010)

For Jeffries, consumers are leading a 'phantasmagoric', life in which the meaning of what they consume is unreal, as is the condition of their minds and social relationships. Federico Chicchi (2016) is a sociologist with an interest in psychoanalysis. He applies both disciplines to consumerism, arguing that capitalism is reliant for its success on the 'phantoms of the commodity'. Capitalism has inserted fictitious significance to the gratuitous collecting of commodities. The phantomisation of the commodity for Chicchi occurs when goods and services are inculcated with fictitious symbolic meanings, chiefly that they bring with them facets of personal freedom. Inciting the amassing of needless goods and services is achieved through mystifying their needlessness. Commodities are inculcated with messages of individualism, distinctiveness, specialness, and autonomy. The reality is, maintains Chicchi, using a mixture of Marxist and Freudian discernments, that the services and goods are saturated with selfishness. They bring to the surface and reinforce inherent narcissistic tendencies. Non-capitalist societies (and even non-unbridled capitalist ones) subdue in childhood through regular socialisation. In less economically exploitative social settings, the child develops into an adult by recognising the needs of others rather than its needs, beyond survival, being paramount.

Chicci also posits, this time using a perspective more reliant on psychoanalytic than Marxist thinking, that commodity fetishism substitutes sexual satisfaction. However, it does not adequately satisfy. The phantom of erotic fulfilment, which is largely occurring as an unconscious process, is that libidinal yearnings and the suffering which stems from their thwarted resolution will be sorted but the pleasure from acquirement is shallow and short-lived.

Given the argument presented above that sex has been commodified, then sexual services or goods specifically tailored for sexual release are available, but these may also provide only temporary and superficial value. The inundation of society with sexuality may offer proliferated expectations but proffer only unrealisable and inadequate consummation.

Hegemonic control has thereby been aided considerably through commodity fetishism, but Jeffries proposes that humanity has been degraded. The paradox of this degradation, points out Jeffries, is that some consumers do discern that they are being conned. But no matter that the consumer may recognise the obscenity of collecting superfluous commodities, the compulsive obsession to buy unnecessarily is too strong to resist.

Critical approaches to consumerism come from other theoretical quarters than those with Marxists leanings. Jean Baudrillard (1970), post-modernist theorist but who was initially influenced by Marx, has put forward a proposition which, as with other critics, attempt to address what it means to those who succumb to consumerism. Writing decades ago, Baudrillard, as the title of his book indicates (*La Société de Consommation:* translated as *The Consumer Society*), that consumerism had become rampant in Western society. He also denotes the level of consumption that had become the norm by the 1970s as a major distorted alteration in human development:

> Today, we are everywhere surrounded by the remarkable conspicuousness of consumption and affluence.... This is now the fundamental mutation in the ecology of the human species.
>
> (Baudrillard, 2001, p. 32)

Consumption has for Baudrillard reached the point of grasping the whole of human life. Human interaction is mediated through inanimate objects rather than meaningful animate exchanges. Again, the reason for excessive acquisitiveness is attributed to people searching for meaning in their lives.

Baudrillard suggests that meaningfulness, of sorts, becomes possible when commodities have what he termed 'sign-value'. The sign-value of a commodity is the extra worth beyond their basic function and/practical merit. The value of what is signalled differs between commodities and between commodity genres. Baked beans have different sign-value to motorcycles, and some brand of baked beans carry a superior sign-value than others, just as there is differentiation in terms of sign value between motorcycles. The grading of sign-value hinges on perceptions of rank. The higher the status of the commodity the more it is desired and once owned the higher the status of the owner, or at least that's what the owner means will be the outcome of her/his procurement. Meaning in this context refers to expected improvement in the quality of lifestyle and pleasure gained from ownership, along with the approbation of those who witness its proprietorship. Self-admiration for the procurement and reactions of admiration from associates and strangers alike swell the sign-value.

Again, however, the question of deceit arises. Baudrillard, as has Jeffries, intonates that the consumer is being conned into gaining meaningfulness from commodities. Baudrillard's post-modernist thinking looks for an alternative explanation of the 'con' to that described by Marx and those adhering to his critique of capitalism. Rather than considering consumerism as the outcome of the powerful (capitalists and their political allies) seeking to commodify everything for their own financial gain and mystify reality whereby the meaning of life is projected to be gainable from owning a heap of ultimately meaningless commodities, a principle of postmodern theorising is free-will. From the postmodern point of view, the old ideological, political, sexual, gender, and lifestyle mantras which steered the performance of individuals, families, and communities, have gone. People have the freedom to choose how they live their live and what they wish to buy. Capitalism, certainly as it has been configured from the 20th century onwards, supplies much from which to choose.

Baudrillard, however, recognises that the freedom to choose is complicated and angst-ridden. If there are 57 varieties of beans from which to choose then which should be chosen? If the many manufactures of motorcycles all proclaim that their vehicles and customer service is second-to-none, then which is the best choice? A further example is that of choosing the best way to reduce the risk of becoming unhappy or suffer serious psychological disturbance. If the latter occurs, then is self-help and the help of friends and family best or should the help of a professional be sought? Should that professional be a psychiatrist, a clinical psychologist, or psychotherapist? If, for example, it is a psychotherapist then which psychotherapeutic approach from a myriad of possibilities would be the most suitable? Having choice is not straightforward. Freedom in the post-modern sense is angst-ridden.

Material ownership ostensibly is pursued willingly and displayed freely to feel and project distinctiveness. Baudrillard, however, points to a deeper and mostly unconscious (or an instance of 'false consciousness') reason for the embracement of consumerism. Rather than exemplifying utter selfishness, consumerism is cosseted to avoid social isolation. The process of choosing, buying, and owning is a communal, and frequently, a mass activity. People are, even if they do so alone, collectively engaged in shopping and displaying the goods they have bought, and mostly engage in using services with other people. This is also the case for one-line consumerism if only because the internet-based corporations use their algorithms to inform their would-be customers that others are making the same choice, and to indicate what fellow customers thought of what they had chosen. Fashionable clothes are worn to be seen, trendy café bars are frequented because attendance is observed. Yet again, however, there is paradox. In the post-modern consumer world, reflects Baudrillard, people become fully alienated. As consumers they live a superfluous and simulated life, one in which needs and wants become conflated, and consuming is all the meaning that life holds.

Those who don't perceive correctly that they are being conned could, should psychiatry deem it apposite clinically and advantageous to its expanding professional arena, regard it as a symptom of mass psychosis. Where there is awareness that commodities are fetishised, yet they are still acquired, then this is analogous to other behaviours which may be classified as neurotic because they have become habitual and detract from other basic human requirements. Obsessive wanting rather than needing is selfish. But, as psychoanalytic psychotherapist Sue Gerhardt submits, obsessively wanting depletes the self of such essential needs as attachment to others and love (Gerhardt, 2010). Although fetishism by itself is not a classified warranting diagnosis in the DSM 5 (American Psychiatric Association, 2013) 'fetishistic disorder' is included. The main indication of this disorder is the persistent and repetitive focusing on inanimate objects for the gratification of sexual urges and fantasies.

Consumerism now encompasses groups of consumers who proclaim and campaign for their rights. There is a multitude of these groups covering a multiplicity of industries and institutions. For example, In Australia the consumer advocacy group Choice (2019) providing reviews of merchandise and amenities to avoid 'dodgy or misleading practices'. The European Consumer Centres Network (2019) offers advice and support regarding on consumer rights and when there are disputes between traders and their customers within the European Union, Norway, and Iceland. 'Psychiatric survivors' are not a united group. For example, there is a split between those who laud status as 'mad' and those who claim that what they experience in form (perhaps hallucinations) are just part of the spectrum of human performance and should not be regarded as special or symptoms of mental disorder. However, the overall impact of decades of campaigning has introduced into the professional and public sphere alternative narratives to those of practitioners, academics, and to the frequently stigmatising views held by the general population (Russo and Sweeney, 2016). For example, some psychiatric survivors have advocated a model of care which focuses on 'recovery' rather than permanent medicalisation and associated stigmatisation (Pilgrim and McCranie, 2013). Some success has been achieved by in asserting their human rights and status as regular citizens, and in moderating, although not removing, the prejudicial stance found in the media and amongst their fellow citizens (Sassatelli, 2007; Dudley, et al., 2012; Rowe, 2015).

The psychiatric survivors' movements have recognised that their input into psychiatric practice could have, and did in many situations, become tokenistic, and their representatives not empowered but incorporated into the institutions and its practice they were meant to be challenging and thereby mollified (Chamberlin, 1978; Adame, 2013; Ocloo and Matthews, 2016). There has also been the danger of psychiatric survivors being used by professionals engaged in occupational advancement, especially those who wish themselves to challenge the power of psychiatrists. However, psychiatric survivors are also designated as 'service-users' and by themselves and the professionals. That is, they have accepted if not extolled their role as consumers and the inevitable if unwitting commodification of their psychological condition and political cause (Esposito and Perez, 2014).

From the twentieth century onwards, consumerism has entered a novel and dynamic realm: the digital world (more about which is discussed in Chapter 6). Increasingly, personal data from consumers and social media users are captured through the technologies used by on-line businesses. It is the contention of, Evgeny Morozov (2018), writer on the implications of technology for people and society, that technology companies are aligned with large corporations who then use this data to increase the sale of their commodities, their profits, and their influence over the lives of their customers (Morozov, 2018). The introduction of technologies using artificial intelligence into this process further fuels further sales, profits, and influence. Governments are also acquiring these technologies, along with artificial intelligence, which could lead to an escalation in their control over the performance of their populations. In an economic system reliant on intensifying the fetishisation of commodities, artificial intelligence is an unprecedentedly powerful tool by which to manage consumption. The management by artificially intelligent technologies intensifying the appetite and passivity of consumers and the vitality of corporations.

An alternative voice to those proclaiming consumerism is the sum of human existence is that of Brendan Canavan (2019), a researcher in the culture of consumption. He argues that consumerism is in terminal decline in the UK and comparative economies throughout the world. According to Canavan, people are buying less often and less overall. Reduced procuring is most apparent in high-street retailing but is also affecting car and mobile-phone (cell-phone) sales. Concerns about the damage to the environment because of rampant consumerism, and an al-be-it small movement to-date towards recycling are partly responsible for this downturn as maybe is a general uncertainty about the state of the world. Furthermore, a 'post-consumer' is emerging notes Canavan. The post-consumer wants 'experiences' to garner her/his identity rather than products. Canavan, however, then undermines his positioning of the environmentally concerned, uncertain, recycling post-consumer, missing the point that plentiful procurement, most of which is ecologically damaging to a greater or lesser extent, is unavoidable for much of modern life. Second-hand goods must be bought in the first place, life has always been uncertain in one way or another, and to engage in 'experiencing', whether that is sharing wine with friends or visiting the Antarctic, products of some sort are being consumed. Moreover, it is Canavan who raises the question of economic sustainability if consumers moderate their inculcated excessive tendencies. Society as it is may fail, intones Canavan.

Canavan also underplays the immense consumerist movement on the internet. He also misses the advance of technology with its prospect of the re-inventing consumerism through its (literally) mind-boggling algorithmic, exploitative capabilities. Nor does Canavan seem to grasp that corporate power will be enhanced hugely by combining both the internet and technology over which they are largely in control.

Such levels of manipulative conduct by corporations, if they were to be the characteristics of individuals, might attract a diagnosis of one of several mental disorders. Indeed, the basic characteristics of capitalism may depict a particularly deep, divisive, and degrading type of societal insanity. Lawyer, writer and film-maker Joel Bakan (2005) argues that the pursuit of profit by big companiesis largely responsible for the pandemic of materialism, commodification, consumerism, which lead to a culture of narcissism.

The insane characteristics of global capitalism and corporate power are conspicuous. Materialism is accentuated and lauded. But, points out Monbiot (2013a; 2013b), a material way of life is associated with depression, anxiety, selfishness, broken relationships, and a lack of social responsibility. For Monbiot, materialism is self-destructive and damages society. There is an over-reliance or inappropriate reliance on financial 'growth' using in the main one specific and contestable measure of gross-domestic-product (Fioramonti, 2017. Moreover, measuring the state of a nation and that of global society based on the state of wealth is dehumanising as it overlooks or discounts qualities such as happiness, health, family and community connections, interpersonal sociability, job satisfaction, engagement in leisure pursuits, the arts, and simply being a good citizen (Castells, 2017; Bowles, 2016). Everything is exposed to commodification, including physical and psychological tribulations. Consumption operates as the pay-off for physically and psychologically unhealthy working and living conditions, longer working lives, and employment/unemployment swings of economic cycles. However, consumption has not paid-off. Heightened and extensive consumerism has coincided with what are claimed to be epochs of anxiety and depression (Horwitz, 2010; LeDoux, 2015; Blazer, 2005; Stosell, 2014; World Health Organisation, 2016). Moreover, rather tackling the insanities of global capitalism and corporate power, the institution of psychiatry has embraced both. Psychiatry has gone 'corporate', most markedly in the USA, due to its long-standing and latterday entrenched participation with pharmaceutical companies. Psychiatry also performs in the interest capitalism and corporatism in its role as an agency of social control, and it its practices whereby a huge collection of human emotions, behaviours, and thoughts are medicalised, and which are commonly treated with corporate capitalism products (Gaylin, 1985; Grohol, 2018; Morrall, 2017).

One highly conspicuous insanity of consumerism is that of 'retail rage'. Examples include video and subsequently broadcast in news programmes and on internet sites fights over products. Violent altercations amongst shoppers competing for discounted products have occurred in France, Britain, and the USA (Atkinson, 2018). A supermarket shop-worker trampled to death in New York when shoppers stampeded into the store during the annual 'Back Friday' sales in which good are discounted heavily (Lee, 2017). But, notwithstanding personal peculiarities which induce participation in a consumer scrum to buy what may be wanted and not be needed, it is a peculiarity of corporate capitalism that creates this frenzied and competitive environment. The deliberate setting-up of situations in which people are liable to become frenzied and maybe violent is more than a peculiarity, however. If it is attributable to individual corporate executives and/or the present shape of the capitalist system, then it is an either a serious personal madness or significant societal insanity. There is, for Monbiot (2017) a form of normalised 'collective madness' whereby consumption has become so pathological that the collection of what he pronounces 'ingenious rubbish' is destroying the planet. The rules of global trade and the requisite for economic growth depend, he insists, on selling utterly useless products.

Criminal psychologist Robert Hare (1999; 2003) is architect of the standard tool for diagnosing psychopathy (otherwise known 'sociopathy', or 'anti-social personality disorder'). Hare's assessment of faults in the personality of an individual which lead an attribution of psychopath can, he intonates, be applied to faults in society. For Hare, some social institutions perform psychopathically. Hare's checklist to aid a diagnosis of psychopathy includes manipulative behaviour, a lack empathy and remorse, and extreme selfishness. Capitalist corporations, for Hare, manipulate to profit financially, show empathy and remorse only to ensure survival and success, and essentially are selfish. For example, Hare argues that the concern shown by corporations over the damage done to the environment in the manufacture and use of their goods and services is manipulative, lacking in genuine empathy and remorse. Corporate programmes of social responsibility may appear to be compassionate and community-spirited, but they are at the core selfish because they are instigated to manipulate public and political opinion:

> Human psychopaths are notorious for their ability to use charm as a mask to hide their dangerously self-obsessed personalities. For corporations, social responsibility may play the same role.
>
> (Hare quoted in Bakan, 2005, p. 56)

Moreover, Bakan (2012) contends that corporations 'ruthlessly' targets children with commodities which are highly profitably but frequently highly unhealthy. Sweets, sugary drinks, fat-laden fast-food, salty snacks, and previously in developed countries and presently in developing countries, tobacco, are advertised as suitable and perhaps largely for children.

Hare and psychologist Paul Babiak claim that corporations, particularly the large ones, are infested with psychopaths in their senior ranks (Babiak and Hare, 2007). These 'snakes in suits' are over-represented in corporate executive positions compared with the incidence of psychopathy in the general population. A successful corporate career, suggest Hare and Babiak, is more likely if the employee is endowed with psychopathic personality traits. These underlying psychopathic traits are used to charm colleagues and impress those with the power to promote. Manipulation, lack of (genuine) empathy and remorse, and selfishness surface as business-orientated performances such as astuteness, high motivation, risk-taking. As Monbiot notes, this can be perceived as ideal corporate stewardship:

The perfect chief executive, from the point of view of the shareholders, is a fully fledged psychopath.

(Monbiot, 2017, p. 185)

But Babiak and Hare add that eventually the fully-fledge psychopathic is not an asset to a business but a drawback. The qualities first perceived as valuable may become the undoing of the business when exorbitant egotism take-over. The more the psychopath has free reign the more the reign becomes freed from the very constraints that keep businesses profitable in the long-run. For example, risk-taking if unfettered will probably result in taking one risk too far and the business failing. Far from astuteness and motivation leading to financial success or other supposed skills without psychopathic connotations, the contention of psychologist and economist Daniel Kahneman is that luck plays a major part (Kahneman, 2012).

Malignancy

The seeds and spectacles of selfishness, as Fromm (1939; 1956) suggests by combining psychological and sociological thinking, can be traced to an intricate societal-psyche interrelationship. However, whilst reflexive convolutions between the psychological make-up of the individual and her/his societal situation remain, the origins and presentations of selfishness have become less to do with personal pathology. In today's globalised society, selfishness is a deeply embedded cultural phenomenon. Like many of the ideas about selfishness already presented in this chapter, Fromm identified capitalism as an economic system which sponsored ego-centrism.

Fromm's combination of Marxist and Freudian ideas led him to the firm conclusion that the societal and personal consequences of capitalism provoked a culture in which individuals were more than expected to be selfish, they were brainwashed so to be, and this inevitably altered their psyche. Fromm, as viewed through his psychological analytical lens, perceived narcissism as benign in some circumstances. He provided the examples of farmers, carpenters and scientists taking pride in their accomplishments. Another example might a mother feeling fulfilled by the birth and accomplishments of her children. In this sense narcissism is normal. Fromm, however, designates narcissism as malignant when it is not connected to a commendable and/or useful achievement:

In the case of malignant narcissism, the object of narcissism is not anything the person does or produces, but something he has; for instance, his body, his looks, his health, his wealth, etc.

(Fromm, 1964, p. 77)

However, there is in Fromm's portrayal of narcissism not only the realisation of how internalised its malignant variant would become. Fromm's malignant narcissism is now not an unusual element of the psyche. Furthermore, the sociological facet of Fromm's imagination did not provide him with prescience about the extent to which the survival of capitalism would require the magnification of the 'self' which has resulted in the normalisation of narcissistic malignance. Nor did Fromm envision the magnificence of capitalism whereby to survive it has invented a plethora of exceedingly impractical but impressively imaginative commodities and implanted its influence across the world.

It is worth repeating that Fromm was not fixated on capitalism and its economic scaffolding but on its malignant effects. Alternative societal systems were identified by Fromm (1942; 1973) which were, for him, also responsible for corrupting humanity. He was vehemently against totalitarianism such as that dispensed by Soviets by the Nazis. Capitalism's speciality is the installation of selfishness and narcissism into the human psyche, whereas totalitarianism, posits Fromm, yields fear, cruelty, and destructiveness across the population.

There are patent and abundant paradoxes in communistic and fascistic societies. For example, the idealistic foundation of communism is 'communality'. But in the case of Union of Soviet Socialist Republics its governance swiftly became dictatorship and oligarchy (Rees, 2004). Nazism in Germany was a 'national socialist' political crusade which purportedly aimed at delivering the 'common good'. But good only came to those who were regarded by the Nazis has having commonality with an exclusive typology, and even then, only for a relatively short period before they too found themselves not in a good situation (Arendt, 1973).

Capitalism, for Fromm, contains less obvious enigmas. Selfishness and narcissism are for Fromm paradoxical symptoms within capitalism because behind the selfishness it furnishes in the individual is not self-fondness but a lack of fondness for herself/himself. This underlying absence of self-love creates constant anxiety about self-worth and personal identity. The (malignant) narcissist has the same sort of internal contradiction, but it is much more potent. Whilst narcissists seem on the surface to be enthralled by their persona and may expound publicly their supposed superior attributes, they are compensating for deep self-loathing:

> [A]n attitude of love for themselves will be found in those who are at least capable of loving others. Hatred against oneself is inseparable from hatred against others, even if on the surface the opposite seems to be the case.
>
> (Fromm, 1939, p. 514)

Fromm (1956) assessment that most people who are caught-up in capitalism to be ultimately incapable of loving themselves and incapable of authentic love for others leads him to propose the rejuvenation of 'the art of loving'. But capitalist society, he realises, does not require love except if sold as a commodity. Neither does it require intellectualism except where intellectualism can further profitable innovation. Humans reaching for the pinnacle of their potential is not perceived by the existing corporate and political elite to be helpful for a materialistic social system. This is especially so if genuine loving becomes a pervasive past-time and the intellect is fully actualised and there is raised collective consciousness about the con of capitalism. What this economic mode does require is the malignancy of self-centred consumption of commodities.

Selfishness is deleterious psychologically and physically. The excessive consumption of processed, fast-food, and 'junk' food is associated with patterns of unhealthy living including a lack of exercise, high intakes of alcohol and use of illegal drugs. In turn, these patterns are linkable to deleterious physical states, including obesity, hypertension, diabetes, heart disease, and cerebral vascular accidents ('strokes') (Kirby, 2015). Materialist values, consumerism, selfishness, and narcissism are associated with low life satisfaction, depression, anxiety, addictions, phobias; obsessive-compulsive disorder; manic-depression; post-traumatic-stress disorder; and personality disorders (Kasser, 2003; Seltzer, 2016; Tweedy, 2016; 2017).

People at an early age become immersed in a culture of consumption. Children are targeted by corporations because they are far more easily conditioned into consumerism than would be adults should they not also have been so acclimatised when they were young. There is evidence, suggests freelance writer and social activist Jennifer Hill (2015), that consumerism is 'eroding childhood'. The erosion occurs because children are increasingly in danger of experiencing low self-esteem, and diagnosable with depression and/ or anxious. An onslaught of advertisements aimed at encouraging children to buy products to improve their appearance, to be smarter, to devour (unhealthy) snacks, and to procure the latest digital communication and entertainment device, and voguish music.

Selfishness, narcissism, and consumerism are insidious when they are inherent to a culture. One generation socialises the next after it has been indoctrinated by political, media, and corporate messages that to be selfish and to consume are normal, indeed desirable, human qualities. A multibillion (USA) dollar industry is perpetually and robustly orchestrating human performance and doing so from 'cradle to grave' (Hill, 2015).

But there is more to selfishness than physical and psychological damage. Selfishness damages the self and society. It's not only that goods and services are acquired, and acquisition seems insatiable, but the desire to acquire turns into what social psychologist Stefano Passini (2013) refers to the 'binge-consuming'. 'Black Friday', the annual retailing event during which many commodities on the High Street and on the internet are massively discounted is a prime example of binge-consuming. But so are the routine shopping events conducted at local shops, out-of-sprawling retail parks, or on-line, which reap collections of new acquisitions to be carried home or by specialised delivery services. Passini argues that a certain compulsion to consume seems to characterise not only how people relate to goods and services, but also how they relate to each other and to institutions. It is a further mark of the harm done to both the self and society when profiteering on the one side and consumers rights on the other constitute the basis of the daily human interchanges.

In the form of excessive consumption, selfishness also maligns the physical environment. However, medical social anthropologist Sandra Carlisle and public health researcher Phil Hanlon (2007) introduce provocative slant on contemporary political and professional campaigns to improve well-being and their environmental effects. They want 'critical and environmental discourses' to be applied to the personal problem and social issues of narcissism which, for them, improving the well-being of individuals embraces. That is, focusing on individuals not only has negative impacts on the individual (for example, using gyms and aeroplanes for self-improving adventures involves the production of environmentally damaging products and pollution). What's more, a focus on individual well-being does little or nothing to tackle the societal antecedents of personal problems such as inequality and violence.

Summary

Selfishness, apart from a fundamental perquisite for the existence and continuation of capitalism, performs a protective task for the economic mode of capitalism. Whilst people concentrate on their individual wants it is improbable that capitalism will be threatened, or at least in any substantial way. Consumerism is an addiction and one which drugs the population into passivity. It weakens the engagement for political action which might lead to major changes in the constitution of society and possibly the end of a capitalism or at least the sort of economics which entrenches selfishness into the culture.

Gerhardt (2010) views Western society as self-interested individuated, and materialistic, and although Gerhardt is concentrates on this part of the world, this description is increasingly applicable globally. She compares her negative appraisal of the West with her idealistic aspiration of an empathic, emotionally mature and literate, unselfish society. This aspiration has much in common with Fromm's (1955) ambition for a sane society. The achievement of this vision writes Gerhardt, requires both personal and political progress. Yet, people and politics seem to be heading in a regressive direction.

To be seen in an expensive car, to own a large house, to dress fashionably and to change fashion repeatedly, to build-up and beautify the body, to help the mind to be mindful and actualise personal potential, to be preoccupied with television, smartphones and social media, to be hooked on eating healthily and walking ten thousand steps or its equivalent recommended daily goal, infatuated with sexual novelty and release, and do everything alone or participate only with those who concur, all come at the cost of sincere interpersonal and community attachment. They also run the risk of entering personal madness and do display societal insanity.

For Fromm people living with the insanity of selfishness, regardless of their plentiful possessions and what are their fictious expressions to the contrary, are profoundly lonely, joyless, and insecure. The consumer society, reasons sociologist Zygmunt Bauman (2007), promises much but does not deliver anything of worth. It fails to what is its primary promise of improving happiness. What it does do, according to Bauman, is produce widespread melancholy, a sense that the self, in seeking satisfaction from consuming, has found only dissociation from itself and from other selves. In industrial society, when society was founded on production not consumption, workers were alienated from what they were producing because of their dissociation from what they were producing. In post-industrial society, founded on consumption, there is similar alienation but this time the whole population is separated from what it consumes because commodities only provide a fleeting and phony meaning for existing. Rather than meaningfulness consumption-oriented economy deepens insecurity.

Insecurity is the insanity offered for consumption in the next chapter.

References

Adame A (2013) There needs to be a place in society for madness. The psychiatric survivor movement and new directions in mental health care. *Journal of Humanistic Psychology*, 22 November. http://journals.sagepub.com/doi/abs/10.1177/0022167813510207 [accessed 4 July, 2019].

American Psychiatric Association (2013) *Diagnostic and Statistical Manual of Mental Disorders, Fifth Edition (DSM-5)*. Arlington, VA: American Psychiatric Association.

Ando V, Claridge G and Clark K (2014) Psychotic traits in comedians. *Br J Psychiatry*, 204(1). http://bjp.rcpsych.org/content/early/2014/01/02/bjp.bp.113.134569. full.pdf+html?sid=a9786822-019f-4f0a-8fa8-59440b75b972 [accessed 19 May, 2014].

Arendt H (1973) *The Origins of Totalitarianism*. Boston, MA: Houghton Mifflin Harcourt.

Atkinson S (2018) Nutella riots: A brief history of shopping scraps. www.bbc.co.uk/news/business-42828256 [accessed 23 May, 2019].

Attwood F (2009) *Mainstreaming Sex: The Sexualisation of Western Culture*. London: Tauris.

Babiak P and Hare R (2007) *Snakes in Suits: When Psychopaths Go to Work*. New York: Harper Collins.

Bakan J (2005) *The Corporation: The Pathological Pursuit of Profit and Power*. London: Constable.

Bakan J (2012) *Childhood Under Siege: How Big Business Ruthlessly Targets Children*. London: Vintage.

Baron-Cohen (2012) *Zero Degrees of Empathy: A New Theory of Human Cruelty*. London: Allen Lane.

Baudrillard J (1970) *La Société de Consommation: Ses Mythes, Ses structures* [The Consumer Society: Myths and Structures]. Paris: Denoël.

Baudrillard J (2001) *Jean Baudrillard: Selected Writings*, 2nd edn. Stanford, CA: Stanford University Press.

Bauer M, Wilkie J, Kim J and Bodenhausen G (2012) Cuing consumerism: Situational materialism undermines personal and social well-being. *Psychological Science*, 23 (5), pp. 517–523.

Bauman Z (2007) *Consuming Life*. Cambridge: Polity.

BBC News (2011) Pope Benedict XVI has attacked the commercialisation of Christmas. www.bbc.co.uk/news/world-europe-16328318 [accessed 10 January, 2019].

Beck U and Beck-Gernsheim E (2001) *Individualization: Institutionalized Individualism and Its Social and Political Consequences*. London: Sage.

Benjamin W (1991) *Gesammelte Schriften* [collected writings]. Frankfurt, Germany: Suhrkamp.

Blazer D (2005) *The Age of Melancholy: "Major Depression" and its Social Origin*. London: Routledge.

Board B and Fritzon K (2005) Disordered personalities at work. *Psychology, Crime & Law*, 11(1), pp. 17–32.

Book of Life (2019) *The Importance of Selfishness. School of Life*. www.theschooloflife.com/thebookoflife/the-importance-of-selfishness/ [accessed 28 May, 2019].

Bowles S (2016) *The Moral Economy: Why Good Incentives are No Substitute for Good Citizens*, New Haven, CT: Yale University Press.

Bridgeman P (2018) Libel actions – here [England and Wales] or the United States? *Law Society Gazette*, 5 November. www.lawgazette.co.uk/libel-actions-here-or-the-united-states/5068173.article [accessed 1 August, 2019].

Canavan B (2019) Consumerism in crisis as millennials stay away from shops. https://theconversation.com/consumerism-in-crisis-as-millennials-stay-away-from-shops-109 827 [accessed 24 May, 2019].

Carlisle S and Hanlon P (2007) Well-being and consumer culture: A different kind of public health problem? *Health Promotion International*, 22(3), pp. 261–268

Castells M (2017) *Another Economy is Possible: Culture and Economy in a Time of Crisis*. Cambridge: Polity.

Chamberlin J (1978) *On Our Own: Patient Controlled Alternatives to the Mental Health System*. New York: Hawthorne.

Chicchi F (2016) Phantasmagoria of the thing: Aporias of the new capitalist discourse. *Política común*, 9. https://quod.lib.umich.edu/p/pc/12322227.0009.003?view=text;rgn=main [accessed 6 July, 2019].

Choice (2019) About us –Who is Choice?www.choice.com.au/about-us [accessed 16 July, 2019].

Comey J (2018) *A Higher Loyalty: Truth, Lies, and Leadership*. London: Macmillan.

Compsto H (2006) *Sexual Liberalization*. New York: Springer.

Dias D (2017) *The Ten Types of Human*. London: Windmill.

Dombek K (2016) *The Selfishness of Others: An Essay on the Fear of Narcissism*. New York: Farrar, Straus and Giroux.

Dudley M, Silove D and Gale F (eds) (2012) *Mental Health and Human Rights: Vision, Praxis, and Courage*. Oxford: Oxford University Press.

Esposito L and Perez F (2014) Neoliberalism and the commodification of mental health. *Humanity and Society*, 38(4), pp. 414–442.

European Consumer Centres Network (2019) Role of the ECC-Net. https://ec.europa.eu/info/live-work-travel-eu/consumers/resolve-your-consumer-complaint/european-consum er-centres-network_en [accessed 16 July, 2019].

Fioramonti L (2017) *The World After GDP: Politics, Business and Society in the Post Growth Era*. Cambridge: Polity.

Fletcher M (2017) The joke's over – How Boris Johnson is damaging Britain's global stature. *New Statesman*, 4 November. www.newstatesman.com/politics/uk/2017/11/joke-s-over-how-boris-johnson-damaging-britain-s-global-stature [accessed 1st August, 2019].

162 *Selfishness*

Freud, S. (1914) *Zur Einführung des Narzißmus* [On Narcissism: An Introduction]. In Strachey, J. (ed.) (2001) *The Standard Edition of the Complete Psychological Works of Sigmund Freud*. London: Vintage.

Fromm E (1939) Selfishness and self-love. *Journal for the Study of Interpersonal Process*, 2, pp. 507–523.

Fromm E (1942) *The Fear of Freedom* [titled in USA 'Escape From Freedom', published 1941]. London: Routledge and Kegan Paul.

Fromm E (1955) *The Sane Society*. New York: Rinehart.

Fromm E (1956) *The Art of Loving*: New York: Harper & Row.

Fromm, E (1964) *The Heart of Man: Its Genius for Good and Evil*. New York: Harper & Row.

Fromm E (1973) *The Anatomy of Human Destructiveness*. New York: Holt, Rinehart & Winston.

Fromm E (1981) *On Disobedience and Other Essays*. New York: Harper & Row.

Gartner J (2017) Mental health professionals declare Trump is mentally ill and must be removed. www.change.org/p/trump-is-mentally-ill-and-must-be-removed [accessed 27 May, 2019].

Gaylin S (1985) The coming of the corporation and the marketing of psychiatry. *Hospital Community Psychiatry*, 36(2), pp. 154–159.

Gerhardt S (2010) *The Selfish Society: How We All Forgot to Love One Another and Made Money Instead*. New York: Simon & Schuster.

Gramsci A (1971) *Prison Notebooks*. London: Lawrence & Wishart.

Grohol J (2018) Top 50 psychiatrists paid by pharmaceutical companies. *PsychCentral*, 8 July. https://psychcentral.com/blog/top-50-psychiatrists-paid-by-pharmaceutical-companies/ [accessed 16 July, 2019].

Hare R (1999) *Without Conscience: The Disturbing World of the Psychopaths Among Us*. New York: Guildford Press.

Hare R (2003) *Hare Psychopathy Checklist-Revised*, 2nd edn. New York: Pearson.

Hill J (2015) *How Consumer Culture Controls Our Kids: Cashing in on Conformity*. Santa Barbara, CA: Praeger.

Hill R (2011) Why consumers in poor countries try harder to 'keep up with the Joneses'. *Forbes*, 16 November. www.forbes.com/sites/onmarketing/2011/11/16/why-consumers-in-poor-countries-try-harder-to-keep-up-with-the-joneses/ [accessed 29 July, 2019].

Horwitz A (2010) How an age of anxiety became an age of depression. *Milbank Quarterly*, 88(1), pp. 112–138.

James O (2007) *Affluenza*. London: Vermillion.

James O (2008) *The Selfish Capitalist*. London: Vermillion.

Jeffries S (2016) The 10 lies about Black Friday's consumerist circle of hell: As we approach the Christmas shopping season finale, what can Neo-Marxist analysis teach us? *The Guardian*, 24 November.

Jeffries S (2017) *Grand Hotel Abyss: The Lives of the Frankfurt School*: London: Verso

Kahneman D (2012) *Thinking, Fast and Slow*. London: Penguin.

Kasser T (2003) *The High Price of Materialism*. Cambridge, MA: Massachusetts Institute of Technology Press.

Kasser T, Rosenblum K, Sameroff A, Deci E, Niemiec C, Ryan R, Árnadóttir O, Bond R, Dittmar H, Dungan N and Hawks S (2013) Changes in materialism, changes in psychological well-being: Evidence from three longitudinal studies and an intervention experiment. *Motivation and Emotion*, 38(1), pp. 1–22.

Kearns M (2018) A joker on Downing Street? *National Review*, 29 October. www.na tionalreview.com/magazine/2018/10/29/a-joker-on-downing-street/ [accessed 12 July, 2018].

Kirby M (2015) *Too much of a good thing? Weight management, obesity, and the healthy body in Britain, 1950–1995* [PhD thesis]. Glasgow: Glasgow University. http://theses.gla.ac.uk/7113/1/2015KirbyMPhD.pdf [accessed 6 July, 2019].

Klein M (2010) Religion & sexuality: Iron Age or Dark Ages? *Psychology Today*, 26 December. www.psychologytoday.com/us/blog/sexual-intelligence/201012/religion-sexua lity-iron-age-or-dark-ages [accessed 18 July, 2019].

Lasch C (1979) *The Culture of Narcissism: American Life in an Age of Diminishing Expectations.* New York: Norton.

Leader D (2013) *Strictly Bipolar.* London: Penguin.

LeDoux J (2015) *Anxious: The Modern Mind in the Age of Anxiety.* London: Oneworld.

Lee B (2017) *The Dangerous Case of Donald Trump.* New York: Thomas Dunne.

Lee B (2018) Trump is now dangerous – that makes his mental health a matter of public interest. *The Observer*, 7 January.

Lee J (2017) Retail rage: Why Black Friday leads shoppers to behave badly. *The Conversation*, 22 November. https://theconversation.com/retail-rage-why-black-friday-leads-shopp ers-to-behave-badly-87647 [accessed 18 July, 2019].

Liddle R (2009) It is the narcissistic middle-aged, not the young, who love Facebook and Twitter. *Spectator*, 15 July.

Liddle R (2014) *Selfish Whining Monkeys: How we Ended Up Greedy, Narcissistic and Unhappy.* London: Fourth Estate.

Lipman F (2009) *Spent: End Exhaustion & Feel Great Again.* London: Hay House.

Monbiot G (2006) *Heat: How to Stop the Planet Burning.* London: Allen Lane.

Monbiot G (2013a) Materialism: A system that eats us from the inside out. *The Guardian*, 9 December.

Monbiot G (2013b) One Rolex short of contentment. 9 December. www.monbiot.com/ 2013/12/09/one-rolex-short-of-contentment / [accessed 26 May, 2019].

Monbiot G (2017) *How Did We Get Into This Mess?: Politics, Equality, Nature.* London: Verso.

Morozov E (2018) Will tech giants move on from the internet, now we've all been harvested? *The Observer*, 28 January.

Morrall P (2006) *Murder and Society.* Chichester: Wiley.

Morrall, P (2008) *The Trouble with Therapy: Sociology and Psychotherapy.* Maidenhead: Open University Press.

Morrall P (2017) *Madness: Ideas about Insanity.* Abingdon-on-Thames: Routledge.

Newman O (2018) *Unhinged: An Insider's Account of the Trump White House*New York: Simon & Schuster.

Ocloo J and Matthews R (2016) From tokenism to empowerment: Progressing patient and public involvement in healthcare improvement. *British Medical Journal Quality & Safety* 25, pp. 626–632.

Ortiz-Ospina E and Roser M (2016) Trust. https://ourworldindata.org/trust [accessed 28 May, 2019].

Page S (2019) *The Matriarch: Barbara Bush and the Making of an American Dynasty.* New York: Twelve.

Passini S (2013) A binge-consuming culture: The effect of consumerism on social interactions in Western societies. *Culture and Psychology*, 19(3), pp. 369–390.

Paul P (2006) *Pornified: How Pornography Is Damaging Our Lives, Our Relationships, and Our Families*. London: St Martins.

Pew Research Centre (2017) Republicans divided in views of Trump's conduct: Democrats are broadly critical. file:///C:/Users/dontb/Downloads/08–29–17-Political-release-final3.pdf [accessed 8 July, 2019].

Pieters R (2013) Bidirectional dynamics of materialism and loneliness: Not just a vicious cycle. *Journal of Consumer Research*, 40(4), pp. 615–631.

Pilgrim D and McCranie A (2013) *Recovery and Mental Health: A Critical Sociological Account*. London: Palgrave.

Pullella P (2018) Remember the poor and shun materialism, Pope says on Christmas Eve. *Reuters*, 24 December. https://uk.reuters.com/article/uk-christmas-season-pope-eve/remember-the-poor-and-shun-materialism-pope-says-on-christmas-eve-idUKKCN1ON15A [accessed 23 May, 2019].

Reade B (2019) Boris Johnson is a shallow, narcissistic, womanising liar. www.mirror.co.uk/news/politics/brian-reade-boris-johnson-shallow-16196976 [accessed 1 August, 2019].

Rees E (ed.) (2004) *The Nature of Stalin's Dictatorship: The Politburo 1928–1953*. London: Palgrave Macmillan.

Ritzer G (1993) *The Mcdonaldization of Society: An Investigation into the Changing Character of Contemporary Social Life*. Newbury Park, CA: Pine Forge.

Ronson J (2012) *The Psychopath Test*. London: Picador.

Rowe M (2015) *Citizenship & Mental Health*. New York: Oxford University Press.

Russo R and Sweeney A (2016) *Searching for a Rose Garden: challenging psychiatry, fostering mad studies*: Ross-on-Wye: PCCS.

Sassatelli R (20007) *Consumer Culture: History, Theory and Politics*. London: Sage.

Schulz W (2009) The "pornification" of human consciousness: Our minds have become "pornified". *Psychology Today*, 26 March. www.psychologytoday.com/blog/genius-and-madness/200903/the-pornification-human-consciousness [accessed 18 July, 2019].

Seltzer L (2016) Self-absorption: The root of all (psychological) evil?: Here's what you should know about obsessing, ruminating, and self-centeredness. *Psychology Today*, 24 August. www.psychologytoday.com/gb/blog/evolution-the-self/201608/self-absorption-the-root-all-psychological-evil [accessed 28 May, 2019].

Simon T (2008) *Dreaming of Jupiter*. London: Abacus.

Stiglitz J (2019) Trump will leave a legacy of selfishness and dishonesty. *The Guardian*, 10 April.

Storr W (2017) *Selfie: How the West Became Self-Obsessed*. London: Picador.

Stosell S (2014) *My Anxious life in an Age of Anxiety*. London: Windmill.

Sword R and Zimbardo P (2017) The elephant in the room: It's time we talked openly about Donald Trump's mental health. *Psychology Today*, 28 February. www.psychologytoday.com/gb/blog/the-time-cure/201702/the-elephant-in-the-room [accessed 27 May, 2019].

Trentmann F (2016) *Empire of Things: How We Became a World of Consumers, from the Fifteenth Century to the Twenty-First*. London: Allen Lane.

Tweedy R (2016) *The Political Self: Understanding the Social Context for Mental Illness*. Abingdon-on-Thames: Routledge.

Tweedy R (2017) A Mad World: Capitalism and the Rise of Mental Illness. *Red Pepper*, 9 August. www.redpepper.org.uk/a-mad-world-capitalism-and-the-rise-of-mental-illness/ [accessed 26 May, 2019].

Twenge J (2014) *Generation Me*. New York: Atria.

Twenge J and Campbell W (2009) *The Narcissism Epidemic: Living in the Age of Entitlement.* Free Press: New York.

Weber M (1930) *The Protestant Ethic and the Spirit of Capitalism.* London: Unwin Hyman.

Whippman R (2016) *America the Anxious: How Our Pursuit of Happiness is Creating a Nation of Nervous Wrecks.* London: St. Martin's Press.

Wolff M (2018) *Fire and Fury: Inside the Trump White House.* London: Little, Brown.

World Health Organisation (2016) Out of the shadows: Making mental health a global development priority. www.who.int/mental_health/advocacy/WB_event_2016/en/ [accessed 4 July, 2019].

Worldwatch Institute (2015) *Vital Signs Volume 22: The Trends That Are Shaping Our Future.* Washington, DC: Island Press.

YouGov (2019) Boris Johnson. https://yougov.co.uk/topics/politics/explore/public_figure/Boris_Johnson [accessed 1 August, 2019].

Young P, Shipley H and Trothen T (2015) *Religion and Sexuality: Diversity and the Limits of Tolerance.* Vancouver, British Columbia: UBC Press.

6 Insecurity

Violence and inequality create insecurity, and selfishness can be coupled with the insanities of specific types of society. Insecurity is a mark of personal madness and regarded as a significant symptom of many types of mental disorder. In today's global society insecurity abounds. It infiltrates much of everyday life and intrudes into the psyche.

Humans have always faced insecurities. The threat of being mauled or devoured by dangerous beasts and attacked by human competitors and their instruments of war, and coping with the vicissitudes of intimate relationships, religious scare-mongering, political tyrannies upheavals, and economic collapses and conversions. The move from an agricultural to industrial mode of production, which also meant the industrialisation of agriculture, caused fundamental and extensive changes in the organisation of society and in the performance of its inhabitants (Stearns, 2018). In those countries which shifted to a post-industrial service-based set-up have seen similar shifts in society and in people (Bell, 1976). From farmers to factory-workers, from factory-workers to the 'gig' economy's pizza deliverers (Partington, 2019). From producers to consumers, and from communitarian. From to an orientation towards community to orientating around the self.

Each era furnishes its own fears. The twenty-first century has inherited many old insecurities, intensified some and concocted dramatic new ones. This chapter first reviews the state of time-worn insecurities whose continued existence are indicative that society is still far from capable of delivering psychological security and in all too many parts of the world not even physical security. These include, anomie, loneliness, and alienation. Far from being resolved, the condition of these hoary human and societal plights have become intensified. Then in this chapter distinctively new insecurities are studied.

Contemporary human insecurity is compounded by the colossal technological contrivances of the twentieth century and their further elaboration in the twenty-first century. But technology is expected to deliver hardly conceivable digital devices and systems and is moving both humanity and society towards a yet to be imagined future. The future may yet be unimaginable, but it will certainly involve considerable proliferation in digitalisation, robotics, automation, and artificial intelligence. Or rather it will be if catastrophe doesn't first befall humanity and its habit.

As Harari notes, things have relatively recently changed dramatically

> [I]n the last few decades we have managed to rein in famine, plague, and war....[T]hey have been transformed from incomprehensible and uncontrollable forces of nature into manageable challenges.
>
> (Harari, 2017, p. 2)

Harari predicts, things will change again relatively soon, dramatically. For Harari there are now new forces, perhaps just as incomprehensible and uncontrollable as had been famine, plague and war. People living in medieval times did not foresee, indeed did not have the conceptual foundations for such foresight, although this is not necessarily true for the intelligentsia of ancient Greco-Roman and Islamic societies. Modifications to the manufacturing and distribution of food, the identification of microbes, sewers and societal situations such as overcrowded cities as harbingers of disease and subsequent social and medical remedies, and the re-evaluation of violence as an unavoidable element of human behaviour, have all come about in a very short segment of human history. Uncontrolled forces with as yet unmanaged challenges for Harari will be released from advances in information technology, robotics, automation, and artificial intelligence, but also from: biotechnology (with the genetic engineering and nanoscience reworking the components of the human body and personality, and what humans eat); cyberspace (where humans increasingly exist in a lawless simulated world), cyborg engineering (the synthesising of the organic and inorganic to manufacture a magnificent human); and 'dataism' (digital information collected and manipulated by the State and corporations using sophisticated and possible irrepressible algorithms). Harari also puts forward the possibility that these forces and challenges may cause the demise of natural selection as well as create blissful and divine immortality. There is a lot about which to feel insecure.

The public issues of violence, inequality, selfishness, are linkable to a morass of psychological private troubles. Moreover, these societal insanities (and many others) may be aggravating in the population at large what past and present social thinkers from various epistemological backgrounds have identified as a personal insecurity which, in differing proportions, is common to all. This common psychological trouble is described, for example as: 'ontological insecurity (Laing, 1961; Giddens, 1991; Browning and Joenniemi, 2016): *La Nausée,* translated as *The Nausea* (Sartre, 1938; 1972); 'existential angst' (Case, 2014; Bauman, 2016); alienation (Marx, 1959; Swain, 2012; Jaeggi, 2016); and anomie (Merton, 1968; Teymoori et al., 2017). These psychological and sociological concepts all relate to the experience of and setting for insecurity. They chime with the experience of rapid social change and fearfulness and uncertainty engendered by perpetual political, economic, and ecological change and markedly when the change is chaotic. Collectively, they subsume the feelings of futility, miserableness, emptiness, perplexity, fuzziness, and chaos, when experiencing the insecurities of *La Nausée,* existential angst, ontological insecurity, and alienation. Those feelings can transform into medicalised psychological states and may be reified as epidemics in mental disorders. Insecurity, therefore is central to the case that society is insane, and a central aspect of personal madness.

Anomie

From the list above of descriptions referring to psychological insecurity it is anomie that resonates most with the sociological imaginativeness. But anomie also deserves to be given pole position ahead of the other topics in this chapter because an anomic state can lead not only to personal madness but suicide.

What is anomie? The idea of anomie as it is used in social science arises from the sociology of Emile Durkheim. Durkheim dabbles with notion in many parts of his written work, but it is from his seminal study of suicide (1951) that anomie is most well-defined. Durkheim's 'suicide' exemplifies pre-eminently how private troubles and social issues are conjoined.

Rapid social change and/or excessive turmoil in society overall or within an individual's community, the absence of social solidarity because of a demise of previous accepted social norms and mores, and a sense of alienation, can lead to the ultimate private trouble of self-murder. This is what Durkheim terms 'anomic suicide'. However, Durkheim refers to three other types of suicide. Egoistic suicide occurs when an individual becomes socially isolated and detached from the norms and mores of society. She/he is incapable of self-regulation and has no other person or social setting to assist in self-regulation. The final act of an unregulated life is to feel that life is not worth living. Altruistic suicide may be committed when there is an allegiance to a cause and an expectation or perception that the cause will be served through its supporter's death. Certain cults, religions, and political factions may induce such suicide. Fatalistic suicide can occur when the social setting restricts severely individual expression and rights, and especially when transgressing the norms and more set by the powerful could lead to harsh, possibly capital, punishment.

There is confusion in Durkheim's work over definitions and overlap between some if not all the types of suicide (Marks, 1974). Moreover, anomie stands out as the type of suicide which is produced by the pathology of society, not the will of the individual; the other three types do contain social causative factors. Social isolation, cults, religions, and political factions, and oppression by the powerful, are all connectible to society as well as the individual. Moreover, all types of anomie, as well as existential angst and ontological insecurity, are the consequences of realising the reality of the chaotic, flawed, pointless, iniquitous, and impermanence of our lives, society, and the universe. That is, anomie is possible when there is a raised consciousness (those of a religious disposition may suggest it false consciousness) about the meaninglessness of life or when societal circumstances are insane such as when violent, iniquitous, and orientated towards selfishness.

Durkheim is aware that not everyone faced with these societal pressures commits suicide. He accepts that anomie, for example, has become normalised in modern society. But through his research comparing different countries with different belief systems and levels of interpersonal integration he concludes that the risk of suicide is raised when the level of anomie is high.

The World Health Organisation (WHO, 2018) records that the annual toll of deaths from suicide is nearly 800,000. Many more, according to WHO, attempt suicide. Suicide occurs across age groups and throughout the world but is more common amongst young people and in countries with low-to-middle average incomes. WHO suggests that there are effective preventative strategies and provides the examples of improved monitoring of suicide attempts and self-harm. What WHO does not provide are tactics for ridding the world of incomprehensible and uncontrollable forces which lead to anomic suicide.

Psychological distress amongst students is also higher than in the general population. The UK university student population in ten years has increased fivefold, reaching approximately 2.3 million each year. The has been an exponential increase in the level of self-reported and help-seeking psychological distress amongst students. Some of this distress becomes diagnosed as mental disorder. Student suicides have also risen. (Thorley, 2017; Jenkins, 2018). Students are vulnerable to psychological distress because of a combination of factors peculiar to their circumstances in this century have become more stressful than experience by their peers in earlier times. The stress has been fuelled by added financial and academic pressures, and the diminishing of employment prospects commensurate with the financial outlay to gain academic credentials.

But is isn't just students whose psychological stability is affected adversely by university system. Independent scholar Liz Morrish (2019) argues that there has been an escalation of anxiety amongst UK university staff because universities have become 'anxiety machines'. Morrish studied the rates of referrals from university staff to counselling services and discovered that between 2009 and 2019 they had risen by 77%. This increase, claims Morrish, is connected to unmanageable workloads and oppressive management regimes, unnecessary bureaucracy, and a growth in precarious contracts of employment. Morrish also mentions the suicide of two university lecturers which have been linked to stressful teaching, disproportionate managerial, and research workloads, and managerial maladroitness in dealing with objections to these amplified expectations.

There are alternative ideas about the unnerved shape of humanity to that of anomie. These alternatives, however, either parallel Durkheim's theory or add extra dimensions. Psychologist Ali Teymoori and his colleagues (Teymoori et al., 2017) outline what they claim is a psychological application of anomie. For them there are two conditions which occur before anomie surfaces. First, the fabric of society must be perceived to have fractured as indicated a momentous lowering of social trust and standards of morality.

Second, a society's leadership must be perceived to also be fracturing with those in power losing legitimacy and effectiveness. Teymoori and his colleagues list what they count as both societal and personal factors which lead to these fractures. These factors include individualism, fetishism of money, a drive to gain personal success, and corruption, all of which are rampant in global society.

The US Army War College use the acronym 'VUCA', which stands for volatility, uncertainty, complexity and ambiguity, when referring to such insecure military situations as occurred following the end of the Cold War in the 1990s (Kan et al., 2018). The concept was used earlier by Warren Bennis and Burt Nanus (1985) who are referring to volatile, uncertain, complex, and ambiguous circumstances as it applies to business leaders. Another leadership theorist, Jeroen Kraaijenbrink (2018), provides a detailed portrayal of each of the four VUCA constituents. Volatility, writes Kraaijenbrink, refers to the fast-moving changes in, for example industry and financial markets, and to how the way the world overall is altering. Kraaijenbrink alludes to the circular economic and societal process of change creating volatility and volatility creating change. Uncertainty for Kraaijenbrink denotes how well the present is understandable and the future can be predicted with any degree of certainty. The world is becoming more complex and ambiguous, explains Kraaijenbrink, and thereby more volatile and uncertain. In this chapter, digitalisation, robotics, automation, and artificial intelligence are the complexities and ambiguities of the present and the future which combine to be interrelated portents of present and future insecurity. Individual performance and interpersonal relationships can be affected, usually detrimentally, by having to navigate such volatile, uncertain, complex, and ambiguous societal situations as wars, poverty, and a culture of selfishness. The four constituents of VUCA are, as Kraaijenbrink realises, linked reflexively.

Volatility and uncertainty, complexity, and ambiguity underlie and overlay Harari's notion of 'uncontrolled forces with as yet unmanaged challenges'. Harari (2015) warns that when the pace at which society's volatility and uncertainty, complexity, and ambiguity accelerates uncontrollably and unmanageably, as it is presently, it manifests in people in the form of anxiety. Anxiety may be both a cause and consequence of what Culpin (2018) refers to as 'an epidemic of sleeplessness' According Culpin (2018), insomnia leads heightened risk of serious physical illness such as coronary disease, cerebra-vascular accidents, diabetes, and cancer, and as well anxiety, depression, and dementia. Culpin's main point, however, is that not sleeping well is bad for careers and business.

On the theme again of (alleged) epidemics, but this time with a pointedly political agenda, Will Hutton demands fundamental changes to society to defeat anxiety. It is young people, observes Hutton, who have become particularly prone to a diagnosis not just of anxiety, but depression, self-harm, attention deficit disorder, and anorexia, and bulimia. Hutton (2016) is a journalist and political economist so it is unsurprising that he sees answers to the apparent epidemic in anxiety at the level of culture – specifically individualism, and the pressure not just to achieve what counts as success in a materialistic free-market world but be happy whilst so doing and to even happier when that goal is reached. Hutton admits that there might be a process of medicalisation operating which has inflated the statistics on mental disorder amongst young people. However, there is still, argues Hutton, a noticeable upsurge in intense psychological suffering in this age group. On the basis that humans are social animals, what Hutton recommends for the achievement of genuine happiness and thereby and reduction in anxiety levels, is more communal contact:

> [T]he building blocks of happiness lie in looking out for each other, acting together, being in teams and pursuing common goals for the common good. Families, schools, colleges, unions, newspapers, sports clubs and even firms should all understand that such commonality should be part of their core DNA.
>
> (Hutton, 2016)

Scott Stossel (2014) is yet another journalist who subscribes to the notion of an anxiety epidemic. So severe is the epidemic today as to warrant the description of 'the age of anxiety'. Stossel writes about his experience of anxiety which he has had since childhood: how ordinary life is interrupted by bouts of extreme fearfulness accompanied by a panoply of physical symptoms including nausea, dizziness, tremors, and difficulties in breathing, swallowing, and walking. On occasions his fear is one of impending death. When not feeling intense dread he still 'buffeted by worry' regarding his health and that of members of his family, finances, work, heading for old age, and dying. His worrying doesn't stop there as he can, he confesses, worry about what might appear to outsiders as extremely and intensely trivial examples of which are rattles in his car and water dripping in his basement. As if that wasn't enough worry, Stossel also suffers from phobias. His inventory of these specific anxieties is lengthy. Some of his phobias are: claustrophobia (fear of entrapment in a closed space); acrophobia (fear of heights); asthenophobia (fear of fainting); bacillophobia (fear of bacteria); aerophobia (fear of flying); emetophobia (fear of vomiting); and turophobia (fear of cheese). He also lists the treatments he has tried. These comprise a host of psychotherapies, anti-anxiety medications, anti-anxiety self-help books, hypnosis, massage, praying, acupuncture, yoga, alcohol, and stoicism.

Stossel questions whether anxiety is a personal trouble best addressed by the profession of medicine, philosophers, psychologists, or religion. On the other hand, Stossel realises that it may be a social issue connected to contemporary culture. He marries the two explanatory strands by settling on a composite answer. For him the sort of anxiety he experiences, and by implication that of all those embraced by the epidemic, is founded in the biology and psychology of the individual and the culture in which she/he exists. Anxiety is a glitch of nature and nurture, a psychological and sociological phenomenon.

As always, it's complicated, but economic insecurity following the aftermath of the 2008/2007 international financial crisis, which came close to destroying the banking basis of capitalism, has been coupled with psychologist distress and suicide (Van Hal, 2015). The complexity arises from mediating components. In the UK the indirect but potent influence on people's ability to remain psychologically sanguine has been (and still is at the time of writing) the prolonged government policy aimed delivering austerity. Austerity in this context means severe restrictions on national and local spending. These restrictions affected the overall profitability of the UK's economy, welfare and health care provision, and wages which have either stagnated or declined (Cribb and Johnson, 2018).

There is substantial empirical evidence supporting the connection (but not definitely causality) between economic failure and frugality and a diagnosis of a multiplicity of mental disorders as well as suicide (WHO, 2011; Frasquilho et al., 2016; Haw et al., 2015). With economic failure and frugality come the insecurities of unemployment, low-paid employment, precarious employment, and employment without union representation and protection to hinder exploitation. A further insecurity is that of not having enough money to pay the rent or mortgage and this can (and does) lead to the loss of a basic human need and right – shelter (Haw et al., 2015). Indebtedness and homelessness should not be common concerns if a society is sane.

It is in these anomic circumstances that people may take their own lives. Those vulnerable to psychological distress and suicide have become affected personally and directly by external forces over which they have no direct control. They could, with hindsight, have voted (in countries where this is allowed) for politicians who might have followed an alternative political ideology and economic policy to that which nearly led to the disintegration of not only the international financial system but global society because global society is founded on that system. With hindsight, politicians, economists, and bankers could, without necessarily changing their fundamental beliefs (in capitalism and a free-market) and motives (to stay in power and/or make money), have refrained from indulging unsustainable financial practices such as subprime mortgage lending.

But this is victim-blaming or, more justifiably, culprit-blaming, and retrospective analysis cannot change what happened which may have in any case been beyond the jurisdiction of any individual or group. According to the Bank of England it is still beyond the jurisdiction of anyone as it will happen again:

> History shows that there are two things we can be sure of when it comes to financial crises: there will be another one, and the next one won't be the same as the last. That's a big problem because they can be very damaging.
>
> (Bank of England, 2019)

It's not just an out-of-control financial system which furnishes insecurity. The Nation State seems to be vulnerable to collapse.

The Nation State has become gradually less important as a societal structure since the process of globalisation began, which is one reason individual governments found the 2007/2008 financial crisis impossible to de-escalate will do when the next one arrives. Novelist and essayist Rana Dasgupta (2018), however, argues that the Nation State is not in a state of a diminishment but demise. There are failing and failed States to be found in North Africa, central Africa, and the Middle-East. But Dasgupta's point is that all National States are doomed to fail because of globalisation. There is the wide-world phenomenon of a country's societal set-up, including its economy and governance, transferring to global systems controlled by global elites.

Globalisation is in the main an economic process built on an ideology which lauds the free-market (and neoliberal capitalism is loudest in lauding unfettered free-marketism). As it is implemented it carries along the cultural accoutrements it requires to function and endure, notably materialism, individualism, consumerism, and a degree of such widespread selfishness the culture overall could be characterised as narcissistic (see Chapter 5). One stark cultural contradiction of a globalised society based on these accoutrements is that individualism and selfishness would appear not to fit with materialistic consumerism whereby similar commodities (whether computers, mobile/cell-phones, cars, clothing, or holidaying in the Caribbean) are admired and acquired by millions of people from across the world. Where global trade appears to dispense dissimilar commodities, these may only be accessed by the few (the discerning or the rich), and the dissimilarity is likely to be marginal. As financial crises demonstrate, the globalised free market also has a fundamental structural fault, and one which surface again and again with the possibly that this economic system will fail completely. Notwithstanding this contradiction and fault (along with other defects) global capitalism has operated effectively enough to be move whole populations in its direction, and today it effectively has all the world's population in its ideological and economic grip. Therefore, as capitalism spread globally it should have spread stability but instead, as worries over employment and housing exemplify, it has furnished insecurity.

There are also countervailing forces to globalisation and standardisation triggering more insecurity. One of those forces is the kick-back against the downfall of the Nation State which has not just been about globalisation but also supra-states, the obvious example being the European Union which in 2016 a majority the British voters wished to leave. As Dasgupta notes, at a time when globalisation was expected to be embedded to the point of no return, threats to societal stability have arisen. These have come in the shape of mass petitions and demonstrations, and in some instances, riots, in Westerns countries including the UK, USA, France, Spain, and Italy. Challenges to 'the old ways' to use Dasgupta's caricature, have also occurred in the shape of both democratic and undemocratic installing of authoritarian regimes or reaffirming already authoritarian governance (Russia). Example of the countries where this has happened are: Russia; China, Rwanda; Venezuela; Thailand; the Philippines; Turkey; Poland; Hungary; and Austria. There is also challenge to the 'old ways' from the upsurge in populist parties and election of populist leaders as happened in the UK in 2019 and USA three years earlier.

There is no single issue upon which civil unrest rests. The petitions, demonstrations, and riots, are campaigns against inequality, unemployment, global warming, and higher taxes on fuel among many other perceived injustices which globalisation has failed either to resolve or has made worse. This extensive and occasionally violent public agitation, however, in part built on another ambiguity, that of making demands for 'new ways' by bringing back the very 'old way' of the Nation State.

It is understandable that there is irrationality amongst the populace of these countries who, according to use Dasgupta, are exhausted, and affected by feelings of hopelessness and futility. Hopelessness and futility are indicators of anomie.

Dasgupta also discerns that the populations of a host of countries not already cited are also in states of discontent. Former colonised parts of the world have erupted. Mass displays civil unrest have managed to change regimes either through shaming their leaders or violence. But many of these countries far from finding new ways which may bring stability, have descended into tribalism, lawlessness, and re-ignited religious fundamentalism. Rather than an enhanced way of life, humanised and effective authority and social institutions have not emerged.

For Dasgupta, the spark that has ignited so much unrest across the world is because the political leadership has lost the moral authority to rule. Injustice is all too apparent. How the rich live a highly privileged life compared to the majority, and how the powerful misuse their power. Dasgupta gives the example continued existence and increased use of tax avoidance and tax havens as having undermined belief in them and the social institutions and social processes which they defend. He also points to what he refers to as 'algorithmic governance' by non-governmental agencies naming Google and Facebook as models of data manipulation, which has led to further feelings of disempowerment. This has all happened as has globalisation unfolded, and the role of the Nation State subsided. What has happened alongside, suggests Dasgupta, is a form of generalised vagrancy. That is, large numbers of people no longer identify with a geographically bounded arena in which there is willing participation in a known and respected culture. Moreover, 'home' has not been replaced with a comparable let alone a better way of life. Dasgupta's prediction is that things will only get worse.

Loneliness

What may not have been good for centuries, and may well get very much worse, is human companionship. Loneliness is yet another contender for the status of epidemic. Joe Smith (2018) journalist and psychologist, suggests that loneliness should be cited as a public health emergency.

Widespread social isolation is damaging for people and society writes Monbiot (2017). Monbiot (2018) writes about how collective action in a small town in England was successful in combating loneliness. Monbiot makes the point, however, that the level of loneliness and damage it does can be lowered. To make this case he refers to what happened in a small English town when a project encompassing collective action was implemented. The target population for the project was people who were suffering physical ill-health and who were socially isolated. The underlying assumption of project was that physical ill-health leads to loneliness because the sufferers are less able to leave their home to mix with others, a situation made worse if they do not have friends or family able or willing to visit them. The supplementary assumption was that as their loneliness exacerbated their physical health deteriorated, and that self-worth worsens, with depression ensuing. Apart from depression, social isolation has been linked specifically with decreased cognitive capability, and raised risk of cardiovascular disease, stroke and hypertension, Alzheimer's disorder, anxiety, alcohol abuse and suicide (Griffin, 2010; Magen, 2018).

The measure used in the Somerset project to test the effectiveness of increased interpersonal contact was the degree to which overall emergency hospital admissions fell. They did fall and they fell dramatically. The main interventions were interpersonal contact, together with help to reach relevant services including community groups such as 'talking cafes' to further increase interaction with others. The core of quality of the contact, however, was kindness:

> The building of compassionate communities makes sense in many contexts... [I]t exercises and demonstrates that essential quality of human kindness which is among our greatest strengths as a species.... [It] emphasises the life-enhancing value of human contact, and thereby generates and affirms a vital sense of meaning and purpose.
>
> (Abel and Clarke, 2018)

Psychiatrist Antony Storr (1988) contradicts the notion that social isolation *per se* is a negative state for humans. For Storr, being with other people can detract from an individual's potential to be creative. Whilst creativity for many theorists coincides with connectivity (see below), being alone allows a greater opportunity to concentrate and thereby potentially generate innovative ideas as well as complete intricate physical tasks. Human fulfilment, therefore, can be achievable through personal effort. The loneliness of the long-distance runner, and many other personal commitments, is conducted primarily in seclusion and only achievable through intentional solitude. Social isolation is not inseparable from human happiness. Isolation is instrumental for many if not most academics, artists, and musicians. Storr recommends spending time alone for all as a technique to improve, not impair, human existence. But, as Storr is aware, there is a huge difference between the unintended and purposeful solitude. Experiencing 'loneliness' infers suffering and there is evidence to suggest that suffering can be extremely serious.

Loneliness is a social condition. That is, the condition of society may bring about loneliness. For example, selfishness, individualism, divorce, living longer but unaccompanied because a partner has died, and more single people there are the greater the demand, and resultant supply, for single occupancy occupation, are circumstances for which society has much responsibility. Furthermore, society overall can be described as 'lonely' when it is replete with isolated individuals (Griffin, 2010). Isolated people can find themselves is an ever-worsening psychological state whereby they become more and more socially isolated. Psychological responses to loneliness can include hypervigilance, aggression, and increased self-centredness. The lonely may then be responded to with avoidance resulting in a downward spiral of insecurities regarding self-esteem (Smith, 2018).

There may also be a neurological and immunological element interplaying with societal and psychological factors. Neuroscientist John Cacioppo and science journalist William Patrick, from research conducted by the former and other colleagues, record that chronic loneliness is associated with the over-production of stress hormones, raise blood pressure, suppression of the immune system by damaging white blood cells. This may then lead to chronic and serious disease, and early death. Extensive periods of loneliness may be as damaging to physical health as obesity and smoking. Loneliness, ostensibly a psychological ailment is also a societal syndrome and biological pathogen (Cacioppo and Patrick, 2009).

In an internet blog, forensic psychologist on anger, madness and destructive behaviour, Stephen Diamo (2014) writes about loneliness and refers to it as a form of alienation. Espousing an existentialist position, Diamo considers human existence as one of perpetual aloneness:

> From the existential perspective, we are born alone and die alone, and live our lives as fundamentally separate beings ultimately isolated and alienated from our fellow creatures.
>
> (Diamo, 2014)

Humans assuage this unavoidable and innate alienation through interpersonal relationships (and it can be added, through attachments to animals). Humans, therefore, engage in sociability for emotional comfort. The emotional consequences without this contact can be devastating especially for infants who, when deprived of adequate human contact, can become extremely emotionally insecure which may affect their physical functioning to such an extent that they die. Depriving adults of interpersonal contact, if prolonged, can also have severe results. Ostracism is used as a punishment in some criminal justice systems and, perhaps with worse cruelty, as torture on captives. Diamo delineates the universal human state of existential aloneness from loneliness which is the consequence of an absence of sociability due to an absence of opportunities, an unwillingness to try, or failed attempts. He points out that whilst loneliness not universal presently it is pervasive.

The title of Diamo's (2014) blog discussed above is *Let's Talk About Loneliness: Alienation in a Linked-Up Age*. Oddly, he makes no attempt to link the digitalisation of much of human communication in the contemporary world, which presumably is what he means by a 'linked-up age', with the pervasiveness of loneliness. The digitalisation of society (which is discussed below) has had a huge impact on humans, including interfering with their existential essence.

Alienation

Alienation has already been referred to concerning loneliness. Loneliness has become a prevalent personal problem and social issue in recent years, however, the experience of being alone spans human history. The meaning of aloneness has altered historically, and loneliness defined as unwanted aloneness may have originated in the sixteenth century when it appeared to signify a dangerous situation whereby an individual had become separated from the protection of her/his compatriots. Alienation, on the other hand, is specific to one period of history and one specific way of structuring of society.

The concept of alienation mostly relates to the organisation and practices of work under capitalism. Understandings of alienation as applied to the organisation of work originates from the early writings of Marx (1959, original 1844). A meta-analysis of research and theorising using the concept of alienated work concludes that it remains a pertinent concept. Employment conditions and employer-employee relations have become highly complex – certainly since Marx first wrote about it – but alienation remains an unwelcome outcome of employment for much of the contemporary workforce (Chiaburu et al., 2014). Marx notes, however, that although workers suffer the most, their employers, the capitalist owners (and today the senior corporate managers), also suffer from alienation only not nearly to the same level as their employees.

Marx's idea of alienation does not appear in his writings as a coherent theory (Swain, 2012). He considers alienation to permeate every aspect of human existence, and that it carries with it major psychological and physical detriments. It also creates a societal situation in which individuals their inherent inclination towards cooperativeness is discarded for the orchestrated impulse of competitiveness. It is alienation as it applied to work within the capitalist mode of economic production that is Marx's focus (1959, original 1844). Humans have become separated from their 'self' and from nature because of alienating working practices installed by capitalism. Marx does not address ecological issues directly, but the alienation of humans from nature can be viewed as having also ruptured nature from its essences (Swain, 2012). Industrialisation, which commenced and flourished during Marx's lifetime, and latterly consumerism, has unglued the necessary ecological ingredients and life-cycle of soil, plants, and precipitation, and annihilated many animal species and is threatening many more.

The separation of humans from nature has caused a dislocation from what Marx regards as a need to be free to produce creatively. An individual's impulse for creativity is stifled, which it is according to Marx for all those unemployed with the capitalist arrangements for work, then an essential element of being human is also suppressed. Therefore, capitalism is dehumanising because it prevents humans from expressing their nature and bifurcates the natural symbioses of human nature and the natural world.

Fromm, using the Marxist strand of his theorising, criticizes the alienation of people in the capitalistic society thus:

> All activities are subordinated to economic goals, means have become ends; man is an automaton – well fed, well clad, but without any ultimate concern for that which is his peculiarly human quality and function.
>
> (Fromm, 1956, p. 133)

Marx claims that the desire for individuals to release their imaginations is not a selfish process. Humans also have an inherent craving for sociability. Some creative production may be executed in private but for the most part human work is naturally a collective activity. People need other people for their psychological well-being but also to help realise their inventiveness. Capitalism replaces authentic cooperation with manufactured competition. Instead of humans working together in mutually satisfying endeavours, they are pitted against each other. Capitalism makes material remuneration, high social status, and power its rewards. Natural human creative production is rewarding because it is a fundamental expression of what it is to be human and is rewarding because it is shared. Ironically, it is not just those who are recruited to work for capitalism (not that there is much choice for most given that capitalism has globalised) who are dehumanised.

The estrangement of workers from their nature is exemplified by the way in which work became compartmentalised in the factory-based industries of the 19th century. Massive profits were made by the owners but the conditions of the working class, at work, at home and in their physical environment between the two, were appalling (Engels, 1969, original 1845). The work was dangerous, repetitive, lengthy, monitored in the minutiae, and insecure for the adults and child employees. No matter how appalling these conditions, losing employment in the factory, which could happen at the whim of a supervisor or boss, meant probable penury. What disconnected the worker from their potential to be creative (but not from their productive value for the owners) was the steady move towards making only part of whatever was being manufactured. Each worker became a cog in the manufacturing process. As such, her/his intellect and skills were limited to what was necessary to make that part. Therefore, the sense of achievement (that is, productive creativity) was also limited or non-existent. Workers did not even need comprehend or witness the completed goods.

At the time Fromm was writing *The Sane Society* (published in 1955), the factories of most of the industrialised world had become assembly lines, and the work had become much more compartmentalised. Today, it is the multitude of battery-hen-like sweatshops, and call centres and many other types of office-base work employing millions globally which today, from the perspective of Marx, which exemplify the estrangement of workers from their nature. The conditions for workers in these jobs are similar to those of previous centuries. They are scripted in minute detail with prescribed outcomes, and supervised intensely, and insecure and stressful (Winch, 2011; Woodcock, 2016; Mezzadri, 2017; War on Want, 2019). Middle-class occupations (including academia and medicine), are prone to such employment specifications, and increasingly so because their activities are increasingly digitalised thereby far more availed to observation by employers (and consumers of their goods and services). More-over, when workers and trade union's demand and better conditions, which had been realised in the twentieth century. But improvements have been under-mined by the growth of the 'gig' economy by the beginning of the twenty-first century, and business made to implement these improvements merely moving to an area of the world where employment protections are absent.

An example of working practices which can be both extremely detrimental to workers and to the physical environment is offered by immunologist Roberta Attanasio (2016). The USA government under the leadership of President Trump is attempting to reverse the decline if that country's coal industry, by for example, changing the rules for power plant emissions to favour the coal industry rather than those industries which do not use fossil fuels (Crooks, 2019). Up until this intervention the coal industry has been in rapid decline. Its operations have devastated landscapes and entire ecosystems, and spread toxic pollutants which have contaminated vast areas of land, the air, and water sup-plies. The coal industry's impact has been linked to cancer, and lung, respira-tory and kidney diseases, and birth defects. Its decline is linkable to the social issue of disconnectedness which in turn is associated with personal troubles such as anxiety, depression, insomnia and substance abuse.

The UK government's Health and Safety Executive (2018) records that for the year 2017–2018 the number of people experiencing work related stress (which encompasses depression and anxiety) was nearly 6,000,000. The amount of working days lost for that period in the UK was 15.4 million. Workload pressures such as tight deadlines and having to take on too many or inappropriate responsibilities, and inadequate support from managers, were reported by sufferers as causing their stress. General medical practitioner and 'TV doctor' Ellie Cannon (2018) suggests that as the conditions of employment are not likely to change for the better (she doesn't supply her reasoning for this prediction), then workers must change themselves. What she suggests is that workers foster defence against stress by indulging in 'healthy interpersonal relationships' in the workplace, and by taking control over aspects of their working day no matter how trivial. Cannon declares that all workers have the ability to feel better at work.

Cannon is also a fan of mindfulness at work. Journalist William Little (2018) argues that the suggestion of workers engaging in mindfulness or similar mediation techniques to deal with work-related stress should provoke anger not nirvana. He points out that it serves employers well to encourage workers to de-stress using what are not too inconvenient (especially is carried-out in the employee's own time) or expense (certainly compared with changing working conditions). He mentions that some of the largest global companies, for example, Google, GlaxoSmithKline and the professional services network KPMG, have realised that these techniques may benefit the individual worker but can also boost productivity.

Mindfulness or 'meeting up' to chat does not reduce alienation at work. But it does reduce the need for employers and politicians to be mindful of the dehumanising effects of not meeting basic human needs

Furthermore, a becalmed workforce more likely to settle for the status quo than demand more holidays, shorter working days, longer breaks at work, and increased wages, let alone lead a revolution.

Digitalisation

Today's society is digitalising. Digitalisation enables opportunities for creativity the quality of which Marx and Fromm could not have predicted. But it does bestow the insecurities on individuals and society that they, along with Durkheim, had already imagined. Human life is increasingly taking place in a digital bubble. Interpersonal communication, consumer-retailer interaction, and exchanges between State institutions and citizens are more-and-more taking place through the internet and digital gadgets. Regular or even constant instant contact is not only possible but easily achieved, but the internet and the gadgets have become the intermediaries for human-to-human and human-to-organisation connections. Digital data is collectable and connectible. Once collected it can be used for the benefit of people and society or to further manipulate and control how both perform. This manipulation and control in the future will not have to rely on human involvement. Algorithmically imbued artificially intelligent systems may act independently, the aftermath of which has only relatively recently a social issue for academic, political and public debate. Digitalisation has speeded connectivity but furthered physical separateness. There are both mind-boggling and mind-altering prospects and penalties for humanity existing in a digital bubble, and potential remarkable progression as well disruptive and destructive consequences for society.

Technology researcher Evgeny Morozov (2013; 2017) reviews the present and potential effects of digitalisation. Technology, observes Morozov, allows consumerism to flourish, has removed the distinction between work and home, has created a new societal arena in which the personal becomes public and novel ways for society to be governed, and has allowed access to an extensive range of leisure and erotic pursuits. There is, therefore, a dramatic reshaping of society and human performance. Morozov then asks if the change is desirable.

Morozov notes that the 'digital turn' in society is tied to capitalism. What Morozov is inferring is that digitalised society's main benefactor and benefiter is big business. Contrived by capitalism, digitalisation has the alienating effects of previous capitalist formations. Digitalisation is not only driving the economy but also the drive for greater productivity and undermines further the relationship workers have with their work. Workers have yet less and less control over what they produce and are more and more controlled. Humans have to engage with digital technology in both manufacturing and service industries, including in academic and medical work.

On the agenda of the 2019 meeting of the World Economic Forum (2019a) was an attempt to understand and the impact of digitalisation on society are happening. The World Economic Forum is the international organization made-up of the influential politicians, bankers, business people, representatives of major non-government agencies, scientists and other experts and campaigners such as the environmental activist Greta Thunberg (who made a video about the climate crisis which was heard at the 2019 meeting). Its mission to encourage 'positive change' by shaping global and local policies (World Economic Forum, 2019b).

The agenda of the meeting indicates that there was a realisation of the profoundly disruptive effect of digitalisation on society. A list of concerns was mentioned. This included employment insecurity. There Forum attendees seemingly appreciated the great uncertainty over how working conditions would be affected. Mention is made of an estimated 2 million to 2 billion job losses because of digitalisation by 2013. Contrarily, digitalisation could create millions of jobs and the examples are provided of the electricity and logistics industries. Another concern for the Forum is that of the insecurity of personal data. Information collected digitally by, for example, corporations and governments is as yet not guaranteed to be retained securely. There is a frank admission from the meeting:

> The truth is that we actually know quite little of what is going to happen. What will the economic impact of innovations be in the future? How will humans interact with machines and algorithms?... How will all of this impact labour markets?
>
> (World Economic Forum, 2019a)

Much earlier than that meeting of the World Economic Forum, Baudrillard was writing about his concerns regarding a digitalised society. Baudrillard, as mentioned in Chapter 5, champions the perspective of postmodernist sociology. For postmodern sociologists, modern society has changed considerably away from respecting authority and the legitimacy of grand narratives whether based on religion, science, or politics. Scepticism is rife in the postmodern world, and 'truth' and reality relative to whoever's narrative is accepted as authentic at that time and in that place (Hicks, 2019).

According to Baudrillard (1970; 1994), postmodern society has yet another characteristic. He argues that people are existing in a 'hypperreal' world for which he uses the term 'simulacra'. In this world real objects and real inter-personal connections have been replaced by simulations or symbols of reality (Tiffin and Nobuyoshi, 2001). As already indicated, 'real' in the postmodern sense does not exist so what is being replaced is an assent to something being real. What people now assent to is a sign. Digital technology furnishes a fantasy world. Regular face-to-face connectivity has been swapped for digitalised means of association. Physical intimacy has been swapped for digitalised relationships (and consumerism similarly segregates and diminishes human contact). Engagement with the simulated world of simulacra occurs through mobile/cell-phone usage (telephoning and texting), and the internet. The latter includes social media communications, buying and selling goods and services including personal banking, playing computer games, watching videos and live or recorded television and radio programmes, and reading news feeds.

What is real and what is hyperreal are no longer distinguishable. Through this process of simulacra, people have become simulations, imitations of humans, and thereby themselves mere objects. (Poster, 2001). Postmodern culture, therefore for Baudrillard, is concocted from a potent artificiality, the hyppereal world of simulacra, whereby its inhabitants can no longer distinguish what is natural from what is a simulation. But simulated existence is not a duplication or imitation of reality. It is a separate existence into which humanity has entered without much indication of awareness or objection that it is so doing.

'Virtual reality' technology offers another entry point into simulacra, only there is a puzzle bordering on paradox in the use of this technology. If the world outside that which is created by this technology is already 'virtual' then what is status of the world created by virtual reality devices? Is it an alternative to simulacra, a competitor to that created postmodern one, or an extended hyperreality, that is a 'super-hyperreality' or 'superimposed hyper-reality'? Furthermore, if people living in simulacra are unaware of the false-ness of their situation this could be described as a form of collective psychosis because they are as distant from knowing what is real as it is contended that those diagnosed as schizophrenic. Otherwise, it is the simulacra-based society which is insane.

For Harari, whilst not claiming everyone is mad and/or society is insane, does claim that there are serious side-effects from spending too much time in the illusory domain of cyberspace (that is, the digital 'ether' generated mainly by the internet) for individuals and society:

> Cyberspace is now crucial to our daily lives, our economy and our security.... [The] Internet is a free and lawless zone that erodes sovereignty, ignores borders, abolishes privacy and poses perhaps the most formidable global security risk.
>
> (Harari, 2017, p. 436)

The House of Commons Science and Technology Committee (2019) also notes the downside of internet usage. Whilst accepting that there is an absence of robust empirical evidence, there are concerns from available research that too much time-consuming social media and text messaging is risky for children. It lists damaging effects as disturbed sleep, becoming a victim of cyber-bullying, sexual grooming, and 'sexting' (receiving or receiving sexual images or messages).

For Harari, there are wider concerns. Brains and 'minds' (already just data-processing algorithmic biological entities) will be re-engineered by those with control over biotechnology and computer algorithms. Eventually, superior computer-based biotechnical algorithms will control the controllers and thereby all organisms to the extent that they will be able to enslave or replace organisms.

In the ninth edition of sociologist George Ritzer's (2018) book containing his seminal thesis 'The McDonaldization of Society', he addresses digitalisation. Ritzer's original idea is that a process of 'rationalisation' is integral to the advance of capitalism, and that process endows working practices and the environments in which people are employed as exemplified by the mind-numbing conditions, uniformity, and questionable quality of fats-food restaurants. Ritzer argued that this style was spreading into many industries and because it was profitable and had the bonus of indoctrinating both workers and consumers into accepting such conditions and associated goods and services. What Ritzer adds to the ninth edition is that despite digital technology replacing the bricks and mortar of capitalist production to a significant extent, control over employees and consumers has remained and may well be enhanced through that shift. That is, the monitoring of workers productivity and the manipulation of consumer choice by the owners of the production process and their political allies has become easier (and more 'rational') through digitalisation.

Journalist, and film-maker Chip Walter (2006) warns that homo sapiens after six million years of evolution (by natural selection) and 200,000 years of occupying the head of the food chain, become 'cyber sapiens' because of digital technology. Harari takes up this theme.

Harari (2017) adopts the term 'dataism' to describe the synchronising of animals (that is, humans) and machines which can come about when both are computed as algorithms. Harari expects that eventually the biological element in this conjoint arrangement will be overtaken by the sophisticated electronic algorithms. At that stage human evolution by natural selection ends. According to Harari, what he refers to as current 'scientific dogma' is to view biological entities in this way. Whether it a human, a giraffe, or a tomato, each is a data processing unit. Collections of data processing units such as beehives, bacteria colonies, forests, and human institutions (schools, the police, and parliament), systems (for example, education, criminal justice, and capitalism), communities, and societies (including global society), are just algorithmic complexities.

Digital technology has produced a race of robots. Robots can carry out routine tasks in the domestic and work places. Harari (2017) points out that the introduction of artificial intelligence into robots could lead to what he describes as 'god-like humans' thereby making humanity redundant. That is, artificial intelligence as it develops replaces human effort but could displace humanity from its top position in the hierarchy or life and ultimately the need to life on earth to have humans in its mix at all.

Internet entrepreneur Andrew Keen (2018), also envisages that humanity's survival is insecure because of digitalisation but has a plan to prevent its demise. For humans to influence the amassing governance of humanity by algorithmic digital technology, there controls must be introduced urgently. Keen recommends first that technological knowledge should be open to no only to expert scrutiny but to that of the public, and there should be communal not private ownership of the outcomes of that knowledge. Second, democracy must be protected by regulating technology corporations which operate in the public domain. This includes companies involved with social media, internet search engines, advertising, music, and videos on the internet.

Kenan Malik (2018) is an academic writer with interests in, for example, neurobiology and the history of science. He argues that rather than worry about intelligent technology and its potential for leading humanity into a dystopian existence of non-existence, concern should be directed at how that worry may impose a self-fulfilling prophecy.

There are, accepts Malik, genuine threats from digital technology. For example, the infecting and hacking of personal, political, and military data and data systems, the use of drones or robots for nefarious purposes, and the positioning of fake (and sometimes real) information, images and videos to cause embarrassment to individuals or to manipulate public opinion for political ends, and criminal activity in cyberspace. What humanity is not at risk from technology insists Malik, is annihilation. Even the most artificially intelligent digital technologies are only 'clever bits of software' that will always remain amenable to human jurisdiction.

Ecological scientist James Lovelock (2006) is famous for his theory of 'Gaia'. What Lovelock proposes is that inorganic and organic environment interacts and behaves as if it were an integrated living organism. As with other organisms, to survive it has self-regulating mechanisms. Earth's homeostatic regulation covers temperature, oxygen and acidity-alkaline levels, and salinity in the seas. Humanity, as with all other life forms, are part of Gaia. But unlike its organic and inorganic fellow participants in the Gaia formulation, humanity has become deregulated. The handiwork of humanity, particularly its industrial and agricultural inventions, by disturbing Gaia are making organic life on earth seriously insecure. The global financial crisis of 2007/2008, Lovelock argues, serves as another example of how major edifices of humanity are vulnerable to collapse and in so doing could cause catastrophic collapse of co-exiting societal and ecological systems (2009).

The period in the history of the earth lasting approximately 300 years during which humans have had most influence over the organic and inorganic environment. The Anthropocene is characterised by the negative consequences of human interference with Gaia, animal and plant extinctions, and contaminated oceans and pollution of the atmosphere. The Anthropocene is coming to an end argues Lovelock (2019).

Contradicting his earlier predictions, however, the end of the Anthropocene may not herald catastrophe. Paradoxically, it is, in his view, a human invention which is coming to the rescue. That invention is artificial intelligence. A new age in which artificial intelligence will come to the fore has already begun, argues Lovelock. He names this new stage in the history of the earth the 'Novacene'. Artificial intelligence will outsmart human thinking and the algorithms of the Anthropocene, according to Lovelock, ten thousand times. By comparison, systems imbued with artificial intelligence in their 'brainpower' will be as different as humans are to plants. They will also have independence.

But far from being a threat to humanity, Lovelock suggests that the humanity, other life forms, and the physical environment can be beneficiaries of the Novocene. Hyperintelligent independent machines need to (re)stabilise Gaia for their own survival. That is, they depend on the earth's stability to enable the elementary resources from which they are made and which allow them to function to continue to be available (even if much of what they require can be produced by their own technologies). They also will depend on the atmosphere remaining a protective shield from the sun's radiation (although, again, some aspects of protection may be self-generated). It is organic life which creates these resources and the shield, explains Lovelock. Therefore, Lovelock concludes, humans (and other living organisms) will not be purged by or become the slaves of artificially intelligent machines but will be their partners.

That humanity and artificial intelligence come together as a new cyborg system which will save the earth from ecological destruction is a mighty leap of hope and a mighty shift from previous prophecies by Lovelock. Rather than seeking to either use its existing intelligence the might of human stupidity is shifting towards devastation not salvation (see Chapter 7).

Social media

Social media, although a component of a digitising society, deserves a special mention. This is because of its pervasive use, particularly by young people, and its potent intoxicating influence on its participants.

There is a long list of social media services with and ever-growing population of users. Example of internet and mobile-phone interpersonal networking, blogging, and data sharing internet websites includes Facebook, YouTube, WhatsApp, Skype, LinkedIn Snapchat, Myspace, Reddit, Flickr, TikTok, Baidu and Sina Weibo (China), VKontakte (Russia), and Gaia

Online (MakeAWebsiteHub.com, 2020). The popularity of these websites will eb and flow, and some will disappear just as new ones will appear. However, social media as a personal and societal artefact seems stable and long-lasting. What may not be as stable, according to physiologist and psychiatrist Igor Pantic (Pantic, 2014; Pantic et al., 2017) is the effect use of this form of interaction will have on the psychological disposition of its users. Pantic notes that whilst there are benefits from belonging from participating with others on line (such as making new – virtual –friends and sharing ideas, news, and solving personal problems) several studies have attributed sustained use of social media by children and adolescents a lowering of self-esteem, narcissistic tendencies, as well as addictive behaviours. A systematic review of empirical evidence relating to the use of social media again by Children and adolescent found that it could be correlated with psychological distress, notably depression and anxiety (Keles et al., 2019).

The Royal Society for Public Health (2017) an independent, multi-disciplinary charity dedicated to the improvement of the public's health and wellbeing, published the results of a survey it conducted examining the effects of social media and young people's mental health and wellbeing. The report refers to rates of anxiety and depression in young people having risen by 70% over the previous 25 years, coinciding with the rise in use of social media whereby presently 91% of 16–24-year-olds use the internet for social networking. It concludes:

- Social media may be more addictive than cigarettes and alcohol.
- Social media use is linked with increased rates of anxiety, depression and poor sleep.
- Cyber bullying is a growing problem amongst people.

However, what is also acknowledged in the report is that social media avails young people to the experiences of others and expert information regarding, for example, issues of health. A further related positive outcome of social media usage is the emotionally support young people receive from their contacts which may lead to maintaining or improving psychological wellbeing.

'Child of our Time' (2019) is an internet blog operated by researchers at University College London conducting and recording empirical evidence from the research of others about the health and happiness of children living in the UK. These researchers have evidence that again links heavy social media use by young people and psychological distress such as depression. What they conclude is that the threat of social media to psychological stability is similar to that of sugar on physical health. Moreover, they found evidence of susceptibility to on-line bullying and harassment, and sleep disturbance. Girls more than boys seem to be susceptible to the harmful influences of social media. In particular, girls experienced lowered self-esteem on average twice as often as boys.

The undesirable effects of social media are a main contributor to those of general use of the internet. There are also complicating factors which are not necessarily known which may mediate these effects. Moreover, the use of social media has become a social norm especially for young people. Separateness and disconnection have stigmatising and isolation consequences. Limited or non-engagement may also cause aspects of psychological distress which could resemble anomie or alienation.

The 2019 World Happiness Report, records Twenge (2019), indicates that happiness and life satisfaction levels among adolescents in the USA, declined after 2012 following a period in which they rose. Both adolescents and adults by 2017 were experiencing much less happy and a markedly less satisfied with life than they had been in the previous decade. Additionally, amongst children and adolescents in the USA and UK there was an increase in the number of incidents of self-harm and suicidal thoughts and diagnoses of depression had risen.

Twenge makes a connection between heightened psychological distress and the growth of digital media. She remarks that the time adolescents were spending on social media, gaming on the internet, and texting on smartphones, had increased gradually over a ten-year period but had accelerated after 2012. By 2018 (the last year the on which the 2019 report has data), the vast majority of USA citizens, including adolescents, had access to the internet and owned a smartphone. On average, 17–18-year-olds are by that year were spending more than six hours a day on digital media activities (internet, social media, and texting). Nearly half of USA adolescents by 2018 were using the internet incessantly.

Adolescents had reduced significantly their time in face-to-face interactions with each other as an outcome of so much time spent in the digital world. They did regularly communicate with friends and 'socialised' but largely indirectly through electronic means. What has also been reduced is reading hard-copy books and magazines, doing homework and sleeping. Twenge cautions that empirical research so far has only provided correlation results. However, the analysis of data from a series of longitudinal and experimental studies does imply that extensive utilisation of digital media and a lowering of psychological well-being are connected causally.

United Kingdom Chief Medical Officers' (Davies et al., 2019) account of empirical research reviews relating to electronic screen-based activities and the psychological well-being of young people including children comes to the similar conclusion to that offered by Twenge. An increased risk of anxiety or depression amongst that age group is cited and of such concern that the Chief Medical Officers' published guidance for parents. This guidance encompasses parents banning the use of mobile/cell phones at mealtimes and bedtime and giving their children more attention.

The poem titled 'God of Gadgets' by Scottish poet Murray McGrath (2019) indicates why Chief Medical officers and parents need to be concerned.

This is an extract from his rhythmical observations of how the digital world breeds obsessiveness:

> I'll worship gizmos, this I vow.
> Connect me, swipe me, link me now.
> Someone will call, email or text,
> I'll call them back, one click, who's next.
> I matter now, at last I know.
> My gadget tells me, it is so.
> Oh God of Gadgets I trust thee,
> My hope and joy, technology.
> My gratitude will overflow,
> With faith in you, I truly know
> That all the world's in touch with me.
> What more in heaven could there be?
> (McGrath, 2019)

The advice of Chief Medical Officers does not encompass the banning of any societal insanities which may be connectible digital obsessiveness and its psychological sequelae or attending to what might make society saner.

Endurance

Insecurity, for Fromm (1942), haunts humans persistently. From the moment of birth, humans seek safety in a world that is intrinsically insecure. The infant human's life depends on obtaining protection and nutrition from its caretakers. These caretakers include parents and older siblings, and eventually friends, family, teachers, and employers. However, Fromm adds that security is also sought from community and society. Becoming an individual, Fromm posits, means, however, engaging in a process of intense anxiety. Reliance on others must converted into self-reliance although humans need both their 'self' to grow in significance whilst not losing attachments to their significant others. There features of the ongoing attachment, however, are different to those required in early life because of the introduction of the individual's desire for autonomy.

What must also be endured are the insecurities of yet more paradoxes. Apart from the insecurity of being born vulnerable and needing the care of others, there is insecurity in seeking separation. The drive to grow into a separate person carries with in yet more uncertainty because it necessitates separation from the very people with whom a strong attachment has for many years meant survival. This separation brings with it a sense of isolation, insignificance, and rekindles feelings of vulnerability which could be considered to encapsulate elements of anomie and alienation and certainly loneliness as discussed in this chapter. Moreover, superimposed onto personal uncertainties are those of a (global) society in a condition of flux through, for example, digitalisation. There is also an angst-provoking discrepancy between growing into an individual and the individualism generated by the requirements of capitalist economics. The latter is an affliction constructed by one type of society, whereas the former is a natural course of human development.

This dialectic between attachment and autonomy is never completely resolved. For Fromm, the psychological task for each human is to accept the insecurities surrounding her/his development from child to adult. Existential and ontological torment for Fromm are lifelong human fears. However, humans experience *La Nausée* in the main sporadically and fearing the freedom that autonomy brings is normal and should be managed not extinguished. The muting, and for some the smothering, of their normal insecurity can be attempted through indulging in alcohol and illegal drugs or taking prescribed pharmaceuticals. Exercise, busyness, holidaying, mind-numbing past-times, are alternative strategies to settle the nausea of living. For others the becalming enticements of, for example, positive psychology or mindfulness might be pursued (see Chapter 7). Religion may also serve to sooth troubled human souls although some may cause more worry if the fires of hell are a prospect. The reason why people either vote for or acquiesce *to autocratic leadership* suggests Fromm, may also be an indirect tactic to quell an individual's angst. A leader whose manifesto is founded on the promise of safety and survival in an insecure world may well be elected or seize power without any or substantial opposition.

Being born and becoming free therefore comes at the price of feeling fearful. Attempting to escape these fears is a deluded endeavour. Ultimately, life ends and no amount of booze, bodybuilding, television ogling and social networking, positive thinking, Buddhist chanting, or totalitarian rulership, can eradicate what either consciously or unconsciously is an underlying personal madness which must be endured. What should not have to be endured, however, are the insecurities which are borne from being born but which are the procreation of society's insanities.

Summary

Humanity is encircled by insecurity. Early homo sapiens groupings had to contend with predators seeking to make them their food whilst also scavenging for their own food, and find shelter to shield them from climatic erratic and severe weather conditions – which much later humans are again facing. Over hundreds of thousands of years, humans have been confronted with wars, genocide, famine, infectious and neoplastic diseases many of which resulted in disability or death, and human-made and natural disasters ranging from volcanic to radioactive eruptions. Contemporary societal uncertainties include the conditions in which the symptoms of anomie, loneliness, and alienation proliferate. Today's digitalising society and tomorrow's promise of an artificially intelligent and robotised world brings yet more imponderables.

Personal uncertainties originate from the psychological substance of being human. As infants become adults, they try to square being reliant on others for their continued existence and welfare with, as they mature, needing to disconnect from others if they are to become sovereign individuals. This incongruity is never alleviated, and for Fromm (1942), should be tolerated not contested.

However, personal management of the private trouble of insecurity when confronted by such social issues as extreme violence, the destitute wing of inequality, a surfeit of selfishness, and artificially intelligent technologies is problematic. It is not conducive to solidifying an individual's psyche which is already struggling to synthesise the dialectic of autonomy and attachment. Under these circumstances it would be abnormal if *La Nausée* did not surface sporadically if not perpetually. Such a surfacing of insecurity may then be liable to interpretation as clinical anxiety, depression, or any of a host of alternative diagnosis in which there are hints at the unavoidable torment of existence.

For Fromm (1956) insecurity is manageable not by escaping from freedom but embracing autonomy and its uncertainties, and by welcoming attachments based on the sureness of love. But coinciding with individual conduct directed at dealing with the dialectic the conduct of insane society needs to be managed.

References

Abel J and Clarke L (2018) Compassionate community project. *Resurgence & Ecologist*, March/April, Issue 307. www.resurgence.org/magazine/article5050-compassion-is-the-best-medicine.html [accessed 1st August, 2019].

Attanasio R (2016) As coal mining declines, community mental health problems linger. *The Conversation*, 2 August. http://theconversation.com/as-coal-mining-declines-community-mental-health-problems-linger-60094 [accessed 30 May, 2019].

Bank of England (2019) Will there be another financial crisis?www.bankofengland.co.uk/knowledgebank/will-there-be-another-financial-crisis [accessed 28 July, 2019].

Baudrillard J (1970) *La Société de Consommation: Ses Mythes, Ses structures* [The Consumer Society: Myths and Structures]. Paris. Denoël.

Baudrillard, J (1994). *Simulacra & Simulation*. Ann Arbor, MI: University of Michigan.

Bauerlein M (2008) *The Dumbest Generation: How the Digital Age Stupefies Young Americans and Jeopardizes Our Future (Or, Don't Trust Anyone Under 30)*. New York: Tarcher/Penguin.

Bauman Z (2016) Trump: A quick fix for existential anxiety. *Social Europe*, 14 November, www.socialeurope.eu/46978 [accessed 29 May, 2019].

Beck U (1992) *Risk Society: Towards a New Modernity*London: Sage.

Bell D (1976) *The Coming of Post-industrial Society*. New York: Basic.

Bennis W and Nanus B (1985) *Leaders: Strategies for Taking Charge*. New York: Harper & Row.

Browning C and Joenniemi P (2016) Ontological security, self-articulation and the securitization of identity. *Cooperation and Conflict* 52(1), pp. 31–47.

Cacioppo J and Patrick W (2009) *Loneliness: Human Nature and the Need for Social Connection*. New York: W. W. Norton & Company.

Cannon E (2018) *Is Your Job Making You Ill?: How to Survive and Thrive When it Happens To You*. London: Piatkus.

Case A (2014) You are your life, and nothing else. *New Philosopher*, 6 January. www.
womankindmag.com/articles/you-are-your-life-and-nothing-else/ [accessed 29 May,
2019].

Chiaburu D, Thundiyil T and Wang J (2014) Alienation and its correlates: A meta-
analysis. *European Management Journal*, 32(1), pp. 24–46.

Child of Our Time (2019) Teenage depression: The potential pitfalls of too much
social media use. http://childofourtimeblog.org.uk/2019/01/teenage-depression-the-p
otential-pitfalls-of-too-much-social-media-use/ [accessed 2 June, 2019].

Cribb J and Johnson P (2018) 10 years on –have we recovered from the financial crisis?
Institute for Fiscal Studies. www.ifs.org.uk/publications/13302 [accessed 28 July, 2019].

Crooks E (2019) Trump administration unveils rules to help coal industry. *Financial
Times*, 19 June. www.ft.com/content/0da01384-92b0-11e9-aea1-2b1d33ac3271 [acces-
sed 2 July 2019].

Culpin V (2018) *The Business of Sleep: How Sleeping Better Can Transform Your
Career*. London: Bloomsbury.

Curran D (2016) *Risk, Power, and Inequality in the 21st Century*. Basingstoke:
Palgrave MacMillan.

Dasgupta R (2018) The demise of the nation state. *The Guardian*, 5 April.

Davies S, Atherton F, Calderwood C, and McBride M (2019) United Kingdom Chief
Medical Officers' commentary on 'Screen-based activities and children and young
people's mental health and psychosocial wellbeing: A systematic map of reviews'.
Department of Health and Social Care. https://assets.publishing.service.gov.uk/gov
ernment/uploads/system/uploads/attachment_data/file/777026/UK_CMO_commentary
_on_screentime_and_social_media_map_of_reviews.pdf. [accessed 30 March, 2019].

Diamo S (2014) Let's talk about loneliness: Alienation in a linked up age. *Psychology
Today*, 24 February. www.psychologytoday.com/gb/blog/evil-deeds/201402/lets-ta
lk-about-loneliness-alienation-in-linked-age [accessed 1 August, 2019].

Durkheim E (1951) *Suicide*. New York: Free Press.

Edwards S and Buzzell L (2008) The waking up syndrome. *Hopedance*, 11(8). www.hop
edance.org/home/soul-news/413-the-waking-up-syndrome [accessed 1 June, 2019].

Engels F (1969, original 1845) *The Condition of the Working Class in England*. St.
Albans: Granada.

Frasquilho D, Matos G, Salonna F, Guerreiro D, Storti C, Gaspar T and Caldas-de-
Almeida J (2016) Mental health outcomes in times of economic recession: A systematic
literature review. *BioMedical Central Public Health*, 16(115). https://bmcpublichealth.
biomedcentral.com/articles/10.1186/s12889-016-2720-y [accessed 1 June, 2019].

Fromm E (1942) *The Fear of Freedom*. London: Routledge and Kegan Paul.

Fromm E (1956) *The Art of Loving*: New York: Harper & Row.

Gazzaley L and Rosen D (2016) *The Distracted Mind: Ancient Brains in a High-Tech
World*. Cambridge, MA: Massachusetts institute of Technology.

Giddens A (1991) *Modernity and Self-Identity*. Cambridge: Polity.

Greengard S (2015) *The Internet of Things*. Cambridge, MA: Massachusetts Institute
of Technology Press.

Griffin J (2010) *The Lonely Society*. London: Mental Health Foundation.

Harari Y (2015) *Sapiens: A Brief History of Humankind*. London: Vintage.

Harari Y (2017) *Homo Deus: A Brief History of Tomorrow*. London: Vintage.

Haw C, Hawton K, Gunnell D and Platt S (2015) Economic recession and suicidal
behaviour: Possible mechanisms and ameliorating factors. *International Journal of
Social Psychiatry*, 61(1), pp. 73–81.

Health and Safety Executive (2018) Work related stress depression or anxiety statistics in Great Britain, 2018. www.hse.gov.uk/statistics/causdis/stress.pdf [accessed 1 June, 2019].

Hicks S (2019) *Explaining Postmodernism: Skepticism and Socialism from Rousseau to Foucault*. Brisbane, Australia: Connor Court.

House of Commons Science and Technology Committee (2019) *Impact of social media and screen-use on young people's health Fourteenth Report of Session 2017–2019*. London: House of Commons.

Hutton W (2016) Only fundamental social change can defeat the anxiety epidemic. *The Guardian*, 8 May.

Internal Displacement Monitoring Centre Disaster (2019) *Displacement: A Global Review, 2008–2018*. Geneva: Internal Displacement Monitoring Centre.

Jaeggi R (2016) *Alienation*. New York: Columbia University Press.

Jenkins P (2018) *Minding Our Future*. London: Universities UK Task Group on Student Mental Health Services, Universities UK.

Jordon M and Hinds J (eds) (2016) *Ecotherapy: Theory, Research and Practice*. London: Palgrave.

Kan P, Whitt J and Hill A (2018) Is "VUCA" a useful term or is it all "VUCA'ED" up? United States Army College War Room. https://warroom.armywarcollege.edu/p odcasts/is-vuca-useful/ [accessed 26 July, 2019].

Keles B, McCrae N and Grealish A (2019) A systematic review: The influence of social media on depression, anxiety and psychological distress in adolescents. *International Journal of Adolescence and Youth*, 21 March. www.tandfonline.com/ doi/full/10.1080/02673843.2019.1590851 [accessed 5 August, 2019].

Keen A (2018) *How to Fix the Future: Staying Human in the Digital Age*. London: Atlantic.

Kraaijenbrink J (2018) What does VUCA really mean? *Forbes*, 19 December. www. forbes.com/sites/jeroenkraaijenbrink/2018/12/19/what-does-vuca-really-mean/#26f80 c3817d6 [accessed 26 July, 2019].

Laing R D (1961) *The Self & Others: Further Studies in Sanity & Madness*. London: Tavistock.

Little W (2018) Mindfulness courses at work? This should have us all in a rage. *The Guardian*, 31 January.

Lovelock J (2006) *The Revenge of Gaia: Earth's Climate Crisis and the Fate of Humanity*. New York: Basic Books.

Lovelock J (2009) *The Vanishing Face of Gaia: A Final Warning*. London: Allen Lane.

Lovelock J (2019) *Novacene: The Coming Age of Hyperintelligence*. London: Allen Lane.

Magen J (2018) Loneliness is bad for your health. *The Conversation*, 26 February. http:// theconversation.com/loneliness-is-bad-for-your-health-90901 [accessed 13 July, 2018].

MakeAWebsiteHub.com (2020) 65+ social networking sites you need to know about. https://makeawebsitehub.com/social-media-sites/ [accessed 9 January, 2020].

Malik K (2018) Worry less about the march of the robots, more about techno panic. *The Observer*, 24 February.

Marks S (1974) Durkheim's theory of anomie. *American Journal of Sociology*, 80(2), pp. 329–363.

Marx K (1959, original 1844) *The Economic and Philosophic Manuscripts*. Moscow: Foreign Languages Publishing House/Progress Publishers.

Marsden J (1999) Cyberpsychosis: The feminization of the postbiological body. In Gordon Lopez A and Parker I (eds) *Cyberpsychology*. New York: Routledge, pp. 59–76.

McGrath M (2019) God of Gadgets published in *Rhymes for Reciting*. Aboyne: Lumphanan Press.

Merton R (1968) *Social Theory and Social Structure*. New York: Free Press.

Mezzadri A (2017) *The Sweatshop Regime: Labouring Bodies, Exploitation, and Garments Made in India*. Cambridge: Cambridge University Press.

Monbiot G (2017) *How Did We Get into This Mess?: Politics, Equality, Nature*. London: Verso.

Monbiot G (2018) The town that's found a potent cure for illness – community. *The Guardian*, 21 February.

Morozov E (2013) *To Save Everything, Click Here: Technology, Solutionism, and the Urge to Fix Problems that Don't Exist*. London: Allen Lane.

Morozov E (2017) The digital hippies want to integrate life and work – but not in a good way. *The Observer*, 3 December.

Morrish L (2019) *Pressure Vessels: The Epidemic of Poor Mental Health Among Higher Education Staff*. Oxford: Higher Education Policy Institute.

Pantic I (2014) Online social networking and mental health. *Cyberpsychology, Behavior and Social Networking*, 17(10), pp. 652–657.

Pantic I, Milanovic A, Loboda B, Błachnio A, Przepiorka A, Nesic D, Mazic S, Dugalic S and Ristic S (2017) Association between physiological oscillations in self-esteem, narcissism and internet addiction: A cross-sectional study. *Psychiatry Research*, 258, pp. 239–243.

Partington R (2019) Gig economy in Britain doubles, accounting for 4.7 million workers. *The Guardian*, 28 June.

Poster M (ed.) (2001) *Jean Baudrillard: Selected Writings*, 2nd edn. Cambridge: UK: Polity.

Ritzer R (2018) *The McDonaldization of Society: Into the Digital Age*, 9th edn. London: Sage.

Royal Society for Public Health (2017) *#Statusofmind Social Media and Young People's Mental Health and Wellbeing*. London: Royal Society for Public Health.

Sartre J-P (1938) *La Nausée* [Nausea]. Paris: Gallimard.

Sartre J-P (1972) *Being and Nothingness: Essay on Phenomenological Ontology* [L'Être et le néant: Essai d'ontologie phénoménologique]. New York: Simon & Schuster.

Siegfried T (2018) Informed wisdom trumps rigid rules when it comes to medical evidence: Systematic reviews emphasize process at the expense of thoughtful interpretation. *Society for Science & the Public*, 23 April. www.sciencenews.org/blog/context/informed-wisdom-trumps-rigid-rules-when-it-comes-medical-evidence?utm_source=email&utm_medium=email&utm_campaign=latest-newsletter-v2 [accessed 1 June, 2019].

Smith J (2018) Loneliness on its way to becoming Britain's most lethal condition. *The Conversation*, 18 April. https://theconversation.com/loneliness-on-its-way-to-becoming-britains-most-lethal-condition-94775 [accessed 1 June, 2018].

Stearns P (2018) *The Industrial Revolution in World History*, 4th edn. New York: Routledge.

Storr A (1988) *Solitude: A Return to the Self*. New York: Free Press.

Stossel S (2014) *My Age of Anxiety*. London: Windmill.

Swain D (2012) *Alienation: An Introduction to Marx's Theory*. London: Bookmarks.

Teymoori A, Bastian B and Jetten J (2017) Towards a psychological analysis of anomie. *Political Psychology*, 38(6), pp. 1009–1023.

Thorley C (2017) *Not by Degrees Improving Student Mental Health in the UK's Universities.* London: Institute for Public Policy Research.

Tiffin J and Nobuyoshi T (eds) (2001) *HyperReality: Paradigm for the Third Millenium.* New York: Routledge.

Twenge J (2019) The sad state of happiness in the united states and the role of digital media. In Helliwell J, Layard R and Sachs J (eds) *World Happiness Report (2019) World Happiness Report. New York: Sustainable Development Solutions Network,* pp. 86–95.

Van Hal G (2015) The true cost of the economic crisis on psychological well-being: A review. *Psychology Research and Behavior Management,* 8, pp. 17–25.

Walter C (2006) *Thumbs, Toes, and Tears.* New York: Walker & Company.

War on Want (2019) Sweatshops in China. https://waronwant.org/sweatshops-china [accessed 30 May, 2019].

Winch G (2011) The last bullying frontier: Call center representatives take a beating. *Psychology Today,* 31 March. www.psychologytoday.com/us/blog/the-squea ky-wheel/201103/the-last-bullying-frontier [accessed 30 May, 2019].

Woodcock J (2016) *Working the Phones: Control and Resistance in Call Centres.* London: Pluto.

World Economic Forum (2019a) Understanding the impact of digitalization on society. http://reports.weforum.org/digital-transformation/understanding-the-impact-of-digitaliza tion-on-society/ [accessed 22 July, 2019].

World Economic Forum (2019b) Our mission. www.weforum.org/about/world-econom ic-forum [accessed 3 August, 2019].

World Health Organisation (WHO) (2011) *Impact of Economic Crises on Mental Health.* Geneva: World Health Organisation.

World Health Organisation (WHO) (2018) Mental health: Suicide data. www.who. int/mental_health/prevention/suicide/suicideprevent/en/ [accessed 1 June, 2019].

Worsley A (2018) History of loneliness. *The Conversation,* 19 March. https://the conversation.com/a-history-of-loneliness-91542 [accessed 2 August, 2019].

7 Stupidity

An academic style of writing usually adheres to conventions of temperate and respectful depictions rather than hard-hitting declarations laced with vitriol (and avoid exclamation marks at all costs). This chapter starts with a deviation from the academic norm: despite much progress in civilising humanity, the continued occurrence if not exacerbation of such societal insanities as violence, inequality, selfishness, and insecurity, along with the climate crisis, cultural inanity, mindless happiness, 'post-truth', and finding faults in individuals rather than society, indicate that humans (including you and I), are unmistakably and unmitigatedly stupid! What's more, this list is limited to a few of humanity's 'super-stupidities'. There is a multitude of mundane follies and to evaluate all of them would require the writing of multi-volume tomes rather than one chapter.

Stupidity is societal insanity when it is collective. That is, when the private trouble of stupidity is rife and patterned it becomes a public issue. However, as has been stated in previous chapters, every social phenomenon is complicated and the features of human absurdity, inanity, and mindlessness, are myriad and tortuous. Beyond the stupidity of continuing if not escalating violence, inequality, selfishness, and insecurity, all of which are linkable directly to personal madness, are superordinate the stupidities mentioned above but not already covered in previous chapters:

- **Crisis**: not preventing, prevaricating about solving, and even denying the actuality of global warming, natural resource exhaustion, decreasing biodiversity, pollution of the land and air, and absence of clean water, starvation in a world of 'nutritional abundance'.
- **Lies**: 'truth' is reconfigured as 'post-truth', reality as relative, everything and everyone as mere socially constructions, and faults in society are segregated into silos of clinical work, academia, and politics instead of being seen as the source and solution for a significant sum of personal madness.
- **Mindlessness**: an exacerbation of crass and corrosive past-times, a plague of inattentiveness, incessant demands for immediate gratification and happiness and ontologically and intellectually fruitless and delusional attempts at escaping the reality of human existence and non-existence.

These overriding three follies foster personal madness indirectly but are primarily indicative of an insane society. Individual participation and acquiescence in such insanity does not just imply stupidity but generalised madness. 'Normality' is in the eye of the beholder but what the observer sees is abnormality should an external vantage point be possible. Fromm (1956) claimed to be an observer of this insanity, and in this book, there is an attempt to witness the stupidity of others without the plenteous personal follies if its author obscuring the view.

The idea that society itself is mad by tolerating violence, inequality and encouraging patterns of human performance geared to fetishising commodities, indulgence in mindless mass media, celebrity, and narcissism, at the expense of intimacy, communality, and aesthetic and intellectual pursuits, is not generally accepted.

Notwithstanding the misleading construing of 'mental health' as a problem rather than 'mental ill-health' (that is, personal madness), philosopher Dan Swain has summarised the central stupidity which underlies the thesis of this book:

> [D]espite widespread agreement on the depth of the problem of mental health, there is a remarkable tendency to ignore the wider social context, to treat these as problems for individuals rather than society as a whole, and to look to solutions in individual therapy or medication.
>
> (Swain, 2012, p. 68)

To regard personal madness as mainly let alone wholly the 'fault' of the individual is both intellectual inept and immoral. To underplay let alone ignore the potency of societal factors such violence, inequality, selfishness, insecurity, and counterparts to this overriding stupidity is indeed a tendency remarkable for its blatant wrongness logically and evidentially. It is also unjust because it blames the victim. By searching mainly or only for miscreant neuro-genes and neuro-chemicals, and neuro-anatomical malefactions, is scientifically indefensible and ethically reprehensible. Psychological distress of primary and secondary victims of interpersonal brutality, armed conflict, murder, terrorism, bullying, and from sadistic entertainments and realistic news broadcasting, should be too apparent to be ignored. What should be too apparent is that poverty, and vast differences in wealth and power, are linkable to psychological suffering. Less obvious because its affects are indirect, is that a culture of selfishness, narcissism, materialism, and consumerism, affects detrimentally what it is to be human but only if genuine happiness, contentment, and altruism are considered desirable qualities and egotism, avarice and the concomitant feelings of 'stress' and inadequacy undesirable.

But, of course, it's complicated. Of course, there are also contradictions.

There is complexity in how scientific endeavour unfolds. Science is a social process (Morrall, 2009). Each scientific discipline, of which there are many, competes for its world view and its methods of testing this view of the world to be worth funding. The provision of funds for scientific research comes, in the main, with utilitarian and/or commercial requirements. Neuroscience and pharmacology, for example, are propositioned as practical and profitable. Neuroscientific and pharmacological research has the added attraction of being able to demonstrate its propositions in the form of tangible technologies and visible data, and whilst their efficacy is controversial both have had success commercially. Moreover, scientific research overall is empirical not theoretical (excepting that all research is propelled by theory or sponsors the development of theory). Psychiatry, and although to a lesser extent clinical psychology and certain psychotherapies, has become saturated with neuroscientific and pharmacological premises and remedies (Rose and Abi-Rached, 2013; Nikolas Rose, 2019; Morrall, 2018). Hence, it is axiomatic that the locus of personal madness is construed as a private trouble. Social issues such as that of societal insanity do not attract funding so easily because research propositions and outcomes are far more ethereal and intangible than neuroscientific and pharmacological studies, and their profitability usually only realisable in the long-term and social rather than financial. The career prospects of clinicians and academics is also influenced by what can be more readily revealed as of value practically and commercially.

The fundamental contradiction in the faulty individual versus faulty society disputation lies in regarding this as a necessary dispute at all. That is, the search for, on the one hand, faults in the biology and psyche of the individual, and on the other faults in societal structures and processes, should not be separate endeavours. Humans, as with most life forms and cultural values and events, are (or course) complex. Rarely can one gene, one biochemical, or anatomical abnormality claim to be the cause of a specific mental disorder, just as rarely can any single societal happenstance be identified as causing personal madness let alone attributed wholly to the insanity of society (Morrall, 2017; Nikolas Rose, 2019).

Crisis

Climate change and its environmental consequences has a generalised negative effect on global society because it increases insecurity at geo-political and personal levels. People and the social fabric of their communities through for example, droughts, wildfires, heatwaves, or the flooding of their locale, are disturbed and in some cases, both living situations and life is destroyed. The consequences of global warming cause physical injuries and allows infectious disease to surface and spread. They also effect psychological stability detrimentally, with an increase in the diagnosis of anxiety, depression, substance abuse, post-traumatic-stress-disorder, and suicide recorded in regions where these consequences have been experienced directly. Moreover, some of these instabilities can become chronic. Higher rates of aggression and violence, and increases in the sense of hopelessness, helplessness, and loss, have also been chronicled in the longer-term following experiences of environmental disaster.

People already diagnosed with mental disorder are vulnerable to a worsening of their (assumed) troublesome psychological condition. Children are also more vulnerable with adverse alterations noted in development, memory, and behaviour (Whitmore-Williams et al., 2017; Jackson and Devadason, 2019).

The language used to describe the conclusions from a wealth of evidence about impending ecological catastrophe changed at the end of the twenty-first century's second decade. Previously, the environmental scientists and activists, had used phrases such as' climate change' and 'global warming'. The presumption was that using an intemperate term would attract more attention from politicians and the public to a social issue already pronounced as the most serious one facing the planet and its life forms. Another reason for altering the nomenclature was that there really is a crisis.

Scholars of disaster preparedness Caleb Redlener, Charlotte Jenkins, and Irwin Redlener highlight the need to call a crisis as crisis:

> Our planet is in crisis. But until we call it a crisis, no one will listen.... There is no longer any doubt that climate change is an unprecedented planetary emergency. And the terms we use to describe this crisis must deliberately reflect an appropriate sense of urgency.
>
> (Redlener et al., 2019)

These scholars add that there is no longer any doubt amongst those scientists studying the earth's climate that the changes that are occurring (and have been since industrialisation began in earnest) are unprecedented and their toxicity of their impact incomparable.

The climate is changing, it is warming, but these are weasel words when the overwhelming incontrovertible evidence is that catastrophe is pending and predicted to befall far earlier than thought previously. 'Crisis' is not intemperate but accurate.

Nevertheless, it waits to seen whether or not the veil of psychological distancing employed by populations in parts of the global population not affected presently by the calamitous weather can be lifted high enough for these people to see and grasp the significance of this crisis. Observation and comprehension, however, is pointless unless followed by substantive action. This action begets a secondary crisis: the need for dramatic alterations in personal performance and the structure of society. Either obliquely or overtly relevant to such an agenda for the transformation of society are the personal troubles and social issues of violence, inequality, selfishness, insecurity, and the parallel stupidities to that of ignoring or repudiating that there is a climate crisis.

The predicament in the earth's climate is not a crisis in the over-used personal or political sense for hiccoughs in relationships or policy failing. The climate is in an authentic crisis because ecological devastation and Anthropocene annihilation is not hyperbole, scaremongering, or survivable. This crisis is a credible prediction that the physical milieu and all humanity may be destroyed – and soon.

A parallel can be drawn between smoking and climate crisis. Mass consumption of cigarettes had begun by the end of the nineteenth century after the tobacco industry mechanised and introduced effective marketing techniques. The causative connection between smoking cigarettes and lung cancer was grasped from the 1940s onwards through multiple epidemiological and experimental studies and analysis of the conduct of cells. At that point there was an epidemic of lung cancer. When the research relating to smoking and cancer began to be published the tobacco industry's representatives denied that there was link. Propaganda campaigns were conducted to convince the public that smoking was safe, and to protect the industry's profits (Proctor, 2012). There is still an epidemic of cancer caused by smoking.

Nearly 80 years after the link was discovered the World Health Organisation (WHO, 2019) published these data:

- 1.1 billion people still engage in smoking (mainly cigarettes), 80% of whom live in low-and middle-income countries.
- Tobacco kills up to half of its users.
- Tobacco kills more than 8 million people each year (most directly from smoking but over 1 million from indirect inhalation)

Coinciding with the start of cigarette mass consumption evidence was accumulating that human activity influenced the climate, although the ancient Greeks had already suspected such a connection. By the late nineteenth century the burning of fossil fuels as prompting a 'greenhouse effect' in the earth's atmosphere (Weart, 2008). One-hundred-and-twenty years later the WHO (2018) was to go way beyond suspicion and declare that climate change is affecting the social and environmental determinants of health, that is clean air, safe drinking water, sufficient food, and secure shelter. The WHO (still using the descriptor 'change' not 'crisis') is also in no doubt about what was on course to happen to humans because of human industriousness, and that the poorest of them would be affected worse:

- Climate change is expected to cause approximately 250,000 additional deaths per year, from malnutrition, malaria, diarrhoea and heat stress, between 2030–2050.
- People living in developing countries are most vulnerable to the adverse health effects caused by air pollution and polluted water, and inadequate food and shelter.

Both physical and psychological well-being, the WHO points out, will be undermined, and predicts that as the climate changes further, so will the rate of diagnosis of a range of infectious diseases and mental disorders. One major calamity because of the climatic crisis is flooding. As the world's temperature and the levels of the seas continue to rise, and precipitation becomes even more unremitting in areas unused to coping with such weather, water and sewage systems are disrupted. Domestic water then is polluted which allows the spread of disease. Flooding also results in people having move and often having so to do in a hurry thereby encouraging the occurrence and spread of misery and anguish.

A direct challenge is made to those who argue either that global warming is not occurring or if it then it is not due to human pursuits from the results of a study conducted by climate researcher Raphael Neukom and colleagues (Neukom et al., 2019). The conclusion of the study is that there is strong evidence that global warming is occurring, that the warming of the world is not only unparalleled in terms of absolute temperatures, but its formation and presentation is unprecedented over the previous two millennia, and that what they refer to as 'anthropogenic' activities are the cause.

The Intergovernmental Panel on Climate Change (IPCC) is the leading international organisation on the impact of global warming and an agency of the United Nations. It assesses the empirical evidence regarding effects and the risks, and suggests how these effects and risks should be managed. As with the WHO, there is no ambiguity in its assessment of these effects and risks. The IPCC (2018) is categorical that global warming is happening. It refers to the consensus among leading climate scientists from across the world that the climate is getting warmer and is so due to human activity. It is not, affirms the IPCC, a natural occurrence with historical equivalents and which will correct itself naturally. Furthermore, the IPCC is witness to the near universal agreement amongst climate scientists that there is little time left to be able to control the rise in the earth's temperature. There is also acceptance amongst these scientists, testifies the IPCC, that the maximum increase temperature after which point large scale environmental disasters will occur is much lower than previously estimated. If the temperature is not controlled, warns the IPCC, then hundreds of millions of people will be exposed to flooding, droughts, extreme heat, and thus further depths of poverty for those already impoverished but also spreading material hardship to a much wider segment of the global population. The IPCC is unequivocal in its warning that unprecedented and urgent changes are necessary to reconfigure global society.

Monbiot continues in the vein of clear-cut comments about the climate crisis by clamming that the earth's living systems are collapsing. He confronts meat-eaters with this hard-hitting statement:

> We [meat-eaters] make no connection in our compartmentalised minds between the beef on our plates and the destruction of rainforests to grow the soya that fed the cattle; between the miles we drive and the oil wells drilled in rare and precious places, and the spills that then pollute them.
>
> (Monbiot, 2017, p. 94)

In scathing assessment of international effort through such organisations as the United Nations, Monbiot refers to the United Nations (and by implication the IPCC) as indulging in a 'phantasm of progress' regarding the managing climate change, with its plethora of 'make-believe' protocols. For Monbiot, the United Nations is indulging in perfunctory planning at a point when the plan needs to alter the set-up of global society profoundly.

Two years after the IPCC (2019) published a protocol which states that the most urgent changes need to be made to food production and consumption in order to reduce greenhouse gases. The world's most urgent problem for the IPCC is the size of the meat diary industries. These industries are destroying the earth's environment more than fossil fuel production and consumption. Meat and dairy, particularly if based on intensified industrial systems, have led to colossal amounts of deforestation and greenhouse gas emissions, and released immense volumes of pollutants into terrestrial ecosystems. The report avoids recommending adherence to vegetarian and vegan diets. It does recommend that governments consider policies and individuals review their eating habits regarding the intake of meat and dairy foodstuffs. The implication of Monbiot's criticism of the United Nations and allied organisations is that they need to be more strident in their verdicts and extremely demanding of governments and individuals to adjust before climatic catastrophe strikes.

The UK-based Institute for Public Policy Research (IPPR, 2019) is a policy think-tank. Researchers from the IPPR do affirm in stark terms that there is a crisis. The physical environment is breaking down (Laybourn-Langton et al., 2019). Inseparable from the primary cause of global warming, what is contributing to the climate crisis is soil infertility and erosion, loss pollinators and many other species, chemicals leaching into the soil, the felling of forests, and the acidification of the oceans. The effect on communities across the world will be disastrous unless the climate is fixed urgently. Economies will become unstable, as will potentially the whole fabric of global society, famines will occur, and large populations of people will be forced to migrate. The IPPR researchers warn that the politics and policies of nations across the world must be directed at dealing with this crisis otherwise a cascade of complex and dynamic tipping points will ensue with devastating effects of nature and humanity.

Humans are putting themselves at risk from each of the tipping points. But the desecration of animal life is a key point over which the earth is tipping, and which may tip humans into oblivion.

There are other crises. The Intergovernmental Science-Policy Platform on Biodiversity and Ecosystem (IBES, 2020) has representatives from 132 governments and 1,000 scientists and is supported by the United Nations. Its aim is to assess the condition of nature and its effect on humans thereby to inform policy-makers about what measures are necessary to sustain the natural world to enable human well-being and 'sustainable development'. The IBES's 2019 Global Report (IBES, 2019) was prepared by leading international climate specialists from the natural and social sciences with contributions from other experts – a total of 350. Over three years, thousands of scientific papers, government reports, and accounts from the public were assessed. It concludes that there is a 'biodiversity crisis', and that although linked it may be worse than that of the climate. Nature is in free-fall because of human development. Nature has been so exploited and spoiled that it may be able to recover. The destruction of forests, sea and soil over-exploitation, pollution of air and water, is resulting in impending extinction for tens of thousands of species which in turn will threaten the necessities for human life – food and water.

Tipping animal species into non-existence means there is little chance of their personal stories being known. If their life is acknowledged, which could be the case if an animal had been kept as a household pet on a small farm, then the story told is unsurprisingly an anthropomorphised version rather than an authentic animal version. Philosopher Peter Singer (1975; 1979) makes the case that animals can express what are the equivalent to human feelings and should have counterpart rights to those of humans. However, an understanding of animal performance is far from the autobiographical and biographical accounts of human performance. What follows is a story of one human (a child) told by other humans (mainly her mother) when the former had tipped too close to one of the elements that threatens all forms of life, pollution.

According to the charity Asthma UK's analysis of data from the Office for National Statistics, nearly 13,000 adults and children died of asthma in England and Wales between the years 2008–2018. This represents a 33% increase during that decade (Asthma UK, 2019). One of the children who died was a nine-year-old girl called Ella Kissi-Debrah (also referred to as Ella Roberta). Ella Kissi-Debrah, however, attracted more media attention than is usual even when the death is that of a child. The reason for the media attention is because for the first time a death from asthma has been associated to environmental pollution. Immuno-pharmacologist Stephen Holgate, who has researched the role of air pollution on asthma, submitted a report to the Attorney General, the UK's chief legal adviser to the government, as evidence for an appeal against the conclusion from an inquest into the girl's death which focused on the disease (acute respiratory failure caused by a severe bronchial spasm) rather than examining extraneous factors. What Holgate found was that there was a notable coincidence of Ella Kissi-Debrah admissions to hospital and spikes in the pollutant nitrogen dioxide as well as toxic minuscule particulate matter in the proximity of her home in Lewisham, a suburb of London. Holgate's evidence was used by the legal team representing Ella Kissi-Debrah's family to ask for a second inquest. This was subsequently granted by the High Court of England and Wales (Dyer, 2019). At the time of writing the second inquest has not taken place. Moreover, Ella Kissi-Debrah's mother points out that living with severe asthma is extremely stressful and at times very frightening (Ella Roberta Family Foundation, 2019). For parents who lose a child for any reason the psychological suffering is likely to be extreme. Parents of children who are more likely to suffer symptoms anxiety, depression, and/or post-traumatic-stress disorder (Field and Behrman, 2003).

Asthma UK reports that many sufferers from asthma associate a worsening of their condition with traffic fumes, smoke or dust particles. The charity also acknowledges that there is already evidence linking asthma in children and adults to long-term exposure to high concentrations of air pollution, and recognises there needs to be much more research conducted into this association. The charity recommends that preventative medicine should be taken regularly to avoid pollution triggering a serious attack of asthma. This advice is understandable when such attacks may result in the loss of life. But linking any disease, especially if life-threatening, to environmental causation demands more action than mere medication.

Stopping deaths from air pollution requires major reorganisation of transport systems, the layout and positioning of residential, working, and leisure areas, and, ultimately, the reconfiguration of global society's reliance on products and energy which fuel pollution. Ironically, many ordinary household products and regular building materials used in the construction of working and leisure facilities may harbour other but just as lethal pollutants (Wilkinson, 2017). That realisation implies a need to reform virtually every aspect of modern life, a prospect yet, and probably never, realisable.

To further champion the case of contrariness is the case of psychological suffering from worrying about the climate crisis. Concern over ecology has brought with it a new branch of psychology, a new psychological syndrome, and a new psychotherapy.

Ecopsychology is of a branch of psychology cultivated by historian Theodore Roszak (1992) which examines the impact of the physical environmental on psychological well-being. Ecotherapy is the therapeutic outcome of ecopsychology which attempts to remedy 'eco-anxiety' and has been developed by eco-therapists Sarah Anne Edwards and Linda Buzzell (2008) Eco-anxiety is a state of psychological distress in which the assumed sufferer feels anxious about the state of the world's ecological condition.

Edwards and Buzzell describe what they consider to the typical process experienced by the eco-anxious as first a stage of denial whereby there a form of psychological distancing from the reality that the earth and its occupants are in trouble. There is so much information and conversation in the public domain about the climate crisis that a position of denial is difficult to maintain. However, argue Edwards and Buzzell, there is still resistance and enter stage two which is characterised subdued awareness of the potential ecological disasters. It is hard to persist with semi-conscious acknowledgement and as with the previous one, according to Edwards and Buzzell, the sufferers of eco-anxiety enter stage three. At this point there is full realisation of actual or potential ecological disaster. There is then, assert Edwards and Buzzell, no return to earlier stages once complete awareness has been reached, but there is yet another psychological phase into which they enter. For Edwards and Buzzell, the eco-anxious having had their consciousness raised inevitably become very anxious. Feelings of despair, hopelessness, and guilt are experienced. But the process is not yet completed. There is a stage five characterised by acceptance of the harm happening to the physical environment, and that personal action to avoid further damage is required. Entry into this final phase, however, is not inevitable.

These stages devised by Edwards and Buzzell are comparable to the phases of psychiatrist Elisabeth Kübler-Ross's model of bereavement. Kübler-Ross (1969) regarded bereavement as a process in which people who had undergone the loss of a loved one or who themselves were dying would experience first denial, then anger, bargaining, depression, and acceptance. Whilst bereavement involves various degrees of anxiety, eco-anxiety implies that being anxious is the overriding emotion. Other indications of eco-anxiety have been noted and include panic attacks, loss of appetite, irritability, substance abuse, obsessive thinking, insomnia, aggression and violence, and suicide (Jordon and Hinds, 2016; Whitmore-Williams et al., 2017). But the overriding feeling is that of existential angst and ontological insecurity medicalised as anxiety. The symptoms of eco-anxiety therefore have more in common with the anxiety states of the DSM-5 (Moffic, 2013). It may be indistinguishable from, for example, the symptomatology of a generalised anxiety or warrant separate categorisation. However, the latter is not an option as eco-anxiety, although recognised by eco-psychologists and eco-psychotherapists, has not been officially medicalised. An 'eco' branch of psychiatry has been in offing since the 1970s (Moffic, 2013). But there is not yet a set of specific eco syndromes sanctified by psychiatry.

Environmental philosopher Glenn Albrecht (2011) uses the phrase 'psychoterratic syndrome' to describe the negative effect on human psychology when the physical environment is perceived to be under threat. He also coined the term 'solastagia' to describe what seems to be an emotion akin to stage four in Edwards and Buzzell's eco-anxiety process. It also resonates with Kübler-Ross's melancholic part of bereavement. For Albrecht, however, solastagia was a synonym for feeling of nostalgia sensed by displaced people such as Australian aborigines when European colonisation disrupted their physical environment to the extent that they had to, or were forced, to move to survive. Angst and melancholy are associable with high levels of homesickness reasoned Albrecht. For Albrecht, solastalgiac angst and melancholy may lead to further psychological harm as well as physical ill-health:

> All people who experience solastalgia are negatively affected by their desolation and likely responses can include the generalised distress ... but can escalate into ... drug abuse, physical illness and mental illness (depression, suicide).
>
> (Albrecht, 2005, p. 46)

All-embracing earthly ecocide may yield a universal extreme version of solastagia which leaves humanity forced to venture into the universe to survive. In the meantime, ecotherapy offers an earthlier remedy. Also in the meantime, most people affected by the climate change do not have access to ecotherapy but are worried because they do not even have access to the basic necessities for life.

Mass forced displacement of people from their homes and geographical locations is happening as a direct consequence of environment hazards, an example of which is flooding nearly all of which is attendant on the climate crisis. Each year more than 17 million people are at risk of being displaced by floods. Desertification associated with changes in the climate, for example in Nigeria, has caused people to move and this has resulted in violence between communities. When people migrate under duress, they tend to lose their assets and income, social contacts, and have difficulties finding essential amenities to sustain their health or life (Internal Displacement Monitoring Centre, 2019).

Lies

The suffering of displaced people is real. As has been indicated above, there is a mountain of evidence supported by a vast number of scientists that what is causing their displacement is real. Yet there is still denial of the reality of a climate crisis. This is a contradiction, but one with particularly pathological cultural characteristics. These characteristics are that truth, and therefore reality, can be malleable, variable, relative, and supplanted. The opposite view to that which considers truth as unstable is that non-truth is miscalculation or calculated misrepresentation. From this point of view, there is no such thing as alternative facts and different actualities. There are only errors and there are only lies.

Philosopher Lee McIntyre (2018) examines the roots of what has become known as 'post-truth'. Post-truth is the terminological rubric which encapsulates the various notions implying that truthfulness is insecure. For McIntyre the post-truth phenomenon has been generated by contemporary technology, and social scientific musings, corporate propaganda, and religion. The internet provides a never-ending flow and persistently available abundance of alternative accounts of any and all personal, societal, and natural events. Hateful, prejudicial, desultory, conciliatory, informed, ill-informed, resolute, desultory, and dissolute narratives and videos can be placed in cyberspace and read or viewed by few or a few billion people with may not have the prudence or the desire to filter the real from the false.

The UK's House of Commons Digital, Culture, Media and Sport Committee (2019) has produced a report on 'disinformation and fake news' in relation to political choice in elections in both the UK and globally. In the report there is acceptance of the sizeable benefits the internet has brought. The internet allows easy admission to enormous amounts knowledge, massive amount of entertainment, instant interpersonal contact, and expedited an interconnected and ingenious system of world trade. The downside of the internet, however, is also sizeable. The House of Commons accuses 'malign forces' of influencing elections causing distortion, disruption, coarsening of political debate, and destabilising political systems and authority. Political propaganda posing as fact is appearing in the news. The influence of these political fabrications is magnified massively because of social and news medias' use of information technology to disseminate stories immediately and extensively, and for it to be retrievable for lengthy periods or indefinitely. Other forms of disinformation and fake information are disseminated similarly resulting in confusion over what is factual and what is fictitious. Commitment to biased positions is also sustained by retrieving and airing what is purported to be truth. The use of phoney data and documentation extends beyond politics. It is used to support views about, for example, health, and the climate crisis. The report calls for greater transparency in the digital sphere over the sources of information and the evidence supporting supposed certainties.

Privacy is another of the House of Common's major concerns. Large technology corporations need to be investigated to reveal how personal digital data is used and who pays for its use. 'Facebook' is named by the committee as exemplifying a 'big data' social media company which tracks its users' activities retains their personal data, profits selling its users' data to advertisers and 'app' developers. The report contains a criticism of Facebook's founder and Chief Executive Officer, Mark Zuckerberg. He is reproached for 'showing contempt' towards the UK Government by not responding personally to invitations to provide evidence to the Committee.

The businesses which benefit from motoring, storing, displaying, and sharing personal data require regulation to prevent commercial misuse as well as misuse by those with malicious intent. The latter includes the politically manipulative but also people intent on defaming or shaming, for example, their peers or ex-partners. 'Hate-speech' directed towards specific beliefs, and ethnic and sexual identity, is another misuse of personal data when openly available on social media platforms, and for which the House of Commons wants reform.

> The big tech companies must not be allowed to expand exponentially, without constraint or proper regulatory oversight. But only governments and the law are powerful enough to contain them.
>
> (House of Commons, 2019, p. 5)

Tristan Harris from the Center for Humane Technology in USA was one of the witnesses called on to provide evidence about the downside of the internet. The report quotes Harris. When referring to the current digital technology he says it is 'hijacking our minds and society' (House of Commons, 2019, p. 8). What the House of Commons advocates is that digital technology be used instead, to free our minds, but this requires regulation. The report contains the warning that without regulation the machines may take charge of people.

McIntyre (2018) contends that the post-truth phenomenon has also been aroused because of its adherents and victims focus on feelings rather than facts. McIntyre gives the examples of the conviction that the universe has been created by an unknown intelligence, the vaccine controversy, and climate crisis denial, whereby feelings have overcome facts. Moreover, McIntyre refers to how the tobacco industry (see above) used the media and political lobbying to submerge the scientific data demonstrating the reality of the harm its products induced. The example of how corporate bosses, with the conscious and unconscious collusion of people in the media and politicians, hid the reality of the lethality of smoking from the public and later disparaged the facts from scientific studies, does not exemplify 'post-truth' but wilful dishonesty. Moreover, smokers were and still are deceptive or self-deceiving, preferring to contest or ignore what in reality is the incontestable and unignorable mass of evidence in the public domain revealing that they are dicing with death but with dice heavily predisposed towards them dying.

Virtually all religious chronicling and practices are driven by belief rather than empirical evidence or robust theorising in the academic sense, and much of what is believed has an emotional content. As such, as the evolutionary biologist Richard Dawkins (2006) has pronounced, religiosity is a delusion – and a dangerous one at that because it undermines faith in truth. For Dawkins, it is only (scientific) truth that humans should be faithful to. Religion for Dawkins (2019) is both delusional and duplicitous. By implication those who believe in an all-powerful deity, intelligent design, or any unverifiable aspect of religiosity, spirituality, or other ethereality, let alone experience visitations from or visualisations of godly figures or their symbols, could be categorised as medically mad. Traditionally, psychiatry considers 'false beliefs' and 'false sensations' as indicative of psychotic disorder (Morrall, 2017).

What may appear to be a paradox in disputations over what is and what isn't truth is the fact that scientific facts cannot in the main be proven completely and they change. But, the central tenets of science are that whilst facts and an understanding of what is real may not be wholly knowable, this does not mean that facts and reality do not exist. What science attempts, through sceptical and critical thinking, and collecting empirical evidence, is to know the facts and reality as well as can be known given available knowledge. As that knowledge develops then a better understanding of what is factual and what is real may be achieved.

For philosopher Simon Blackburn (2005; 2017) the scientific method is a far better option on which to base human civilisation that cynicism, relativism, or nihilism. Those who scorn truth, those who consider truth to be wholly culturally contained, and those who exult in nothingness, are likely to use real mobile/cell phones, watch real television, switch on real computers using real power sources, travel in real cars, motorcycles, and aeroplanes, and have real medical investigations and take real medicines when really ill. Every one of these facets of today's global society have arisen from scientifically informed technologies. What irks both Blackburn and Dawkins particularly, is the social scientific fetish for postmodernism whereby everything is considered to be a social construct and thereby susceptible to deconstruction. They accuse adherents to postmodernist ideas of hypocrisy because they construct their intellectual lives around real objects. Academic careers and personal well-being for postmodernists as for mathematicians, physicists, philosophers, and evolutionary biologists, require the aforementioned real accoutrements of the modern world.

Cognitive psychologist Stephen Pinker (2018) is also scathing about the idea that science is based merely on the beliefs of a specific culture and at a set time. Smallpox has been cured, and humans have gone into space using techniques that are somewhat more substantial than if they were merely socially constructed. Moreover, he also implies that morality can be factual rather than always created and bound by cultural norms. For example, slavery, genital mutilation, and the subjugation of women, are considered normal in certain cultures but the basis of these practices can be contested rationally and the facts of their harm highlighted.

Truth, predictably, given how often the issue of complexity has already surfaced regarding the subject matter of this book, is complex. Fixing factuality is rarely easy because knowledge is constantly improving. Julian Baggini (2018), philosopher and journalist, argues that despite the complexity of truth it cannot be left to the deconstruction inclinations of postmodernists. Baggini reasons, as do Blackburn, Dawkins, and Pinker, that truth is worth defending. What is crucial, however, is not just identifying truths but how and by whom what purports to be knowledge is established. The meaning of madness (and mental disorder) is influenced by cultural ideas about acceptable and unacceptable human performance but it also refers to real personal suffering expressed by real people. The meaning of madness is also swayed by the societal necessity of ensuring personal safety and mechanisms of social control, and by the technologies and discourses of a host of professions, and by media and public opinion. Rather than concluding that such influences mean that there is no meaning to madness, it means that the real meaning of madness cannot be understood easily because of these influences. Finding the truth of madness may not come about from postmodernist deconstructive compulsions, and nor may it be found in the wiring of the brain. It may never be found. But the search for and maintenance of truth has value especially when that truth may mean relief from suffering and/or social acceptance.

In 2017, thousands of scientists and their supporters went on a march through the capital of the USA to defend scientific truth (St Fleur, 2017). They have continued their campaign under the name 'March For Science' using the slogan 'Science Not Silence' (March for Science, 2019). Similar protests are reported as occurring in hundreds of other USA cities, and in Europe and Asia. Their reason marching is given as the policies President Donald Trump. Trump's polices are regarded by these scientists as politicising science by undermining scientific evidence such as that which points to the crisis in the climate. When the leader of the most powerful country in the world is accused of misusing the truth by a multitude of scientists whose *raison d'être* is to try to establish the truth then this is insanity. The insanity of post-truth has become a fact when a leading USA newspaper accuses openly President Donald Trump of making over 12,000 false or misleading claims since assuming office (*Washington Post*, 2019).

Mindlessness

Blackburn (2005) refers to the soggy ideas behind the 'anything goes' regard of truth. He suggests it is easy to be frightened by what is happening in the world. Among the most frightening of things to feel frightened about, Blackburn continues, is what is going on people's minds, making them behave the way they do. Applying Blackburn's reasoning to the topics of this book, tolerating, ignoring or contributing to violence, inequality, selfishness, insecurity, global warming, and the lies underpinning political leadership, all point to an epidemic of mindlessness. It's not that there aren't reasons to be cheerful. But there are also reasons not to be cheerful.

There are many techniques available for making the worried more contented which attempt to make readjusts to what Blackburn fears is going on in people's minds. Clinical psychologists and psychotherapists have various remedies for coping with psychological distress presumed to stem from living in a distressed world. One of these, is ecotherapy which, as noted above, is designed to assuage apprehensions about the climate crisis. But by far the most prolific therapeutic approach radiates from the 'happiness industry' embodied by positive psychology and its serenity-generating offshoots such as mindfulness.

Martin Seligman is one of the architects of psychology's positive outgrowth. Seligman's 'scientific' assumption is that humans want to be happy. What Seligman (2002) designates as 'authentic happiness' is achievable if the individual's potential for 'lasting fulfilment' is realised, and positive psychology provides the means by which fulfilment and hence happiness is attained.

> Positive Psychology is the scientific study of the strengths that enable individuals and communities to thrive. The field is founded on the belief that people want to lead meaningful and fulfilling lives, to cultivate what is best within themselves, and to enhance their experiences of love, work, and play.
>
> (Positive Psychology Center, 2019)

Life becomes worth living, for the positive psychologists, when individuals adopt techniques aimed at savouring and acting on constructive thoughts and emotions rather than dwelling on angst and misery. A primary technique used in the constructing constructiveness is thinking about events that have brought some degree of pleasure. These experiences of positiveness can then be logged in memory or as a tangible record, perhaps a diary. Once logged they can be remembered or re-read so that they can be savoured repeatedly. Another technique is for the person seeking positiveness to inform family members, friends, and colleagues, or even strangers, of her/his gratitude for any contribution they may have made helping her/him triumph over cheerlessness. The Positive Psychology Center advertises books, courses, videos, and on-line programmes to enable a more co-ordinated process to be followed on the path to positiveness.

For political economist Will Davies (2016), the processing of people into cheerfulness, which began long before the invention of positive psychology, is now highly commercialised. Those buying the books, courses, videos, and on-line programmes are consuming the commodities of yet another capitalist industry centred on servicing self-centredness. In the process, yet another human emotion has become colonised by politicians the bosses of big business. Happiness scoring is used to assess and ameliorate workers' productiveness. The happiness quotient is adopted in political mantras to offset the unpopularity with purely economic measurement of a country's well-being. Happiness is promised to help 'nudge' people towards accepting social policies which they might otherwise snub. The happiness industry therefore for Davies is not interested in genuine happiness but in profit and power.

Reaching for happiness in a world riddled with unbridled cruelty, unyielding discrimination, unrestrained competitiveness fetishised consumption, anomie, alienation, loneliness, and known and unknown threats from digitalisation, to resolve what at root are not only private troubles but also public issues is the epitome of mindlessness.

People who suffer from a lack of appreciation of the mess in the world warrant the designation of personal madness. This tag applies to much of the public, but expressly to those professionals who deal with the consequences of a faulty society by mainly or only focusing on the renovation of the thinking, emotions, and behaviour of individuals. Those promoting (and selling) and (buying) positiveness and mindfulness are engaging in senseless consumerism other in the sense of profit for the purveyor and yet another of what sociologists Stan Cohen and Laurie Taylor (1992) described as 'escape attempts' from reality. That reality is not only an elemental existential angst and ontological insecurity but the anguish from society's insanities.

The meditative method of mindfulness has become mainstream and millions of people are carrying-out mindful manoeuvring by not moving (Purser et al., 2016). An array of organisations in Western countries, including schools, prisons, and military and government agencies, are utilising this pacifying practice which has its origins in the Eastern countries.

Self-described 'mindful cranks' Ron Purser and David Loy (2019) use the slogan 'where using your mind is not necessarily a bad thing' on their website which houses information relating to the adaptation and adopting of Buddhism in the West. Purser, a scholar in management studies, and Loy, a Zen teacher, are in favour of Buddhism being practised in the West. However, they point to a shadow side of the West's embracement of mindfulness.

Purser and Loy suggest what they refer to as the 'mindfulness revolution' has come about on the promise it offers a panacea for resolving nearly all personal troubles. What has also come about, observe Purser and Loy, is a series of profitable small businesses supplying training in the technique and related relaxing products including meditation cushions, crystals, scents, benches and stones, and singing bowls. Moreover, large corporations are engaged with the mindful revolution. Mindfulness business consultants are being recruited on the promise that their meditative skills will increase a company's productivity by reducing its employees' anguish a large part of which is likely to be a consequence of their working conditions:

> [C]orporations have jumped on the mindfulness bandwagon because it conveniently shifts the burden onto the individual employee: stress is framed as a personal problem, and mindfulness is offered as just the right medicine to help employees work more efficiently and calmly within toxic environments.
>
> (Purser and Loy, 2013)

Pursor and Loy are scathing about the quality of mindfulness which is being delivered to both the public and corporations. The marketisation of mindfulness has resulted in a dilution of its Buddhist underpinnings. There is what they describe as a 'denaturing' of mindfulness when it is used to relieve headaches, reducing blood pressure, or for simple relaxation. Its use by corporations is hardly adhering to the spiritual basis of an ancient religious tradition but is adhering to the spirit of capitalism which they denote as 'McMindfulness' (Purser and Loy, 2013; Pursor, 2019).

The promotion of positive thinking and mindfulness as ideal human strategies to achieve what is conjured as the ideal human goal of happiness is misleading and malign because it diverts attention from the societal causes of negativity and from unhappiness as an emotion which can drive inventiveness including ways of changing society for the better (Ehrenreich, 2010; Burkeman, 2013; Davies, 2016). The commodification of positiveness and mindfulness is a contemporary cultural inanity. But there are many more.

People have become so engrossed in mindlessness that stupidity has become normalised. Human stupidity, contends Fromm (1955), is exemplified by a surfeit in everyday inanities. Western culture become dumbed-down through commodification and consumerism. The low-level and alienating requirements of factory assembly line and office work have replaced the highly-skilled and satisfying work of artisanship and craftsmanship with low-level skills.

Mass entertainments have, observed Fromm, replaced personalised, interpersonal, and community-based pleasures and learning opportunities. Although literacy and numeracy amongst Western populations had become nearly universal by the 1950s, and access to books, newspapers, radio, television, and film could provide levels of intellectual and creative stimulation unparalleled in human history, the masses were provided with and deliberately sought mediocrity, tawdriness, shallowness, and idleness. Sitting in front of the television for hours daily gazing at programmes with content centred on frivolity and ferocity typifies Fromm's assessment that even in the 1950s society was riddled with cultural garbage.

Over the decades since Fromm wrote about the insanity of society inanity has increased markedly and is set to intensify. Since the 1950s there has been a commodification of virtually everything (including the virtual world) and the inculcation of consumerism as a fundamental, routine, and socially acceptable if not applaudable human activity. Work and leisure pursuits are now affected equally with workers deskilled due to the rise of the low-brow requirements of the service industry, automation of manufacturing, and industrialisation of agriculture. Digitalisation – with its concomitants, robotics and artificial intelligence – will further reduce the need for human acumen in the workplace and increase the obtuse obsessiveness with electronic gadgetry. Recreation is now replete with cognitively stupefying social media forums, 'reality' television shows the essence of which is human humiliation, magazines which prevail only on malicious gossip about celebrities, films, videos, and computer games which revel in sadism and slaughter, binge alcohol consumption, corporate sport, and readily available and wide-ranging pornographic material via the internet.

Summary

Human society is not wholly uncivilised, human culture is not wholly inane, and humans are not completely stupid (more about which in the Conclusion). Had Fromm been alive today he might well have been amazed at the extent of scientific and technological innovation which enables instant communication across continents, journeys to be made from one side of the world to the other in one day, cancer to be cured, and how easily titanic quantities of knowledge can be retrieved by anyone with a computer or 'smart' telephone which for much of the world's population is obtainable (although not always affordable).

That said, Fromm may also have been saddened at how stupid humanity has become by still partaking in interpersonal savagery and lethality, wars and genocide, by the extent of the gap between the rich and the poor, the proliferation of commodification, consumerism, and egotism, and by the level of psychological distress caused by old and new insecurities.

Fromm might have been saddened but it is unlikely he would have stunned because by the time he died (1980) the atrocities of the Vietnam War and Khmer Rouge's genocide in Cambodia had occurred, countries such as the UK had undergone serious economic, political, and industrial woes in the 1970s, selfishness was flourishing not diminishing, and humanity continued to threatened by nuclear conflict. But he assuredly would be startled that human stupidity had reached the stage of allowing the climate to be near catastrophe, was allowing lies to be taken as truths, and at the paradox that commendable human cleverness was also responsible for the invention of its own insanities.

References

Albrecht G (2005) 'Solastalgia': A new concept in health and identity. *PAN 3*, pp. 41–55.
Albrecht G (2011) Chronic environmental change: Emerging 'psychoterratic' syndromes. In Weissbecker I (ed.) *Climate Change and Human Well-Being. International and Cultural Psychology*. New York: Springer, pp. 43–56.

Asthma UK (2019) Asthma death toll in England and Wales is the highest this decade. www.asthma.org.uk/about/media/news/press-release-asthma-death-toll-in-england-and-wales-is-the-highest-this-decade/ [accessed 12 August, 2019].

Baggini J (2018) *A Short History of Truth: Consolations for a Post-Truth World.* London: Quercus.

Blackburn S (2005) *Truth: A Guide for the Perplexed.* London: Penguin

Blackburn S (2017) *Truth: Ideas in Profile.* London: Profile Books

Burkeman O (2013) *The Antidote: Happiness for People Who Can't Stand Positive Thinking.* Edinburgh: Canongate.

Cohen S and Taylor L (1992) *Escape Attempts: The Theory and Practice of Resistance in Everyday Life,* 2nd edn. London: Routledge.

Davies W (2016) *The Happiness Industry: How the Government and Big Business Sold Us Well-Being.* New York: Verso.

Dawkins R (2006) *The God Delusion.* London: Bantam Press.

Dawkins R (2019) *Outgrowing God: A Beginner's Guide.* London: Bantam Press.

Dyer C (2019) Mother is granted new inquest over daughter's death from asthma. *British Medical Journal,* 364, p. 1192. www.bmj.com/content/364/bmj.l1192 [accessed 12 August, 2019].

Edwards S and Buzzell L (2008) The waking up syndrome. *Hopedance,* 11(8). www.hopedance.org/home/soul-news/413-the-waking-up-syndrome [accessed 12 January, 2020].

Ehrenreich B (2010) *Smile or Die: How Positive Thinking Fooled America and the World.* London: Granta.

Ella Roberta Family Foundation (2019) About the Foundation. http://ellaroberta.org/about-the-foundation/ [accessed 12 August, 2019].

Field M and Behrman R (eds) (2003) *When Children Die: Improving Palliative and End-of-Life Care for Children and Their Families.* Washington, DC: National Academies Press.

Fromm E (1955) *The Sane Society.* New York: Rinehart.

Fromm E (1956) *The Art of Loving.* New York: Harper & Row.

House of Commons Digital, Culture, Media and Sport Committee (2019) *Disinformation and 'Fake News': Final Report.* London: House of Commons.

Institute for Public Policy Research (2019) About us. Institute for Public Policy Research. www.ippr.org/about [accessed 12 August, 2019].

Intergovernmental Panel on Climate Change (IPCC) (2019) *Climate Change and Land: An IPCC Special Report on Climate Change, Desertification, Land Degradation, Sustainable Land Management, Food Security, and Greenhouse Gas Fluxes in Terrestrial Ecosystem* [Summary for policymakers]. Geneva, Switzerland: The Intergovernmental Panel on Climate Change. www.ipcc.ch/site/assets/uploads/2019/08/4.-SPM_Approved_Microsite_FINAL.pdf [accessed 12 August, 2019].

Intergovernmental Science-Policy Platform on Biodiversity and Ecosystem (2019) Global report: Summary for policymakers of the global assessment report on biodiversity and ecosystem services. Intergovernmental Science-Policy Platform on Biodiversity and Ecosystem. www.ipbes.net/global-assessment-report-biodiversity-ecosystem-services [accessed 12 January, 2020].

Intergovernmental Science-Policy Platform on Biodiversity and Ecosystem (IBES) (2020) What is IPBES? Intergovernmental Science-Policy Platform on Biodiversity and Ecosystem. www.ipbes.net/about [accessed 12 January, 2020].

Intergovernmental Panel on Climate Change (IPCC) (2018) *Global Warming of 1.5°.* Geneva: World Meteorological Organization/United Nations.

Internal Displacement Monitoring Centre (2019) *2019 Global Report on Internal Displacement*. Geneva, Switzerland: Internal Displacement Monitoring Centre.

Jackson L and Devadason C (2019) *Climate Change, Flooding and Mental Health*. Oxford: Rockefeller Foundation Economic Council on Planetary Health at the Oxford Martin School.

Jordan M and Hinds J (eds) (2016) *Ecotherapy: Theory, Research and Practice*. London: Macmillan.

Kübler-Ross, E. (1969) *On Death and Dying*, London: Routledge.

Laybourn-Langton L, Rankin L and Baxter D (2019) *This is a Crisis: Facing Up to the Age of Environmental Breakdown*. London: Institute for Public Policy Research.

March For Science (2019) Science not silence. https://marchforscience.com/ [accessed 14 August, 2019].

McIntyre L (2018) *Post-Truth*. Cambridge, MA: Massachusetts Institute of Technology.

Moffic H (2013) Eco-psychiatry: Why we need to keep the environment in mind [transcript from the 2013 American Psychiatric Association Conference]. *Psychiatric Times*, 19 May. www.psychiatrictimes.com/apa2013/eco-psychiatry-why-we-need-keep-environment-mind [accessed 12 August, 2019].

Monbiot G (2017) *How Did We Get Into This Mess?: Politics, Equality, Nature*. London: Verso.

Morrall P (2009) *Sociology and Health: An Introduction*, 2nd edn. London: Routledge.

Morrall P (2017) *Madness: Ideas about Insanity*. Abingdon-on-Thames: Routledge.

Morrall P (2018) Sociology of and in psychotherapy: The seventh sin. In Cohen B (ed.) *Handbook of Critical Theory and Mental Health*. London: Routledge, pp. 235–243.

Neukom R, Steiger N, Gómez-Navarro J, Wang J and Werner J (2019) No evidence for globally coherent warm and cold periods over the preindustrial Common Era. *Nature* [research letter], 24 July, 571, pp. 550–554.

Pinker S (2018) *Enlightenment Now*. London: Allen Lane.

Positive Psychology Center (2019) Welcome: The mission of the Positive Psychology Center. https://Ppc.Sas.Upenn.Edu/ [accessed 15 August, 2019].

Proctor R (2012) The history of the discovery of the cigarette lung cancer link: Evidentiary traditions, corporate denial, global toll. *British Medical Journal: Tobacco Control*, 21(2), pp. 87–91.

Pursor R (2019) *McMindfulnes: How Mindfulness Became the New Capitalist Spirituality*. London: Penguin.

Purser R, Forbes D and Burke A (2016) *Handbook of Mindfulness: Culture, Context and Social Engagement*. New York: Springer.

Purser R and Loy D (2013) Beyond McMindfulness. *Huffington Post*, 31 August. www.huffingtonpost.com/ron-purser/beyond-mcmindfulness_b_3519289.html [accessed 15 August, 2019].

Purser R and Loy D (2019) Meet the cranks. www.mindfulcranks.com/meet-the-cranks [accessed 15 August, 2019].

Redlener C, Jenkins C and Redlener I (2019) Our planet is in crisis. But until we call it a crisis, no one will listen. *The Guardian*, 31 July.

Rose N (2019) *Our Psychiatric Future: The Politics of Mental Health*. Cambridge: Polity.

Rose N and Abi-Rached J (2013) *Neuro: The New Brain Sciences and the Management of the Mind*. Princeton, NJ: Princeton University Press.

Roszak T (1992) *The Voice of the Earth*. New York: Simon & Schuster.

Seligman M (2002) *Authentic Happiness: Using the New Positive Psychology to Realize Your Potential for Lasting Fulfillment*. New York: Simon and Schuster.

Singer P (1975) *Animal Liberation: A New Ethics for Our Treatment of Animals*. London: HarperCollins.

Singer P (1979) *Practical Ethics*. Cambridge: Cambridge University.

St Fleur N (2017) Scientists, feeling under siege, march against Trump policies. *New York Times*, 22 April. www.nytimes.com/2017/04/22/science/march-for-science.html?_r=0 [accessed 23 July, 2019].

Swain D (2012) *Alienation: An Introduction to Marx's Theory*. London: Bookmarks.

Washington Post (2019) Fact checker: In 928 days, President Trump has made 12,019 false or misleading claimswww.washingtonpost.com/graphics/politics/trump-claims-database/?utm_term=.cf70878818f3&tid=a_inl_manual [accessed 14 August, 2019].

Weart S (2008) *The Discovery of Global Warming*. Cambridge, MA: Harvard University Press.

Whitmore-Williams S, Manning C, Krygsman K and Speiser M (2017) *Mental Health and Our Changing Climate: Impacts, Implications, and Guidance*. Washington, DC: American Psychological Association, and ecoAmerica.

Wilkinson C (2017) Healthy homes: The hidden toxins in everyday building materials. *Financial Times*, 2 June. www.ft.com/content/5411fd18-409c-11e7-82b6-896b95f30f58 [accessed 12 August, 2019].

World Health Organisation (WHO) (2018) *Climate Change and Health*. Geneva: World Health Organisation. www.who.int/news-room/fact-sheets/detail/climate-change-and-health [accessed 9 August, 2019].

World Health Organisation (WHO) (2019) *Tobacco: Key Facts*. Geneva: World Health Organisation, 26 July. www.who.int/news-room/fact-sheets/detail/tobacco [accessed 9 August, 2019].

8 Conclusion

A mass of incidents of personal madness[1] has been mentioned in this book. Most of the madness has not been diagnosed as mental disorder either because it hasn't passed by the clinical gaze of the medical profession, or because it does not fit or warrant psychiatric classification. Where madness has been medicalised (and at times epidemics proclaimed) this may be a consequence of accurate psychiatric and justifiable diagnosis or the increasing medicalisation of personal troubles.

Personal troubles are social issues. Madness is a personal trouble that gains much of its context from its society. Its meaning and direction are shaped by social attitudes (which may be tolerant or prejudicial) and social institutions (the main one of which is the biologically biased subdivision of the profession of medicine – psychiatry). Society contributes or causes many personal troubles. Together with the input of imaginative insights from sociology, the idea from Fromm (1955) that the more society has lost grip on its sanity the more personal madness will occur has been applied to five social issues which are indubitably personally troubling. Violence, inequality, selfishness, insecurity, and stupidity have been presented as societal insanities directly or indirectly linkable to psychological distress.

Emphasising societal factors in the making of madness is not intended to discount, devaluate, or denounce biological and psychological contributions. But in this book, there is an emphasis on correcting the imbalance between evaluating madness on the basis that the individual has faults and society is at fault. To put it forthrightly, to ignore or underplay the effects of society on the psychological (and physical) make-up of humans is madness (and stupid).

It has been claimed for decades and remains a claim that sociologists and other societally attuned academics have the capability to work with psychiatrists and psychologists, and collectively they are more capable of fathoming personal madness (Eisenberg, 1977; 1986; Eisenberg and Kleinman, 1980; Wessely, 2013; Nikolas Rose, 2018). Simon Wessely, President of the Royal College of Psychiatrists from 2014–2017, is unequivocal in his support for the marrying of biology, psychology, and social(logical) knowledge and practices:

In order to help the understanding, treatment and support of those with mental disorders, psychiatry brings together in equal measure the biological, psychological and social. Remove any one of these three, and I'm not sure what you would have, but it's not psychiatry.

(Wessely, 2016)

There is marrying of academics and clinicians working in the speciality tagged 'social neuroscience' (Cacioppo and Berntson, 1992; Todorov et al., 2014). Its nomenclature signifies the synthesis of nurture and nature regarding human performance. The neuroscientist David Eagleman (2015) is a protagonist of another speciality in which there is a marring of nature and nurture, 'social neuroscience'. Eagleman recognises that humans are 'social creatures'.

If humans are social animals and the 'social' side of humanity is suspect in the making of madness, then is follows that it is society that needs the equivalent of medication or possibly surgery. If the treatment is successful, then what then the condition of the cured 'patient'?

The teenage daughter of economist, former Greek Minister of Finance, and academic Yanis Varoufakis asks her father 'Is humanity that stupid?' (Varoufakis, 2017, p. 7). Xenia Varoufakis is referring to inequality, but her question could apply equally to violence, selfishness, insecurity, and most surely to the super-stupidity of ecological destruction. Her father decides to answer his daughter's question by writing a book titled *Talking With My Daughter* in which he argues for a more democratic, just, and rational society. In this book he also advises his daughter to maintain her outrage but to use it tactically, when the time is right.

Personal action might lead to societal change or at least be a significant element in a momentum of change brought about by historical and cultural forces not under the control of individuals. Unusual examples of individual and collective political action surfaced in 2019. Thousands of school children deserted their classrooms and marched in cities across the world to draw attention to the climate crisis (*BBC News*, 2019). They are reported to have gained their inspiration to protest from the campaigning of teenage Swedish climate activist, Greta Thunberg (see, for example, Thunberg, 2019). This inspirational young person says she has suffered from depression, obsessive-compulsive-disorder, selective mutism, and is diagnosed with a form of autism, Asperger's Syndrome (Thunberg, 2018). Greta Thunberg points to a paradox pertinent to her activism and autism:

I think in many ways that we autistic are the normal ones, and the rest of the people are pretty strange, especially when it comes to the sustainability crisis, where everyone keeps saying climate change is an existential threat and the most important issue of all, and yet they just carry on like before.

(Thunberg, 2018)

Perhaps, paradoxically, personal madness may make society saner. Perhaps, para-doxically, if masses of individuals (including sociologists, psychiatrists, psycholo-gists, and psychotherapists) get madder they might not just carry on like before.

But it's more complex. Individual action is only part of the solution.

Individuals are to some degree masters/mistresses of their own fate but a fate which is conditional on how their society operates. How society operates is conditional on what individuals, either separately or grouped, decide to think, feel, and act. Individual volition and societal pressure are in a push-and-pull myriad of complex arrangements which it is problematic to untangle. When the structure of that (global) society is massively and manifestly unjust then the pulls and pushes will be preferential for some and disadvantaging for many. When the ideology of a society sanctions cruelty, poverty, materialism, consumerism, narcissism, uncertainty, and stupidity, then insanity sits outside the individual. Repositioning society from insanity to sanity requires more than acclaiming or even acting on the positions of individuals.

Moreover, individuals are involved in a similarly multifaceted interplay with the various constituents of their biology and psychology. Some people do manage to escape from the chains of their social system and act, feel, and think differently from the 'insane' inculcations of society. Some people will become mad no matter what the structure and ideology of society. That is, a sane society is not a cure-all for all insanity. Therefore, there is a resolution to the discrepancy in Fromm's work whereby personal madness and the insanity of society are coupled. Fromm does not provide an assurance that if society becomes sane then personal madness and societal insanity will be decoupled. If madness (or mental disorder) has biological, psychological, and societal facets then sorting only one of these components still leaves the influence of other two. The concomitant conundrum of 'in an insane society is everyone mad?' is also resolvable but not only because some people have biological and psychological resilience to combat the negative effects from violence, inequality, selfishness, insecurity and stupidity, but they may also or instead be invigorated by the 'sociological imagination' as was Fromm.

Most assuredly humanity has improved much of its lot since the very brief and extremely precarious days of living in caves and human society has matured since the culturally incestuous, rigidly ruled, and noxious days of the middle-ages and even the Victorian period. But the proposition of improvements is only valid if, as posited by Pinker (2018) and Gates (2017), the trajectory of development is measured over thousands of years. If increases in life-span, decreasing violence, fantastic and exotic scientific, technological, and medical innovations, are judged against continuing, current, and prospective atavistic, regressive, unedifying, and idiotic aspects of human performance and societal circumstances then human and societal progress does not appear so pronounced. In 2019 the viral infection COVID-19 (a coronavirus) was discovered. By March of 2020 this virus had spread across the world and further indicated the precariousness of progress. In a joint statement by the International Chamber of Commerce and World Health Organisation (2020) COVID-19 is described as a 'global health and societal emergency'. On the personal level, there is panic, fear, and anxiety about contamination, and worry and misery because of employment and financial insecurity, social isolation, and perceived scarcity of food and toilet paper (McKeever, 2020). There is also an expected exacerbation of existing psychological distress amongst those already diagnosed with mental disorder (Moukaddam and Asim, 2020). At the level of society, the fragility and folly of national and international economic, medical, and care systems, has been laid bare by a variety of the common cold (Evans, 2020).

To move society from insanity to sanity Fromm proposes what he describes as 'humanistic communitarian socialism'. Social sanity can be restored, Fromm (1955) suggests, by curtailing acquisitiveness, encouraging human compassion, comradeship, compromise, empathy, and love, and involvement in edifying and in the main shared activities such as art, music, and meaningful mental or physical work. Monbiot ideal society seems to replicate much of that wished by Fromm:

> To seek enlightenment, intellectual or spiritual; to do good; to love and to be loved; to create and to teach; these are the highest purposes of humankind. If there is meaning in life, it lies here.
>
> (Monbiot, 2017, p. 48)

Academics and clinicians, I argue, have a social and professional responsibility to take 'moral action', perhaps taking their inspiration from these school children, to make society saner. Indeed, the need for political activism amongst clinicians and academics is acknowledged by both (Hilary Rose and Steven Rose, 2016; Flood et al., 2013; Choudry, 2015). But what is also required is the initiation of a revolutionary and revelatory idea, a 'fourth way' to surpass the old ideas of capitalism, communism, and communitarianism. If the 'sociological imagination' has taught me anything, then this idea will only come to fruition when relevant and complex historical and cultural forces have ripened. Until then barbarianism is more likely than Fromm's bohemianism, climatic catastrophe more credible than cooperation to cool this planet, and clear-cut epidemics of madness and additional societal insanities more probable than an outbreak of psychological stability and society becoming sane.

Paradoxically, it may be that severity of the insanities of violence, inequality, selfishness, insecurity, and stupidity are indicative that society will soon ripen into sanity. But it may also be that human society will have to first succumb to full-blown insanity.

Note

1 To remind the reader, synonyms for personal madness are used in this book (for example, 'psychological distress', 'psychological suffering', and 'psychological instability'). The term 'mental disorder' pertains to a medicalised psychological state. 'Insanity' is used to describe a condition of society.

References

BBC News (2019). Climate strikes spread worldwide as students call for action. www.bbc.co.uk/news/world-47581585 [accessed 15 March, 2019].

Cacioppo J and Berntson G (1992). Social psychological contributions to the decade of the brain: Doctrine of multilevel analysis'. *American Psychologist*. 47(8), pp. 1019–1028.

Choudry A (2015) *Learning Activism: The Intellectual Life of Contemporary Social Movements*. Toronto, Canada: University of Toronto.

Gates B (2017) Bill Gates's 7 predictions for our future. World Economic Forum, 8 May. www.weforum.org/agenda/2017/05/bill-gates-is-pretty-good-at-predicting-the-future-this-is-what-he-thinks-will-happen-next1 [accessed 9 July, 2018].

Eagleman D (2015) *The Brain: The Story of You*. Edinburgh: Canongate.

Eisenberg L (1977) Psychiatry and society: A sociobiologic synthesis. *New England Journal of Medicine*, 296(16), pp. 903–910.

Eisenberg L (1986) Mindlessness and brainlessness in psychiatry. *The British Journal of Psychiatry*, 148(5), pp. 497–508.

Eisenberg L and Kleinman A (eds) (1980) *The Relevance of Social Science for Medicine*. New York: Springer.

Evans O (2020) Socio-Economic Impacts of Novel Coronavirus: The Policy Solutions. BizEcons Quarterly, Strides Educational Foundation, volume 7, pp. 3–12. http://bequarterly.rysearch.com/wp-content/uploads/2020/03/Evans-2020-Socioeconomic-impacts-of-novel-coronavirus-The-policy-solutions.pdf [accessed 23 March, 2020].

Flood, M, Martin, B. and Dreher, T. (2013) Combining academia and activism: common obstacles and useful tools. *Australian Universities Review*, 55(1), pp. 17–26.

Fromm E (1955) *The Sane Society*. New York: Rinehart.

International Chamber of Commerce and World Health Organisation (2020) ICC-WHO Joint Statement: An unprecedented private sector call to action to tackle COVID-19. https://www.who.int/news-room/detail/16-03-2020-icc-who-joint-statement-an-unprecedented-private-sector-call-to-action-to-tackle-covid-19 [accessed 21 March, 2020].

Mason P (2019) *Clear Bright Future: A Radical Defence of the Human Being*. London: Allen Lane.

McKeever A (2020) Coronavirus is Spreading Panic. Here's the Science Behind Why. National Geographic, 12 March 2020. https://www.nationalgeographic.com/history/reference/modern-history/why-we-evolved-to-feel-panic-anxiety/ [accessed 21 March, 2020].

Monbiot G (2017) *How Did We Get Into This Mess?: Politics, Equality, Nature*. London: Verso.

Moukaddam N and S Asim (2020) Psychiatrists Beware! The Impact of COVID-19 and Pandemics on Mental Health. *Psychiatric Times*, 15 March 2020, 37(3). https://www.psychiatrictimes.com/psychiatrists-beware-impact-coronavirus-pandemics-mental-health [accessed 21 March, 2020].

Pinker S (2018) *Enlightenment Now: The Case for Reason, Science, Humanism, and Progress*. London: Allen Lane.

Rose H and Rose S (2016) *Can Neuroscience Change Our Minds?* Cambridge: Polity.

Rose N (2018) *Our Psychiatric Future: The Politics of Mental Health*. Cambridge: Polity.

Rose N and Abi-Rached J (2013) *Neuro: The New Brain Sciences and the Management of the Mind*. Princeton, NJ: Princeton University Press.

Thunberg G (2018) The disarming case to act right now on climate change. TED: Ideas Worth Spreading. www.ted.com/talks/greta_thunberg_the_disarming_case_to_act_right_now_on_climate/transcript [accessed 17 August, 2019].

Thunberg G (2019) Greta Thunberg full speech at extinction rebellion protest in London. www.youtube.com/watch?v=hKMX8WRw3fc [accessed 17 August, 2019].

Todorov A, Fiske A and Prentice D (eds) (2014) *Social Neuroscience: Toward Understanding the Underpinnings of the Social Mind.* Oxford: Oxford University Press.

Varoufakis Y (2017) *Talking with my Daughter. A Brief History of Capitalism.* London: Vintage.

Wessely S (2016) Fuller picture of modern psychiatry. *The Guardian*, 26 February. www.theguardian.com/society/2016/feb/26/a-fuller-picture-of-modern-psychiatry [accessed 17 August, 2019].

Wessely S and James O (2013) Do we need to change the way we are thinking about mental illness? *The Observer*, 12 May.

Index